Clinical
Epidemiology
The Essentials

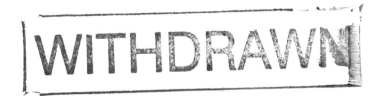

614.
4

FLE

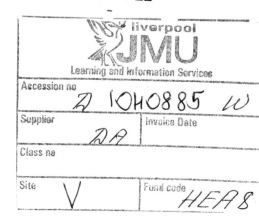

Clinical Epidemiology

The Essentials

Fifth Edition

Robert H. Fletcher, MD, MSc

Professor Emeritus
Department of Population Medicine
Harvard Medical School
Boston, Massachusetts

Adjunct Professor
Departments of Epidemiology and Social Medicine
The University of North Carolina at Chapel Hill
Chapel Hill, North Carolina

Suzanne W. Fletcher, MD, MSc

Professor Emerita
Department of Population Medicine
Harvard Medical School
Boston, Massachusetts

Adjunct Professor
Departments of Epidemiology and Social Medicine
The University of North Carolina at Chapel Hill
Chapel Hill, North Carolina

Grant S. Fletcher, MD, MPH

Assistant Professor of Medicine
The University of Washington School of Medicine
Seattle, Washington

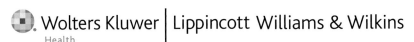
Wolters Kluwer | Lippincott Williams & Wilkins
Health

Philadelphia • Baltimore • New York • London
Buenos Aires • Hong Kong • Sydney • Tokyo

Acquisitions Editor: Susan Rhyner
Product Manager: Catherine Noonan
Marketing Manager: Joy Fisher-Williams
Designer: Teresa Mallon
Compositor: Aptara, Inc.

Fifth Edition

351 West Camden Street   Two Commerce Square
Baltimore, MD 21201   2001 Market Street
                                Philadelphia, PA 19103

Printed in China

9 8 7 6 5 4

Library of Congress Cataloging-in-Publication Data

Fletcher, Robert H.
  Clinical epidemiology : the essentials / Robert H. Fletcher, Suzanne
W. Fletcher, Grant S. Fletcher. – 5th ed.
      p. ; cm.
  Includes bibliographical references and index.
  ISBN 978-1-4511-4447-5 (alk. paper)
  I. Fletcher, Suzanne W.   II. Fletcher, Grant S.   III. Title.
  [DNLM: 1. Epidemiologic Methods. WA 950]

  614.4–dc23
                                  2012022346

DISCLAIMER

Care has been taken to confirm the accuracy of the information present and to describe generally accepted practices. However, the authors, editors, and publisher are not responsible for errors or omissions or for any consequences from application of the information in this book and make no warranty, expressed or implied, with respect to the currency, completeness, or accuracy of the contents of the publication. Application of this information in a particular situation remains the professional responsibility of the practitioner; the clinical treatments described and recommended may not be considered absolute and universal recommendations.

The authors, editors, and publisher have exerted every effort to ensure that drug selection and dosage set forth in this text are in accordance with the current recommendations and practice at the time of publication. However, in view of ongoing research, changes in government regulations, and the constant flow of information relating to drug therapy and drug reactions, the reader is urged to check the package insert for each drug for any change in indications and dosage and for added warnings and precautions. This is particularly important when the recommended agent is a new or infrequently employed drug.

Some drugs and medical devices presented in this publication have Food and Drug Administration (FDA) clearance for limited use in restricted research settings. It is the responsibility of the health care provider to ascertain the FDA status of each drug or device planned for use in their clinical practice.

To purchase additional copies of this book, call our customer service department at **(800) 638-3030** or fax orders to **(301) 223-2320**. International customers should call **(301) 223-2300**.

Visit Lippincott Williams & Wilkins on the Internet: http://www.lww.com. Lippincott Williams & Wilkins customer service representatives are available from 8:30 am to 6:00 pm, EST.

This book is for clinicians—physicians, nurses, physicians' assistants, psychologists, veterinarians, and others who care for patients—who want to understand for themselves the strength of the information base for their clinical decisions. Students of epidemiology and public health may also find this book useful as a complement to the many excellent textbooks about epidemiology itself.

To reach full potential, modern clinicians should have a basic understanding of clinical epidemiology for many reasons.

First, clinicians make countless patient care decisions every day, some with very high stakes. It is their responsibility to base those decisions on the best available evidence, a difficult task because the evidence base is vast and continually changing. At the simplest level, responsible care can be accomplished by following carefully prepared recommendations found in evidence-based guidelines, review articles, or textbooks, but patient care at its best is far more than that. Otherwise, it would be sufficient to have it done by technicians following protocols. Sometimes the evidence is contradictory, resulting in "toss-up" decisions. The evidence may be weak, but a decision still needs to be made. Recommendations that are right for patients on average need to be tailored to the specific illnesses, behaviors, and preferences of individual patients. Expert consultants may disagree, leaving the clinicians with primary responsibility for the patient in the middle. Special interests—by for-profit companies or clinicians whose income or prestige is related to their advice—may affect how evidence is summarized. For these reasons, clinicians need to be able to weigh evidence themselves in order to meet their responsibilities as health care professionals.

Second, clinical epidemiology is now a central part of efforts to improve the effectiveness of patient care worldwide. Clinicians committed to research careers are pursuing formal postgraduate training in research methods, often in departments of epidemiology. Grants for clinical research are judged largely by the principles described in this book. Clinical epidemiology is the language of journal peer review and the "hanging committees" that decide whether research reports should be published and the revisions necessary to make them suitable. Local "journal clubs" now carefully evaluate pivotal articles rather than survey the contents of several journals. The National Library of Medicine now includes search terms in MEDLINE for research methods, such as randomized controlled trial and meta-analysis. In short, clinical medicine and epidemiology are making common cause. "Healing the schism" is what Kerr White called it.

Third, the care of patients should be fun. It is not fun to simply follow everyone else's advice without really knowing what stands behind it. It is exhausting to work through a vast medical literature, or even a few weekly journals, without a way of quickly deciding which articles are scientifically strong and clinically relevant and which are not worth bothering with. It is unnerving to make high-stakes decisions without really knowing why they are the right ones. To capture all the enjoyment of their profession, clinicians need to be confident in their ability to think about evidence for themselves, even if someone else has done the heavy lifting to find and sort that evidence, by topic and quality, beforehand. It is fun to be able to confidently participate in discussions of clinical evidence regardless of whether it is within one's specialty (as all of us are nonspecialists in everything outside our specialty).

In this book, we have illustrated concepts with examples from patient care and clinical research, rather than use hypothetical examples, because medicine is so deeply grounded in practical decisions about actual patients. The important questions and studies have evolved rapidly and we have updated examples to reflect this change, while keeping examples that represent timeless aspects in the care of patients and classic studies.

As clinical epidemiology becomes firmly established within medicine, readers expect more from an entry-level textbook. We have, therefore, added new topics to this edition. Among them are comparative effectiveness, practical clinical trials, noninferiority trials, patient-level meta-analyses, and modern concepts in grading evidence-based recommendations. We have also discussed risk, confounding, and effect modification in greater depth.

Modern research design and analyses, supported by powerful computers, make it possible to answer clinical questions with a level of validity and generalizability not dreamed of just a few years ago. However, this often comes at the cost of complexity, placing readers at a distance from the actual data and their meaning. Many of us may be confused as highly specialized research scientists debate alternative meanings of specific terms or tout new approaches to study design and statistical analyses, some of which seem uncomfortably like black boxes no matter how hard we try to get inside them. In such situations, it is especially valuable to remain grounded in the basics of clinical research. We have tried to do just that with the understanding that readers may well want to go on to learn more about this field than is possible from an introductory textbook alone.

Clinical epidemiology is now considered a central part of a broader movement, evidence-based medicine. This is in recognition of the importance, in addition to judging the validity and generalizability of clinical research results, of asking questions that can be answered by research, finding the available evidence, and using the best of that evidence in the care of patients. We have always considered these additional competencies important, and we give them even more attention in this edition of the book.

We hope that readers will experience as much enjoyment and understanding in the course of reading this book as we have in writing it.

Robert H. Fletcher
Suzanne W. Fletcher
Grant S. Fletcher

Acknowledgments

We are fortunate to have learned clinical epidemiology from its founders. Kerr White was Bob and Suzanne's mentor during postgraduate studies at Johns Hopkins and convinced us that what matter are "the benefits of medical interventions in relation to their hazards and costs." Alvan Feinstein taught a generation of young clinician–scholars about the "architecture of clinical research" and the dignity of clinical scholarship. Archie Cochrane spent a night at our home in Montreal when Grant was a boy and opened our eyes to "effectiveness and efficiency." David Sackett asserted that clinical epidemiology is a "basic science for clinical medicine" and helped the world to understand. Many others have followed. We are especially grateful for our work in common with Brian Haynes, founding editor of *ACP Journal Club*; Ian Chalmers, who made the Cochrane Collaboration happen; Andy Oxman, leader of the Rocky Mountain Evidence-Based Healthcare Workshop; Peter Tugwell, a founding leader of the International Clinical Epidemiology Network (INCLEN); and Russ Harris, our long-time colleague at the interface between clinical medicine and public health at the University of North Carolina. These extraordinary people and their colleagues have created an exciting intellectual environment that led to a revolution in clinical scholarship, bringing the evidence base for clinical medicine to a new level.

Like all teachers, we have also learned from our students, clinicians of all ages and all specialties who wanted to learn how to judge the validity of clinical observations and research for themselves. Bob and Suzanne are grateful to medical students at McGill University (who first suggested the need for this book), the University of North Carolina and Harvard Medical School; fellows in the Robert Wood Johnson Clinical Scholars Program, the International Clinical Epidemiology Network (INCLEN), and the Harvard General Medicine Fellowship; CRN Scholars in the Cancer Research Network, a consortium of research institutes in integrated health systems; and participants in the Rocky Mountain Evidence-Based Healthcare Workshops. They were our students and now are our colleagues; many teach and do research with us. Over the years, Grant has met many of these people and now learns from medical students, residents, and faculty colleagues as he teaches them about the care for patients at Harborview Hospital and the University of Washington.

While editors of the *Journal of General Internal Medicine* and *Annals of Internal Medicine*, Bob and Suzanne learned from fellow editors, including members of the World Association of Medical Editors (WAME), how to make reports of research more complete, clear, and balanced so that readers can understand the message with the least effort. With our colleagues at *UpToDate*, the electronic information source for clinicians and patients, we have been developing new ways to make the best available evidence on real-world, clinical questions readily accessible during the care of patients and to make that evidence understandable not just to academicians and investigators, but to full-time clinicians as well.

Ed Wagner was with us at the beginning of this project. With him, we developed a new course in clinical epidemiology for the University of North Carolina School of Medicine and wrote the first edition of this book for it. Later, that course was Grant's introduction to this field, to the extent he had not already been introduced to it at home. Ed remained a coauthor through three editions and then moved on to leadership of Group Health Research Institute and other responsibilities based in Seattle. Fortunately, Grant is now on the writing team and contributed his expertise with the application of clinical epidemiology to the current practice of medicine, especially the care of very sick patients.

We are grateful to members of the team, led by Lippincott Williams & Wilkins, who translated word processed text and hand-drawn figures into an attractive, modern textbook. We got expert, personal attention from Catherine Noonan, who guided us in the preparation of this book throughout; Jonathan Dimes, who worked closely with us in preparing illustrations; and Jeri Litteral, who collaborated with us in the copy editing phase of this project.

We are especially grateful to readers all over the world for their encouraging comments and practical suggestions. They have sustained us through the rigors of preparing this, the fifth edition of a textbook first published 30 years ago.

Contents in Brief

Contents

Introduction

We should study "the benefits of medical interventions in relation to their hazards and costs."

—Kerr L. White
1992

KEY WORDS

Clinical epidemiology
Clinical sciences
Population sciences
Epidemiology
Evidence-based
    medicine
Health services
    research
Quantitative decision
    making
Cost-effectiveness
    analyses
Decision analyses
Social sciences
Biologic sciences
Variables
Independent variable

Dependent variable
Extraneous variables
Covariates
Populations
Sample
Inference
Bias
Selection bias
Measurement bias
Confounding
Chance
Random variation
Internal validity
External validity
Generalizability
Shared decision
    making

Example

A 51-year-old man asks to see you because of chest pain that he thinks is "indigestion." He was well until 2 weeks ago, when he noticed tightness in the center of his chest after a large meal and while walking uphill. The tightness stopped after 2 to 3 minutes of rest. A similar discomfort has occurred several times since then, sometimes during exercise and sometimes at rest. He gave up smoking one pack of cigarettes per day 3 years ago and has been told that his blood pressure is "a little high." He is otherwise well and takes no medications, but he is worried about his health, particularly about heart disease. He lost his job 6 months ago and has no health insurance. A complete physical examination and resting electrocardiogram are normal except for a blood pressure of 150/96 mm Hg.

This patient is likely to have many questions. Am I sick? How sure are you? If I am sick, what is causing my illness? How will it affect me? What can be done about it? How much will it cost?

As the clinician caring for this patient, you have the same kinds of questions, although yours reflect greater understanding of the possibilities. Is the probability of serious, treatable disease high enough to proceed immediately beyond simple explanation and reassurance to diagnostic tests? How well do various tests distinguish among the possible causes of chest pain: angina pectoris, esophageal spasm, muscle strain, anxiety, and the like. For example, how accurately will an exercise stress test be in either confirming or ruling out coronary artery disease? If coronary artery disease is found, how long can the patient expect to have the pain? How likely is it that other complications—congestive heart failure, myocardial infarction, or atherosclerotic disease of other organs—will occur? Will the condition shorten his life? Will reduction of his risk factors for coronary artery disease (from cigarette smoking and hypertension) reduce his risk? Should other possible risk factors be sought? If medications control the pain, would a coronary revascularization procedure add benefit—by preventing a future heart attack or cardiovascular death? Since the patient is unemployed and without health insurance, can less expensive diagnostic work-ups and treatments achieve the same result as more expensive ones?

Clinical Questions and Clinical Epidemiology

The questions confronting the patient and doctor in the example are the types of clinical questions at issue in most doctor–patient encounters: What is "abnormal"? How accurate are the diagnostic tests we use? How often does the condition occur? What are the risks for a given disease, and how do we determine the risks? Does the medical condition usually get worse, stay the same, or resolve (prognosis)? Does treatment really improve the patient or just the test results? Is there a way to prevent the disease? What is the underlying cause of the disease or condition? and How can we give good medical care most efficiently? These clinical questions and the epidemiologic methods to answer them are the bedrock of this book. The clinical questions are summarized in Table 1.1. Each is also the topic of specific chapters in the book.

Clinicians need the best possible answers to these kinds of questions. They use various sources of information: their own experiences, the advice of their colleagues, and reasoning from their knowledge of the biology of disease. In many situations, the most credible source is clinical research, which involves the use of past observations on other similar patients to predict what will happen to the patient at hand. The manner in which such observations are made and interpreted determines whether the conclusions reached are valid, and thus how helpful the conclusions will be to patients.

Health Outcomes

The most important events in clinical medicine are the health outcomes of patients, such as symptoms (discomfort and/or dissatisfaction), disability, disease, and death. These patient-centered outcomes are sometimes referred to as "the 5 Ds" (Table 1.2). They are the health events patients care about. Doctors should try to understand, predict, interpret, and change these outcomes when caring for patients. The 5 Ds can be studied directly only in intact humans and not in parts of humans (e.g., humeral transmitters, tissue

Table 1.1

Clinical Issues and Questions[a]

Issue	Question
Frequency (Ch. 2)	How often does a disease occur?
Abnormality (Ch. 3)	Is the patient sick or well?
Risk (Chs. 5 and 6)	What factors are associated with an increased risk of disease?
Prognosis (Ch. 7)	What are the consequences of having a disease?
Diagnosis (Ch. 8)	How accurate are tests used to diagnose disease?
Treatment (Ch. 9)	How does treatment change the course of disease?
Prevention (Ch. 10)	Does an intervention on well people keep disease from arising? Does early detection and treatment improve the course of disease?
Cause (Ch. 12)	What conditions lead to disease? What are the origins of the disease?

[a]Four chapters—Risk: Basic Principles (4), Chance (11), Systematic Reviews (13), and Knowledge Management (14)—pertain to all of these issues.

cultures, cell membranes, and genetic sequences) or in animals. Clinical epidemiology is the science used to study the 5 Ds in intact humans.

In modern clinical medicine, with so much ordering and treating of lab test results (for such things as plasma glucose levels, hematuria, troponins, etc.), it is difficult to remember that laboratory test results are not the important events in clinical medicine. It

Table 1.2

Outcomes of Disease (the 5 Ds)[a]

Death	A bad outcome if untimely
Disease[b]	A set of symptoms, physical signs, and laboratory abnormalities
Discomfort	Symptoms such as pain, nausea, dyspnea, itching, and tinnitus
Disability	Impaired ability to go about usual activities at home, work, or recreation
Dissatisfaction	Emotional reaction to disease and its care, such as sadness or anger

[a]Perhaps a sixth D, destitution, belongs on this list because the financial cost of illness (for individual patients or society) is an important consequence of disease.
[b]Or illness, the patient's experience of disease.

becomes easy to assume that if we can change abnormal lab tests toward normal, we have helped the patient. This is true only to the extent that careful study has demonstrated a link between laboratory test results and one of the 5 Ds.

Example

The incidence of type 2 diabetes mellitus is increasing dramatically in the United States. Diabetics' risk of dying from heart disease is two to four times greater than that among people without diabetes, and cardiovascular disease accounts for approximately 70% of all deaths in diabetic patients. New pharmacologic efforts to control diabetes have produced a class of drugs, thiazolidinediones, that increase insulin sensitivity in muscle, fat and the liver. Several studies showed that these drugs lower hemoglobin A1C levels in diabetic patients. One such drug, rosiglitazone, was approved for use in 1999. However, over the ensuing years, several follow-up studies demonstrated a surprising result: Patients on the drug were likely to experience more, not less, heart trouble, with different studies showing increases in heart attacks, heart failure, stroke, and cardiovascular or all-cause mortality (1–3). Because many of the studies demonstrating positive results of the drug on glucose and hemoglobin A1C levels were not originally designed to examine longer-term cardiovascular results, most follow-up studies were not rigorous trials. Nevertheless, enough concern was raised that, in 2010, the U.S. Food and Drug Administration restricted use of rosiglitazone; in Europe, sales of the drug were suspended.

During their training, clinicians are steeped in the biology of disease, the sequence of steps that leads from subcellular events to disease and its consequences. Thus, it seemed reasonable to assume that an intervention that lowered blood sugar in diabetics would help protect against heart disease. However, although very important to clinical medicine, these biologic mechanisms cannot be substituted for patient outcomes unless there is strong evidence confirming that the two are related. (In fact, the results of studies with several different medications are raising the possibility that, in type 2 diabetes,

aggressively lowering levels of blood sugar does not protect against heart disease.) Establishing improved health outcomes in patients is particularly important with new drugs because usually pharmacologic interventions have several clinical effects rather than just one.

THE SCIENTIFIC BASIS FOR CLINICAL MEDICINE

Clinical epidemiology is one of the basic sciences that clinicians rely on in the care of patients. Other health sciences, summarized in Figure 1.1, are also integral to patient care. Many of the sciences overlap with each other.

Clinical epidemiology is the science of making predictions about individual patients by counting clinical events (the 5 Ds) in groups of similar patients and using strong scientific methods to ensure that the predictions are accurate. The purpose of clinical epidemiology is to develop and apply methods of clinical observation that will lead to valid conclusions by avoiding being misled by systematic error and the play of chance. It is an important approach

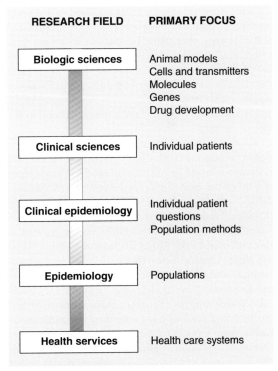

Figure 1.1 ■ The health sciences and their complementary relationships.

to obtaining the kind of information clinicians need to make good decisions in the care of patients.

The term "clinical epidemiology" is derived from its two parent disciplines: clinical medicine and epidemiology. It is "clinical" because it seeks to answer clinical questions and to guide clinical decision making with the best available evidence. It is "epidemiology" because many of the methods used to answer questions about how to best care for patients have been developed by epidemiologists and because the care of individual patients is seen in the context of the larger population of which the patient is a member.

Clinical sciences provide the questions and approach that can be used to care for individual patients. Some biologic sciences, such as anatomy and physiology, are "clinical" to the extent that they provide sound information to guide clinical decisions. For example, knowing the anatomy of the body helps determine possibilities for diagnosis and treatment of many symptoms.

The population sciences study large groups of people. Epidemiology is the "study of disease occurrence in human populations" (4) by counting health-related events in people in relation to the naturally occurring groups (populations) of which they are members. The results of many such studies are directly applicable to the care of individual patients. For example, epidemiology studies are used as the basis for advice about avoiding behaviors such as smoking and inactivity that place patients at increased risk. Other epidemiologic studies, such as those showing harmful effects of passive smoking and other environmental and occupational hazards, are the basis for public health recommendations. Clinical epidemiology is a subset of the population sciences useful in the care of patients.

Clinicians have long depended on research evidence to some extent, but understanding clinical evidence is more important in modern times than it was in the past for several reasons. An extraordinary amount of information must be sorted through. Diagnostic and therapeutic interventions have the potential for great effectiveness, as well as risk and cost, so the stakes in choosing among them are high. Clinical research at its best has become stronger and, thus, can be a sounder basis for clinical decisions. Nevertheless, the credibility of clinical research continues to vary from study to study, so clinicians need to have a method for sorting out strong from weak evidence.

Evidence-based medicine is a modern term for the application of clinical epidemiology to the care of patients. It includes formulating specific "answerable" clinical questions, finding the best available research

Table 1.3

Factors Other Than Evidence-Based Medicine That May Influence Clinical Decisions

Eminence-based medicine	Senior colleagues who believe experience trumps evidence
Vehemence-based medicine	Substitution of volume and stridency for evidence
Eloquence (or elegance)-based medicine	Sartorial elegance and verbal eloquence
Providence-based medicine	The decision is best left in the hands of the Almighty
Diffidence-based medicine	Too timid to make any medical decision
Nervousness-based medicine	Fear of litigation is a powerful stimulus to overinvestigation and overtreatment
Confidence-based medicine	Bravado

Adapted from Isaacs D, Fitzgerald D. Seven alternatives to evidence-based medicine. BMJ 1999;319:1618.

evidence bearing on those questions, judging the evidence for its validity, and integrating the critical appraisal with the clinician's expertise and the patient's situation and values (5). This book deals with several aspects of evidence-based medicine, especially critically appraising the evidence about clinical questions.

In real-life clinical settings, other kinds of "evidence" compete for clinicians' attention and can influence medical decisions. Table 1.3 describes some of them in a parody of evidence-based medicine that was published some years ago, but is still true today. Probably all clinicians have experienced at least one of these factors during their training years! Another factor, not so humorous but very relevant, has been described as level IV evidence (6). Clinicians tend to remember cases when things go terribly wrong in the care they give an individual patient and are more likely to change practice after such an experience than after reading a well-done study. Less valid alternatives to evidence-based medicine can be very compelling at the emotional level and may provide a convenient way of coping with uncertainty, but they are a weak substitute for good research evidence.

Health services research is the study of how non-biologic factors (e.g., clinical workforce and facilities, how care is organized and paid for, and clinicians' beliefs and patients' cooperation) affect patients' health. Such studies have shown, for example, that medical care differs substantially from one small geographic area to another (without corresponding differences in patients' health); that surgery in hospitals that often perform a specific procedure tends to have better outcomes than hospitals in which the procedure is done infrequently; and that aspirin is underutilized in the treatment of acute myocardial infarction, even though this simple practice has been shown to reduce the number of subsequent vascular events by about 25%. These kinds of studies guide clinicians in their efforts to apply existing knowledge about the best clinical practices.

Other health services sciences also guide patient care. Quantitative decision making includes cost-effectiveness analyses, which describe the financial costs required to achieve a good outcome such as prevention of death or disease and decision analyses, which set out the rational basis for clinical decisions and the consequences of choices. The social sciences describe how the social environment affects health-related behaviors and the use of health services.

Biologic sciences, studies of the sequence of biologic events that lead from health to disease, are a powerful way of knowing how clinical phenomena may play out at the human level. Historically, it was primarily the progress in the biologic sciences that established the scientific approach to clinical medicine, and they continue to play a pivotal role. Anatomy explains nerve entrapment syndromes and their cause, symptoms, and relief. Physiology and biochemistry guide the management of diabetic keto-acidosis. Molecular genetics predicts the occurrence of diseases ranging from common cardiovascular diseases and cancer to rare inborn errors of metabolism, such as phenylketonuria and cystic fibrosis.

However, understanding the biology of disease, by itself, is often not a sound basis for prediction in intact humans. Too many other factors contribute to health and disease. For one thing, mechanisms of disease may be incompletely understood. For example, the notion that blood sugar in diabetic patients is more affected by ingestion of simple sugars (sucrose or table sugar) than by complex sugars such as starch (as in potatoes or pasta) has been dispelled by rigorous studies comparing the effect of these foods on blood glucose. Also, it is becoming clear that the effects of genetic abnormalities may be modified by complex physical and social environments such as diet and exposure to infectious and chemical agents. For example, glucose-6-phosphate dehydrogenase (G6PD) is an enzyme that protects red blood cells against oxidant injury leading to hemolysis. G6DP deficiency is the most common enzyme deficiency

in humans, occurring with certain mutations of the X-linked G6PD gene. However, males with commonly occurring genetic variants of G6PD deficiency are usually asymptomatic, developing hemolysis and jaundice only when they are exposed to environmental oxidant stresses such as certain drugs or infections. Finally, as shown in the example of rosiglitazone treatment for patients with type 2 diabetes, drugs often have multiple effects on patient health beyond the one predicted by studying disease biology. Therefore, knowledge of the biology of disease produces hypotheses, often very good ones, about what might happen in patients. But these hypotheses need to be tested by strong studies of intact human beings before they are accepted as clinical facts.

In summary, clinical epidemiology is one of many sciences basic to clinical medicine. At best, the various health-related sciences complement one another. Discoveries in one are confirmed in another; discoveries in the other lead to new hypotheses in the first.

Example

In the 1980s, clinicians in San Francisco noticed unusual infections and cancers in homosexual men, conditions previously seen only in profoundly immunocompromised patients. The new syndrome was called "acquired immune deficiency syndrome" (AIDS). Epidemiologists established that the men were suffering from a communicable disease that affected both men and women and was transmitted not only by sexual activity but also by needle sharing and blood products. Laboratory scientists identified the human immunodeficiency virus (HIV) and have developed drugs specifically targeting the structure and metabolism of this virus. Promising drugs, often developed based on understanding of biological mechanisms, have been tested for effectiveness in clinical trials. A new clinical specialty, in the care of patients with HIV infection, has arisen. Public health workers have promoted safe sex and other programs to prevent HIV infection. Thus, clinicians, epidemiologists, laboratory scientists, and public health officers have all contributed to the control of this new disease, especially in more developed countries, leading to a major increase in survival and improvement in quality of life of HIV-infected individuals

BASIC PRINCIPLES

The purpose of clinical epidemiology is to foster methods of clinical observation and interpretation that lead to valid conclusions and better patient care. The most credible answers to clinical questions are based on a few basic principles. Two of these—that observations should address questions facing patients and clinicians, and results should include patient-centered health outcomes (the 5 Ds)—have already been covered. Other basic principles are discussed below.

Variables

Researchers call the attributes of patients and clinical events variables—things that vary and can be measured. In a typical study, there are three main kinds of variables. One is a purported cause or predictor variable, sometimes called the independent variable. Another is the possible effect or outcome variable, sometimes called the dependent variable. Still, other variables may be part of the system under study and may affect the relationship between the independent and dependant variables. These are called extraneous variables (or covariates) because they are extraneous to the main question, though perhaps very much a part of the phenomenon under study.

Numbers and Probability

Clinical science, like all other sciences, depends on quantitative measurements. Impressions, instincts, and beliefs are important in medicine too, but only when added to a solid foundation of numerical information. This foundation allows better confirmation, more precise communication among clinicians and between clinicians and patients, and estimation of error. Clinical outcomes, such as occurrence of disease, death, symptoms, or disability, can be counted and expressed as numbers.

In most clinical situations, the diagnosis, prognosis, and results of treatment are uncertain for an individual patient. An individual will either experience a clinical outcome or will not, and predictions can seldom be so exact. Therefore, a prediction must be expressed as a probability. The probability for an individual patient is best estimated by referring to past experience with groups of similar patients—for example, that cigarette smoking more than doubles the risk of dying among middle-aged adults, that blood tests for troponins detect about 99% of myocardial infarctions in patients with acute chest pain, and that 2% to 6% of patients undergoing elective surgery for abdominal aortic aneurysm will die

within 30 days of the procedure, as opposed to 40% to 80% when emergency repair is necessary.

Populations and Samples

Populations are all people in a defined setting (such as North Carolina) or with certain defined characteristics (such as being age >65 years or having a thyroid nodule). Unselected people in the community are the usual population for epidemiologic studies of cause. On the other hand, clinical populations include all patients with a clinical characteristic such as all those with community-acquired pneumonia or aortic stenosis. Thus, one speaks of the general population, a hospitalized population, or a population of patients with a specific disease.

Clinical research is ordinarily carried out on a sample or subset of people in a defined population. One is interested in the characteristics of the defined population but must, for practical reasons, estimate them by describing the characteristics of people in a sample (Fig. 1.2). One then makes an inference, a reasoned judgment based on data, that the characteristics of the sample resemble those of the parent population.

The extent to which a sample represents its population, and thus is a fair substitute for it, depends on how the sample was selected. Methods in which every member of the population has an equal (or known) chance of being selected can produce samples that are extraordinarily similar to the parent population, at least in the long run and for large samples. An everyday example is opinion polls using household sampling based on census data. In our own clinical research, we often use a computer to select a representative sample from all patients in our large, multispecialty group practice, each of which has the same chance of being selected. On the other hand, samples taken haphazardly or for convenience (i.e., by selecting patients who are easy to work with or happen to be visiting the clinic when data are being collected) may misrepresent their parent population and be misleading.

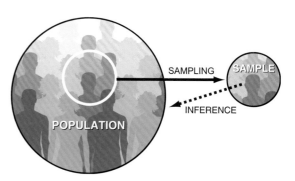

Figure 1.2 ■ Population and sample.

Bias (Systematic Error)

Bias is "a process at any stage of inference tending to produce results that depart systematically from the true values" (7). It is "an error in the conception and design of a study—or in the collection, analysis, interpretation, publication, or review of data—leading to results or conclusions that are systematically (as opposed to randomly) different from the truth" (8).

Example

Patients with inguinal hernia who get laparoscopic repair seem to have less postoperative pain and more rapid return to work than those who get the traditional, open surgery. The careful clinician asks, "Are the results of laparoscopic surgery really better or might they only appear better as a result of biases in the way the information was collected?" Perhaps laparoscopic repair is offered to patients who are in better health or who seem to have better tissue strength because of age or general health. Perhaps surgeons and patients are more inclined to think that the procedure should cause less pain, because it is new and the scar is smaller, and so the patients report less pain and the surgeons are less likely to ask about it or are less likely to record pain in the medical record. Perhaps patients who get laparoscopic surgery are usually instructed to return to work earlier than those who get open surgery. If any of these were so, the favorable results could be related to systematic differences in how patients were selected for the laparoscopic procedure, how they reported their symptoms, or how they were told what they can do—rather than a true difference in success rates. As discussed in Chapter 5, there are ways to protect against these potential biases. Studies that avoided these biases have found that patients who undergo laparoscopic surgery do in fact experience less pain after surgery (but only early on) and a more rapid return to work by a few days. But laparoscopic surgery takes longer, and several studies found more serious complications in patients receiving it, as well as a higher rate of recurrence, especially among older men (9,10). In summary, careful studies found that the choice between the two procedures is not clear cut.

Table 1.4

Bias in Clinical Observation	
Selection bias	Occurs when comparisons are made between groups of patients that differ in determinates of outcome other than the one under study.
Measurement bias	Occurs when the methods of measurement are dissimilar among groups of patients
Confounding	Occurs when two factors are associated (travel together) and the effect of one is confused with or distorted by the effect of the other

Observations on patients (whether for patient care or research) are particularly susceptible to bias. The process tends to be just plain untidy. As participants in a study, human beings have the disconcerting habit of doing as they please and not necessarily what would be required for producing scientifically rigorous answers. When researchers attempt to conduct an experiment with them, as one might in a laboratory, things tend to go wrong. Some people refuse to participate, whereas others drop out or choose another treatment. In addition, clinicians are inclined to believe that their therapies are successful. (Most patients would not want a physician who felt otherwise.) This attitude, which is so important in the practice of medicine, makes clinical observations particularly vulnerable to bias.

Although dozens of biases have been defined (11), most fall into one of three broad categories (Table 1.4).

Selection Bias

Selection bias occurs when comparisons are made between groups of patients that differ in ways other than the main factors under study, ones that affect the outcome of the study. Groups of patients often differ in many ways—age, sex, severity of disease, the presence of other diseases, the care they receive, and so on. If one compares the experience of two groups that differ on a specific characteristic of interest (e.g., a treatment or a suspected cause of disease) but are dissimilar in these other ways and the differences are themselves related to outcome, the comparison is biased and little can be concluded about the independent effects of the characteristic of interest. In the herniorrhaphy example, selection bias would have occurred if patients receiving the laparoscopic procedure were healthier than those who had open surgery.

Measurement Bias

Measurement bias occurs when the method of measurement leads to systematically incorrect results.

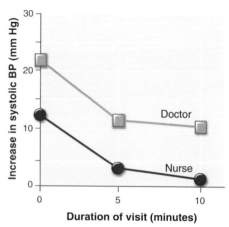

Figure 1.3 ■ **White coat hypertension.** Increase in systolic pressure, determined by continuous intraarterial monitoring, as the blood pressure is taken with a sphygmomanometer by an unfamiliar doctor or nurse. (Redrawn with permission from Mancia G, Parati G, Pomidossi G, et al. Alerting reaction and rise in blood pressure during measurement by physician and nurse. Hypertension 1987;9: 209–215.)

Example

Blood pressure levels are powerful predictors of cardiovascular disease. However, multiple studies have shown that taking a blood pressure measurement is not as simple as it seems (12). Correct measurement requires using appropriate procedures, including using a larger cuff size for overweight and obese adults, positioning the patient so that the upper arm is below the level of the right atrium and so the patient does not have to hold up the arm, and taking the measurement in a quiet setting and multiple times. If any of these procedures is not done correctly, the resulting measurements are likely to be artificially and systematically elevated. Another factor leading to systematically higher blood pressure readings, sometimes called "white coat hypertension" (Fig. 1.3), occurs when blood pressure is measured by physicians, suggesting that visits to the doctor cause anxiety in patients. However, clinicians who deflate the blood pressure cuff faster than 2 to 3 mm/sec will likely underestimate systolic (but overestimate diastolic) blood pressure. Studies have also shown a tendency for clinicians to record values that are just at the normal level in patients with borderline high blood pressures. Systematic errors in blood pressure measurements can, therefore, lead to overtreatment or undertreatment of patients in clinical practice. Clinical research based on blood pressure measurements taken during routine patient care can lead to misleading results unless careful standardized procedures are used. These kinds of biases led to the development of blood pressure measurement instruments that do not involve human ears and hands.

Confounding

Confounding can occur when one is trying to find out whether a factor, such as a behavior or drug exposure, is a cause of disease in and of itself. If the factor of interest is associated or "travels together" with another factor, which is itself related to the outcome, the effect of the factor under study can be confused with or distorted by the effect of the other.

Example

Supplements of antioxidants, such as vitamins A, C, and E, are popular with the lay public. Laboratory experiments and studies of people who choose to take antioxidants suggested that antioxidants prevent cardiovascular disease and certain cancers. However, careful randomized studies, which are able to avoid confounding, routinely found little effect of antioxidants (13,14). In fact, when results of these studies were combined, use of antioxidants, especially at high doses, was associated with small increases, not decreases, in death rates. How could the results of early studies be reconciled with the opposite findings of later, carefully controlled, trials? Confounding has been suggested, as illustrated in Figure 1.4. People who take antioxidants on their own are likely to do other things differently than those who do not take antioxidants—such as exercise more, watch their weight, eat more vegetables, and not smoke—and it may be these activities, not antioxidants, that led to lower death rates in the studies not randomizing the intervention.

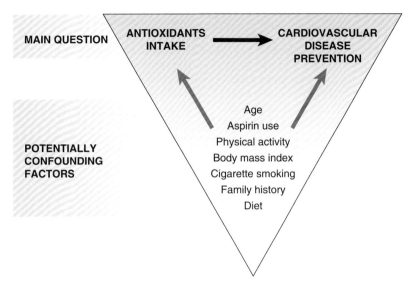

Figure 1.4 ■ Confounding. The relationship between antioxidant intake and cardio-vascular risk is potentially confounded by patient characteristics and behaviors related to both antioxidant use and development of cardiovascular disease.

Most clinical research studies, especially studies that observe people over time, routinely try to avoid confounding by "controlling" for possible confounding variables in the analysis (see Chapter 5). Variables such as age, sex, and race are almost always analyzed for confounding because so many health outcomes vary according to them. Studies that involve human behavior (such as taking antioxidants regularly), are especially prone to confounding because human behavior is so complex that it is difficult to analyze for all the factors that might influence it.

A variable does not have to be a cause of the disease or other condition of interest in order to be a confounding variable. It may just be related to the condition in a particular set of data at hand, because of selection bias or chance, but not related in nature. Whether just in the data or in nature, the consequences are the same: the mistaken impression that the factor of interest is a true, independent cause when it is not.

Selection bias and confounding are related. They are described separately, however, because they present problems at different points in a clinical study. Selection bias is an issue primarily when patients are chosen for investigation and it is important in the design of a study. Confounding must be dealt with during analysis of the data, once the observations have been made.

A study may involve several types of biases at the same time.

Example

Concerns have been raised that caffeine consumption during pregnancy may lead to adverse fetal outcomes. It would be unethical to determine if caffeine is dangerous to fetuses by an experiment assigning some pregnant women to drink high levels of caffeine, and others not, so researchers have usually studied what happens during pregnancy according to the amount of caffeine ingested. However, several biases have been demonstrated in many of these studies (15). Measurement bias could have occurred because most studies relied on self-reported intake of caffeine. One study demonstrated recall bias, a type of measurement bias that refers to differential recall in people with an adverse outcome compared to those with a normal outcome. An association was found between caffeine consumption and miscarriage when women were interviewed after they miscarried, but not when women were questioned about caffeine consumption before miscarriage (16). If some women were recruited for caffeine studies during prenatal visits (women who are likely to be particularly health conscious) and others recruited toward the end of their pregnancy, the different approaches to recruitment could lead to selection bias that might invalidate the results. Finally, heavy coffee consumption is known to be associated with cigarette smoking, lower socio-economic levels, greater alcohol consumption, and generally less health consciousness, all of which could confound any association between caffeine and adverse fetal outcomes.

The potential for bias does not mean that bias is actually present in a particular study or, if present, would have a big enough effect on the results to matter. For a researcher or reader to deal effectively with bias, it is first necessary to know where and how to look for it and what can be done about it. But one should not stop there. It is also necessary to determine whether bias is actually present and how large it is likely to be, and then decide whether it is important enough to change the conclusions of the study in a clinically meaningful way.

Chance

Observations about disease are ordinarily made on a sample of patients because it is not possible to study all patients with the disease in question. Results of unbiased samples tend to approximate the true value. However, a given sample, even if selected without bias, may misrepresent the situation in the population as a whole because of chance. If the observation were repeated on many such patient samples from the same population, results for the samples would cluster around the true value, with more of them close to, rather than far from, the true value. The divergence of an observation on a sample from the true population value, due to chance alone, is called random variation.

All of us are familiar with chance as an explanation for why a coin does not come up heads exactly 50% of the time when it is flipped, say, 100 times. The same effect, random variation, applies when comparing the effects of laparoscopic and open repair of inguinal hernia, discussed earlier. Suppose all biases were removed from a study of the effects of the two procedures. Suppose, further, that the two procedures are, in reality, equally effective in the amount of pain caused, each followed by pain in 10% of patients. Because of chance alone, a single study with small numbers of patients in each treatment group might easily find that patients do better with laparoscopy than with open surgery (or vice versa).

Chance can affect all the steps involved in clinical observations. In the assessment of the two ways of repairing inguinal hernia, random variation occurs in the sampling of patients for the study, the selection of treatment groups, and the measurements of pain and return to work.

Unlike bias, which tends to distort results in one direction or another, random variation is as likely to result in observations above the true value as below it. As a consequence, the mean of many unbiased observations on samples tends to approximate the true value in the population, even though the results of individual small samples may not. In the case of inguinal hernia repair, multiple studies, when evaluated together, have shown laparoscopic repair results in less pain in the first few days after surgery.

Statistics can be used to estimate the extent to which chance (random variation) accounts for the results of a clinical study. Knowledge of statistics can also help reduce the role of chance by helping to create a better design and analyses. However, random variation can never be eliminated totally, so chance should always be considered when assessing the results of clinical observations. The role of chance in clinical observations will be discussed in greater depth in Chapter 11.

The Effects of Bias and Chance Are Cumulative

The two sources of error—bias and chance—are not mutually exclusive. In most situations, both are present. The relationship between the two is illustrated in Figure 1.5. The measurement of diastolic blood pressure on a single patient is taken as an example; each dot represents an observation on that patient. True blood pressure, which is 80 mm Hg for this patient, can be obtained by an intra-arterial cannula, but this method is not feasible for routine measurements. Blood pressure is ordinarily measured indirectly, using a sphygmomanometer (blood pressure cuff). As discussed in

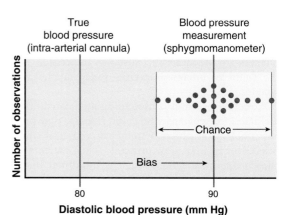

Figure 1.5 ■ **Bias and chance.** True blood pressure by intra-arterial cannula and clinical measurement by sphygmomanometer.

an earlier example, the simpler instrument is prone to error or deviations from the true value. In the figure, the error is represented by all of the sphygmomanometer readings falling to the right of the true value. The deviation of sphygmomanometer readings to higher values (bias) may have several explanations (e.g., the wrong cuff size, patient anxiety, or "white coat hypertension"). Individual blood pressure readings are also subject to error because of random variation in measurement, as illustrated by the spread of the sphygmomanometer readings around the mean value (90 mm Hg).

The main reason for distinguishing between bias and chance is that they are handled differently. In theory, bias can be prevented by conducting clinical investigations properly or can be corrected during data analysis. If not eliminated, bias often can be detected by the discerning reader. Most of this book is about how to recognize, avoid, or minimize bias. Chance, on the other hand, cannot be eliminated, but its influence can be reduced by proper design of research, and the remaining effect can be estimated by statistics. No amount of statistical treatment can correct for unknown biases in data. Some statisticians would go so far as to suggest that statistics should not be applied to data that are vulnerable to bias because of poor research design, for fear of giving false respectability to fundamentally misleading work.

Internal and External Validity

When making inferences about a population from observations on a sample, clinicians need to make up their minds about two fundamental questions. First, are the conclusions of the research correct for the people in the sample? Second, if so, does the sample represent fairly the patients the clinician is most interested in, the kind of patients in his or her practice, or perhaps a specific patient at hand (Fig. 1.6)?

Internal validity is the degree to which the results of a study are correct for the sample of patients being studied. It is "internal" because it applies to the conditions of the particular group of patients being observed and not necessarily to others. The internal validity of clinical research is determined by how well the design, data collection, and analyses are carried out, and it is threatened by all of the biases and random variation discussed earlier. For a clinical observation to be useful, internal validity is a necessary but not sufficient condition.

External validity is the degree to which the results of an observation hold true in other settings. Another term for this is generalizability. For the individual clinician, it is an answer to the question, "Assuming that the results of a study are true, do they apply to my patients as well?" Generalizability expresses the

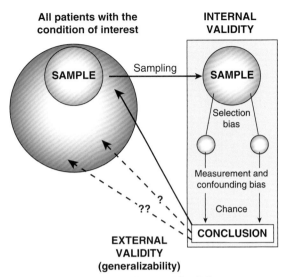

Figure 1.6 ■ Internal and external validity.

validity of assuming that patients in a study are similar to other patients.

Every study that is internally valid is generalizable to patients very much like the ones in the study. However, an unimpeachable study, with high internal validity, may be totally misleading if its results are generalized to the wrong patients.

Example

What is the long-term death rate in anorexia nervosa, an eating disorder mainly afflicting young women? In a synthesis of 42 studies, estimated mortality was 15% over 30 years (17). These studies, like most clinical research, were of patients identified in referral centers where relatively severe cases are seen. A study of all patients developing anorexia in a defined population provided a different view of the disease. Researchers at the Mayo Clinic were able to identify all patients developing this disease in their city, Rochester, Minnesota, from 1935 to 1989 (Fig. 1.7) (18). All-cause mortality at 30 years was 7%, half that of reported studies. The predicted mortality in people without anorexia nervosa of the same age and sex was about the same, 6%. Therefore, although some patients do die of anorexia nervosa, most published studies greatly overestimate the risk, presumably because they report experience with relatively severe cases.

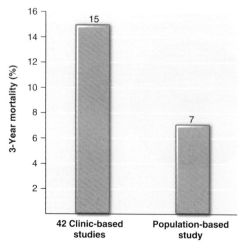

Figure 1.7 ■ Sampling bias. Thirty-year mortality from all causes in patients with anorexia nervosa. Comparison of a synthesis of 42 published studies, mainly from referral centers, and a study of all patients with anorexia in the population. (Data from Sullivan PF. Mortality in anorexia nervosa. Am J Psychiatry 1995;152:1073–1074; and Korndorter SR, Lucan AR, Suman VJ, et al. Long-term survival of patients with anorexia nervosa: a population-based study in Rochester, Minn. Mayo Clin Proc 2003;78:278–284.)

The generalizability of clinical observations, even those with high internal validity, is a matter of personal judgment about which reasonable people might disagree. A situation often occurs when clinicians must decide whether to use the results of a well-done study for a patient who is older than those in the study, a different gender, or sicker. It might be that a treatment that works well in young healthy men does more harm than good in older, sicker women.

Generalizability can rarely be dealt with satisfactorily in any one study. Even a defined, geographically based population is a biased sample of other populations. For example, hospital patients are biased samples of county residents, counties of states, states of regions, and so on. The best a researcher can do about generalizability is to ensure internal validity, have the study population fit the research question, describe the study patients carefully, and avoid studying patients who are so unusual that experience with them generalizes to few others. It then remains for other studies, in other settings, to extend generalizability.

INFORMATION AND DECISIONS

The primary concerns of this book are the quality of clinical information and its correct interpretation. Making decisions is another matter. True, good decisions depend on good information, but they involve

a great deal more as well, including value judgments and weighing competing risks and benefits.

In recent years, medical decision making has become a valued discipline in its own right. The field includes qualitative studies of how clinicians make decisions and how the process might be biased and can be improved. It also includes quantitative methods such as decision analysis, cost-benefit analysis, and cost-effectiveness analysis that present the decision-making process in an explicit way so that its components and the consequences of assigning various probabilities and values to them can be examined.

Patients and clinicians make clinical decisions. At best, they make decisions together, a process called shared decision making, recognizing that their expertise is complementary. Patients are experts in what they hope to achieve from medical care, given their unique experiences and preferences. They may have found a lot of information about their condition (e.g., from the Internet) but are not grounded in how to sort out credible from fallacious claims. Doctors are experts in whether and how likely patients' goals can be achieved and how to achieve them. For this, they depend on the body of research evidence and the ability, based on the principles of clinical epidemiology, to distinguish stronger from weaker evidence. Of course, clinicians also bring to the encounter experience in how disease presents and the human consequences of care, such as what it is like to be intubated or to have an amputation, with which patients may have little experience. For clinicians to play their part on this team, they need to be experts in the interpretation of clinically relevant information.

Patients' preferences and sound evidence are the basis for choosing among care options. For example, a patient with valvular heart disease may prefer the possibility of long-term good health that surgery offers, even though surgery is associated with discomfort and risk of death in the short term. A clinician armed with critical reading and communication skills can help the patient understand how big those potential benefits and risks are and how surely they have been established.

Some aspects of decision analysis, such as evaluation of diagnostic tests, are included in this book. However, we have elected not to go deeply into medical decision making itself. Our reason is that decisions are only as good as the information used to make them, and we have found enough to say about the essentials of collecting and interpreting clinical information to fill a book.

ORGANIZATION OF THIS BOOK

In most textbooks on clinical medicine, information about each disease is presented as answers to traditional clinical questions: diagnosis, clinical course, treatment, and the like. However, most epidemiology books are organized around research strategies such as clinical trials, surveys, case-control studies, and the like. This way of organizing a book may serve those who perform clinical research, but it is often awkward for clinicians.

We have organized this book primarily according to the questions clinicians encounter when caring for patients (Table 1.1). Figure 1.8 illustrates how these questions correspond to the book's chapters, taking HIV infection as an example. The questions relate to

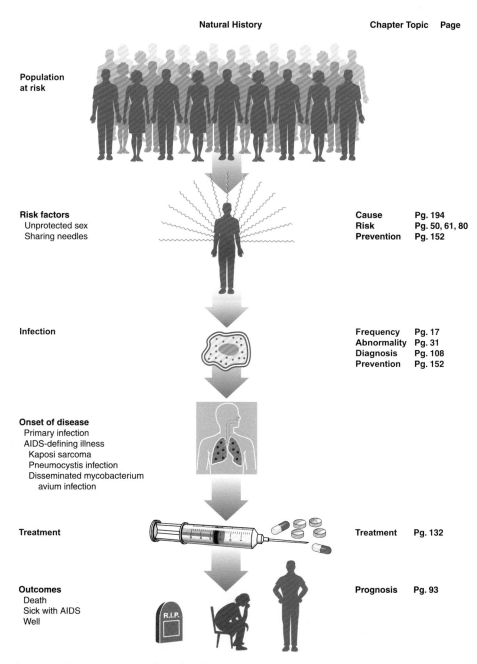

Natural History

Chapter Topic   Page

Population at risk

Risk factors
  Unprotected sex
  Sharing needles

Cause   **Pg. 194**
Risk   **Pg. 50, 61, 80**
Prevention   **Pg. 152**

Infection

Frequency **Pg. 17**
Abnormality **Pg. 31**
Diagnosis **Pg. 108**
Prevention **Pg. 152**

Onset of disease
  Primary infection
  AIDS-defining illness
    Kaposi sarcoma
    Pneumocystis infection
    Disseminated mycobacterium
      avium infection

Treatment

Treatment **Pg. 132**

Outcomes
  Death
  Sick with AIDS
  Well

Prognosis **Pg. 93**

Figure 1.8 ■ **Organization of this book in relation to the natural history of human immunodeficiency virus (HIV) infection.** Chapters 11, 13, and 14 describe cross-cutting issues related to all points in the natural history of disease.

the entire natural history of disease, from the time people without HIV infection are first exposed to risk, to when some acquire the disease and emerge as patients, through complications of the disease, AIDS-defining illness, to survival or death.

In each chapter, we describe research strategies used to answer that chapter's clinical questions.

Some strategies, such as cohort studies, are useful for answering several different kinds of clinical questions. For the purposes of presentation, we have discussed each strategy primarily in one chapter and have simply referred to the discussion when the method is relevant to other questions in other chapters.

Review Questions

Questions 1.1–1.6 are based on the following clinical scenario.

A 37-year-old-woman with low back pain for the past 4 weeks wants to know if you recommend surgery. You prefer to base your treatment recommendations on research evidence whenever possible. In the strongest study you can find, investigators reviewed the medical records of 40 consecutive men with low back pain under care at their clinic—22 had been referred for surgery, and the other 18 patients had remained under medical care without surgery. The study compared rates of disabling pain after 2 months. All of the surgically treated patients and 10 of the medically treated patients were still being seen in the clinic throughout this time. Rates of pain relief were slightly higher in the surgically treated patients.

For each of the following statements, circle the one response that best represents the corresponding threat to validity.

1.1. Because there are relatively few patients in this study, it may give a misleading impression of the actual effectiveness of surgery.

   A. Selection bias
   B. Measurement bias
   C. Confounding
   D. Chance
   E. External validity (generalizability)

1.2. The results of this study may not apply to your patient, a woman, because all the patients in the study were men.

   A. Selection bias
   B. Measurement bias
   C. Confounding
   D. Chance
   E. External validity (generalizability)

1.3. Fewer patients who did not have surgery remained under care at the clinic 2 months after surgery.

   A. Selection bias
   B. Measurement bias
   C. Confounding
   D. Chance
   E. External validity (generalizability)

1.4. The patients who were referred for surgery were younger and fitter than those who remained under medical care.

   A. Selection bias
   B. Measurement bias
   C. Confounding
   D. Chance
   E. External validity (generalizability)

1.5. Compared with patients who had medical care alone, patients who had surgery might have been less likely to report whatever pain they had and the treating physicians might have been less inclined to record pain in the medical record.

   A. Selection bias
   B. Measurement bias
   C. Confounding
   D. Chance
   E. External validity (generalizability)

1.6. Patients without other medical conditions were both more likely to recover and more likely to be referred for surgery.

   A. Selection bias
   B. Measurement bias
   C. Confounding
   D. Chance
   E. External validity (generalizability)

For questions 1.7–1.11, select the best answer.

1.7. Histamine is a mediator of inflammation in patients with allergic rhinitis ("hay fever"). Based on this fact, which of the following is true?

   A. Drugs that block the effects of histamines will relieve symptoms.
   B. A fall in histamine levels in the nose is a reliable marker of clinical success.
   C. Antihistamines may be effective, and their effects on symptoms (e.g., itchy nose, sneezing, and congestion) should be studied in patients with allergic rhinitis.
   D. Other mediators are not important.
   E. If laboratory studies of disease are convincing, clinical research is unnecessary.

1.8. Which of the following statements about samples of populations is incorrect?

   A. Samples of a populations may have characteristics that differ from the population even though correct sampling procedures were followed.
   B. Samples of populations are the only feasible way of studying the population.
   C. When populations are correctly sampled, external validity is ensured.
   D. Samples of populations should be selected in a way that every member of the population has an equal chance of being chosen.

1.9. You are making a treatment decision with a 72-year-old man with colon cancer. You are aware of several good studies that have shown that a certain drug combination prolongs the life of patients with colon cancer. However, all the patients in these studies were much younger. Which of the statements below is correct?

   A. Given these studies, the decision about this treatment is a matter of personal judgment.
   B. Relying on these studies for your patient is called internal validity.
   C. The results in these studies are affected by chance but not bias.

1.10. A study was done to determine whether regular exercise lowers the risk of coronary heart disease (CHD). An exercise program was offered to employees of a factory, and the rates of subsequent coronary events were compared in employees who volunteered for the program and those who did not volunteer. The development of CHD was determined by means of regular voluntary checkups, including a careful history, an electrocardiogram, and a review of routine health records. Surprisingly, the members of the exercise group developed higher rates of CHD even though fewer of them smoked cigarettes. This result is least likely to be explained by which of the following?

   A. The volunteers were at higher risk for developing CHD than those not volunteering before the study began.
   B. The volunteers did not actually increase their exercise and the amount of exercise was the same in the two groups.
   C. Volunteers got more check-ups, and silent myocardial infarctions were, therefore, more likely to have been diagnosed in the exercise group.

1.11. Ventricular premature depolarizations are associated with an increased risk of sudden death from a fatal arrhythmia, especially in people with other evidence of heart disease. You have read there is a new drug for ventricular premature depolarizations. What is the most important thing you would like to know about the drug before prescribing it to a patient?

   A. The drug's mechanism of action.
   B. How well the drug prevents ventricular premature depolarizations in people using the drug compared to those who do not use the drug.
   C. The rate of sudden death in similar people who do and do not take the drug.

Questions 1.12–1.15 are based on the following clinical scenario.

Because reports suggested estrogens increase the risk of clotting, a study compared the frequency of oral contraceptive use among women admitted to a hospital with thrombophlebitis and a group of women admitted for other reasons. Medical records were reviewed for indication of oral contraceptive use in the two groups. Women with thrombophlebitis were found to have been using oral contraceptives more frequently than the women admitted for other reasons.

For each of the following statements, select the one response that represents the corresponding threat to validity.

1.12. Women with thrombophlebitis may have reported the use of contraceptives more completely than women without thrombophlebitis because they remembered hearing of the association.

    A. Selection bias
    B. Measurement bias
    C. Confounding
    D. Chance
    E. External validity (generalizability)

1.13. Doctors may have questioned women with thrombophlebitis more carefully about contraceptive use than they did those without thrombophlebitis (and recorded the information more carefully in the medical record) because they were aware that estrogen could cause clotting.

    A. Selection bias
    B. Measurement bias

    C. Confounding
    D. Chance
    E. External validity (generalizability)

1.14. The number of women in the study was small.

    A. Selection bias
    B. Measurement bias
    C. Confounding
    D. Chance
    E. External validity (generalizability)

1.15. The women with thrombophlebitis were admitted to the hospital by doctors working in different neighborhoods than the physicians of those that did not have thrombophlebitis.

    A. Selection bias
    B. Measurement bias
    C. Confounding
    D. Chance
    E. External validity (generalizability)

Answers are in Appendix A.

REFERENCES

1. Home PD, Pocock SJ, Beck-Nielsen H, et al. Rosiglitazone evaluated for cardiovascular outcomes in oral agent combination therapy for type 2 diabetes (RECORD): a multicentre, randomized, open-label trial. Lancet 2009;373:2125–2135.
2. Lipscombe LL, Gomes T, Levesque LE, et al. Thiazolidinediones and cardiovascular outcomes in older patients with diabetes. JAMA 2007;298:2634–2643.
3. Nissen SE, Wolski K. Effect of rosiglitazone on the risk of myocardial infarction and death from cardiovascular causes. N Engl J Med 2007;356:2457–2471.
4. Friedman GD. Primer of Epidemiology, 5th ed. New York: Appleton and Lange; 2004.
5. Straus SE, Richardson WS, Glasziou P, et al. Evidence-Based Medicine: How to Practice and Teach EBM, 4th ed. New York: Churchill Livingstone; 2011.
6. Stuebe AM. Level IV evidence—adverse anecdote and clinical practice. N Engl J Med 2011;365(1):8–9.
7. Murphy EA. The Logic of Medicine. Baltimore: Johns Hopkins University Press; 1976.
8. Porta M. A Dictionary of Epidemiology, 5th ed. New York: Oxford University Press; 2008.
9. McCormack K, Scott N, Go PM, et al. Laparoscopic techniques versus open techniques for inguinal hernia repair. Cochrane Database Systematic Review 2003;1:CD001785. Publication History: Edited (no change to conclusions) 8 Oct 2008.
10. Neumayer L, Giobbie-Hurder A, Jonasson O, et al. Open mesh versus laparoscopic mesh repair of inguinal hernia. N Eng J Med 2004;350:1819–1827.
11. Sackett DL. Bias in analytic research. J Chronic Dis 1979;32: 51–63.
12. Pickering TG, Hall JE, Appel LJ, et al. Recommendations for blood pressure in humans and experimental animals. Part 1: Blood pressure measurement in humans. A statement for professionals from the Subcommittee of Professional and Public Education of the American Heart Association Council on High Blood Pressure Research. Circulation 2005;111: 697–716.
13. Bjelakovic G, Nikolova D, Gluud LL, et al. Mortality in randomized trials of antioxidant supplements for primary and secondary prevention: systematic review and meta-analysis. JAMA 2007; 297(8):842–857.
14. Vevekananthan DP, Penn MS, Sapp SK, et al. Use of antioxidant vitamins for the prevention of cardiovascular disease: meta-analysis of randomized trials. Lancet 2003;361: 2017–2023.
15. Norman RJ, Nisenblat V. The effects of caffeine on fertility and on pregnancy outcomes. In: Basow DS, ed. UpToDate. Waltham, MA: UpToDate; 2011.
16. Savitz DA, Chan RL, Herring AH, et al. Caffeine and miscarriage risk. Epidemiology 2008;19:55–62.
17. Sullivan PF. Mortality in anorexia nervosa. Am J Psychiatry 1995;152:1073–1074.
18. Korndorfer SR, Lucas AR, Suman VJ, et al. Long-term survival of patients with anorexia nervosa: a population-based study in Rochester, Minn. Mayo Clin Proc 2003;78: 278–284.

Chapter 2

Frequency

Here, it is necessary to count.
—*P.C.A. Louis*[†]
1787–1872[a]

KEY WORDS

Numerator
Denominator
Prevalence
Point prevalence
Period prevalence
Incidence
Duration of disease
Case fatality rate
Survival rate
Complication rate
Infant mortality rate
Perinatal mortality
  rate
Prevalence studies
Cross-sectional studies
Surveys
Cohort

Cohort studies
Cumulative
  incidence
Incidence density
Person-time
Dynamic population
Population at risk
Random sample
Probability sample
Sampling fraction
Oversample
Convenience samples
Grab samples
Epidemic
Pandemic
Epidemic curve
Endemic

Chapter 1 outlined the questions that clinicians need to answer as they care for patients. Answers are usually in the form of probabilities and only rarely as certainties. Frequencies obtained from clinical research are the basis for probability estimates for the purposes of patient care. This chapter describes basic expressions of frequency, how they are obtained from clinical research, and how to recognize threats to their validity.

[†]A 19th Century physician and proponent of the "numerical method" (relying on counts, not impressions) to understand the natural history of diseases such as typhoid fever.

Example

A 72-year-old man presents with slowly progressive urinary frequency, hesitancy, and dribbling. A digital rectal examination reveals a symmetrically enlarged prostate gland and no nodules. Urinary flow measurements show a reduction in flow rate, and his serum prostate-specific antigen (PSA) is not elevated. The clinician diagnoses benign prostatic hyperplasia (BPH). In deciding on treatment, the clinician and patient must weigh the benefits and hazards of various therapeutic options. To simplify, let us say the options are medical therapy with drugs or surgery. The patient might choose medical treatment but runs the risk of worsening symptoms or obstructive renal disease because the treatment is less immediately effective than surgery. Or he might choose surgery, gaining immediate relief of symptoms but at the risk of operative mortality and long-term urinary incontinence and impotence.

Decisions such as the one this patient and clinician face have traditionally relied on clinical judgment based on experience at the bedside and in the clinics. In modern times, clinical research has become sufficiently strong and extensive that it is possible to ground clinical judgment in research-based probabilities—frequencies. Probabilities of disease, improvement, deterioration, cure, side effects, and death are the basis for answering most clinical questions. For this patient, sound clinical decision making requires accurate estimates of how his symptoms and complications of treatment will change over time according to which treatment is chosen.

ARE WORDS SUITABLE SUBSTITUTES FOR NUMBERS?

Clinicians often communicate probabilities as words (e.g., usually, sometimes, rarely) rather than as numbers. Substituting words for numbers is convenient and avoids making a precise statement when one is uncertain about a probability. However, words are a poor substitute for numbers because there is little agreement about the meanings of commonly used adjectives describing probabilities.

Example

Physicians were asked to assign percentage values to 13 expressions of probability (1). These physicians generally agreed on probabilities corresponding to adjectives such as "always" or "never" describing very likely or very unlikely events but not on expressions associated with less extreme probabilities. For example, the range of probabilities (from the top to the bottom tenth of attending physicians) was 60% to 90% for "usually," 5% to 45% for "sometimes," and 1% to 30% for "seldom." This suggests (as authors of an earlier study had asserted) that "difference of opinion among physicians regarding the management of a problem may reflect differences in the meaning ascribed to words used to define probability" (2).

Patients also assign widely varying probabilities to word descriptions. In another study, highly skilled and professional workers outside of medicine thought "usually" referred to probabilities of 35% to 100%; "rarely" meant to them a probability of 0% to 15% (3).

Thus, substituting words for numbers diminishes the information conveyed. We advocate using numbers whenever possible.

PREVALENCE AND INCIDENCE

In general, clinically relevant measures of frequency are expressed as proportions, in which the numerator is the number of patients experiencing an event (cases) and the denominator is the number of people in whom the

event could have occurred (population). The two basic measures of frequency are prevalence and incidence.

Prevalence

Prevalence is the fraction (proportion or percent) of a group of people possessing a clinical condition or outcome at a given point in time. Prevalence is measured by surveying a defined population and counting the number of people with and without the condition of interest. Point prevalence is measured at a single point in time for each person (although actual measurements need not necessarily be made at the same point in calendar time for all the people in the population). Period prevalence describes cases that were present at any time during a specified period of time.

Incidence

Incidence is the fraction or proportion of a group of people initially free of the outcome of interest that develops the condition over a given period of time. Incidence refers then to *new* cases of disease occurring in a population initially free of the disease or new outcomes such as symptoms or complications occurring in patients with a disease who are initially free of these problems.

Figure 2.1 illustrates the differences between incidence and prevalence. It shows the occurrence of

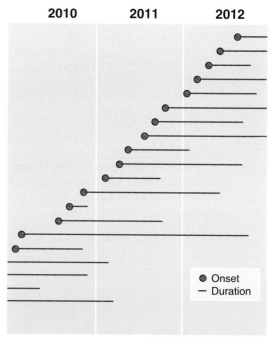

Figure 2.1 ■ Incidence and prevalence. Occurrence of disease in 10,000 people at risk for lung cancer, 2010 to 2012.

lung cancer in a population of 10,000 people over the course of 3 years (2010–2012). As time passes, individuals in the population develop the disease. They remain in this state until they either recover or die—in the case of lung cancer, they usually die. Four people already had lung cancer before 2010, and 16 people developed it during the 3 years of observation. The rest of the original 10,000 people have not had lung cancer during these 3 years and do not appear in the figure.

To calculate prevalence of lung cancer at the beginning of 2010, four cases already existed, so the prevalence at that point in time is 4/10,000. If all surviving people are examined at the beginning of each year, one can compute the prevalence at those points in time. At the beginning of 2011, the prevalence is 5/9,996 because two of the pre-2010 patients are still alive, as are three other people who developed lung cancer in 2010; the denominator is reduced by the 4 patients who died before 2011. Prevalence can be computed for each of the other two annual examinations and is 7/9,992 at the beginning of 2011 and 5/9,986 at the beginning of 2012.

To calculate the incidence of new cases developing in the population, we consider only the 9,996 people free of the disease at the beginning of 2010 and what happens to them over the next 3 years. Five new lung cancers developed in 2010, six developed in 2011, and five additional lung cancers developed in 2012. The 3-year incidence of the disease is all new cases developing in the 3 years (16) divided by the number of susceptible individuals at the beginning of the follow-up period (9,996), or 16/9,996 in 3 years. What are the annual incidences for 2010, 2011, and 2012? Remembering to remove the previous cases from the denominator (they are no longer at risk of developing lung cancer), we would calculate the annual incidences as 5/9,996 in 2010, 6/9,991 in 2011, and 5/9,985 in 2012.

Prevalence and Incidence in Relation to Time

Every measure of disease frequency necessarily contains some indication of time. With measures of prevalence, time is assumed to be instantaneous, as in a single frame from a motion picture film. Prevalence depicts the situation at that point in time for each patient, even though it may, in reality, have taken several months to collect observations on the various people in the population. However, for incidence, time is the interval during which susceptible people were observed for the emergence of the event of interest. Table 2.1 summarizes the characteristics of incidence and prevalence.

Why is it important to know the difference between prevalence and incidence? Because they answer two entirely different questions: on the one hand, "What proportion of a group of people has a condition?"; and on the other, "At what rate do new cases arise in a defined population as time passes?" The answer to one question cannot be obtained directly from the answer to the other.

RELATIONSHIPS AMONG PREVALENCE, INCIDENCE, AND DURATION OF DISEASE

Anything that increases the duration of disease increases the chances that the patient will be identified in a prevalence study. Another look at Figure 2.1 will confirm this. Prevalent cases are those that remain affected, to the extent that patients are cured, die of their disease, or leave the population under study, they are no longer a case in a prevalence survey. As a result, diseases of brief duration will be more likely to be missed by a prevalence study. For example, 15% of all deaths from coronary heart disease occur outside the hospital within an hour of onset and without prior symptoms of heart disease. A prevalence

Table 2.1

Characteristics of Incidence and Prevalence

a. Characteristic	b. Incidence	c. Prevalence
Numerator	New cases occurring during a period of time among a group initially free of disease	Existing cases at a point or period of time
Denominator	All susceptible people without disease at the beginning of the period	All people examined, including cases and non-cases
Time	Duration of the period	Single point or period
How measured	Cohort study (see Chapter 5)	Prevalence (cross-sectional) study

study would, therefore, miss nearly all these events and underestimate the true burden of coronary heart disease in the community. In contrast, diseases of long duration are well represented in prevalence surveys, even when their incidence is low. The incidence of inflammatory bowel disease in North America is only about 2 to 14 per 100,000/year, but its prevalence is much higher, 37 to 246/100,000, reflecting the chronic nature of the disease (4).

The relationship among incidence, prevalence and duration of disease in a steady state, in which none of the variables is changing much over time, is approximated by the following expression:

$$\text{Prevalence} = \text{Incidence} \times \text{Average duration of the disease}$$

Alternatively,

$$\text{Prevalence/Incidence} = \text{Duration}$$

Example

The incidence and prevalence of ulcerative colitis were measured in Olmstead County, Minnesota, from 1984 to 1993 (5). Incidence was 8.3/100,000 person-years and prevalence was 229/10,000 persons. The average duration of this disease can then be estimated as 229/100,000 divided by 8.3/100,000 = 28 years. Thus, ulcerative colitis is a chronic disease consistent with a long life expectancy. The assumption of steady state was met because data from this same study showed that incidence changed little during the interval of study. Although rates are different in different parts of the world and are changing over longer periods of time, all reflect a chronic disease.

Similarly, the prevalence of prostate cancer on autopsy is so much higher than its incidence that the majority of these cancers must never become symptomatic enough to be diagnosed during life.

SOME OTHER RATES

Table 2.2 summarizes some rates used in health care. Most of them are expressions of events over time. For example, a case fatality rate (or alternatively, the survival rate) is the proportion of people having a disease who die of it (or who survive it). For acute diseases such as Ebola virus infection, follow-up time may be implicit, assuming that deaths are counted over a long enough period of time (in this case, a few weeks) to account for all of them that might have occurred. For chronic diseases such as cardiovascular disease or cancer, it is more usual to specify the period of observation (e.g., the 5-year survival rate). Similarly, complication rate, the proportion of people with a disease or treatment who experience complications, assumes that enough time has passed for the complications to have occurred. These kinds of measures can be underestimations if follow-up is not really long enough. For example, surgical site infection rates have been underreported because they have been counted up to the time of hospital discharge, whereas some wound infections are first apparent after discharge (6).

Other rates, such as infant mortality rate and perinatal mortality rate (defined in Table 2.2) are approximations of incidence because the children in the numerator are not necessarily those in the denominator. In the case of infant mortality rate for a given year, some of the children who die in that year were born in the previous year; similarly, the last children to be born in that year may die in the following year. These rates are constructed in this way to make measurement more feasible, while providing a useful approximation of a true rate in a given year.

Table 2.2

Some Commonly Used Rates

Case fatality rates	Proportion of patients who die of a disease
Complication rate	Proportions of patients who suffer a complication of a disease or its treatment
Infant mortality rate	Number of deaths in a year of children <1 *year of age* / Number of live births in the same year
Perinatal mortality rate (World Health Organization definition)	Number of stillbirths and deaths in the first week of life per 1,000 live births
Maternal mortality rate	Number of maternal deaths related to childbirth in a given year / Number of live births in the same population during the same year

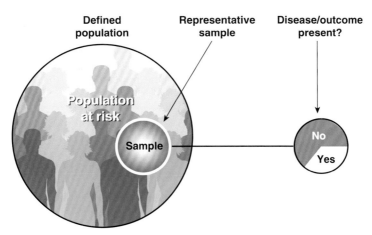

Figure 2.2 ■ The design of a prevalence study.

STUDIES OF PREVALENCE AND INCIDENCE

Prevalence and incidence are measured by entirely different kinds of studies.

Prevalence Studies

In prevalence studies, people in a population are examined for the presence of the condition of interest. Some members of the population have the condition at that point in time, whereas others do not (Fig. 2.2). The fraction or proportion of the population that has the condition (i.e., cases) constitutes the prevalence of the disease.

Another term for prevalence studies is cross-sectional studies because people are studied at a "cross-section" of time. Prevalence studies are also called surveys if the main measurement is a questionnaire.

The following is an example of a typical prevalence study.

Example

The World Health Organization created a research consortium to study the cross-national prevalence of depression. More than 37,000 people, randomly selected from the general population, were interviewed in 10 countries in North America, Latin America, Europe, and Asia. Major depressive episodes were diagnosed by face-to-face interviews, using an instrument designed to give consistent results in different languages and cultures. Response rates were 57% to 90%. Thirty-day prevalence (actually a period prevalence but a good estimate of point prevalence because of the narrow time window) ranged from a high of 4.6% in the United States to a low of 0.9% in Japan. Period prevalence was higher; for example, in the United States, the 12-month prevalence was 10.0% and the lifetime prevalence was 16.9%. The authors concluded that "major depressive episodes are a commonly occurring disorder that usually has a chronic-intermittent course" (7).

Incidence Studies

The population under examination in an incidence study is a cohort, which is defined as a group of people having something in common when they are first assembled and are then followed over time for the development of outcome events. For this reason, incidence studies are also called cohort studies. A sample of people free of the outcome of interest is identified and observed over time to see whether an outcome event occurs. Members of the cohort may be healthy at first and then followed forward in time for the emergence of disease—for example, from being cancer-free until the onset (or not) of pancreatic cancer. Or, all of them may have a recently diagnosed disease (such as pancreatic cancer) and then be followed forward in time to outcomes such as recurrence or death. Incidence studies will be discussed in greater detail in Chapters 5 and 7.

Cumulative Incidence

To this point, the term "incidence" has been used to describe the rate of new events in a group of people of fixed size, all members of which are observed over a period of time. This is called cumulative incidence because new cases are accumulated over time.

Incidence Density (Person-Years)

Another approach to studying incidence is to measure the number of new cases emerging in an ever-changing population, one in which individuals are under study and susceptible for varying lengths of time. The incidence derived from studies of this type is called incidence density because it is, figuratively speaking, the density of new cases in time and place.

Clinical trials often use the incidence density approach. Eligible patients are enrolled over a period of time so that early enrollees are treated and followed up for longer periods than late enrollees. In an effort to keep the contribution of individual patients commensurate with their follow-up interval, the denominator of an incidence density measure is not persons at risk for a specific time period but person-time at risk for the outcome event. A patient followed for 10 years without an outcome event contributes 10 person-years, whereas one followed for 1 year contributes only 1 person-year to the denominator. Incidence density is expressed as the number of new cases per total number of person-years at risk.

The person-years approach is especially useful for estimating the incidence of disease in dynamic populations, those in which some individuals in the population are entering and others leaving it as time passes. Incidence studies in large populations typically have an accurate count of new cases in the population (e.g., from hospital records or disease registries), but the size and characteristics of the population at risk can only be estimated (from census and other records) because the people in it are entering and leaving the region continually. This approach works because the proportion of people who enter or leave is small, relative to the population as a whole (Fig. 2.3), so the population is likely to be relatively stable over short periods of time.

all care provided to county residents was provided within the county and most residents had agreed to let their records be used for research. The population of the county was estimated from census data at approximately 175,000. Incidence of herpes zoster, adjusted to the age and sex of the U.S. adult population, was 3.6 per 1,000 person-years and rose with age. Pain after the herpes attack occurred in 18% of these patients.

Incidence of herpes zoster infection was described in person-years in a dynamic population, whereas pain after infection was a cumulative incidence in which all patients with herpes zoster were followed up.

A disadvantage of the person-years approach is that it lumps together different lengths of follow-up. A small number of patients followed for a long time can contribute as many person-years as a large number of patients followed for a short time. If patients with long follow-up are systematically different from those with short follow-up—perhaps because outcome events take a long time to develop or because patients with especially bad risk tend to leave the population—the resulting incidence density will depend on the particular combination of number of patients and follow-up times. For example, the latency period between exposure to carcinogen and onset of cancer is at least 10 years for most cancers. It might be possible to see an increase in cancer rates

Example

A study of the incidence of herpes zoster infections ("shingles") and its complications provides and example of both incidence density and cumulative incidence. Investigators in Olmstead County, Minnesota reviewed medical records of adult residents of the county (8). Other studies showed that more than 98% of

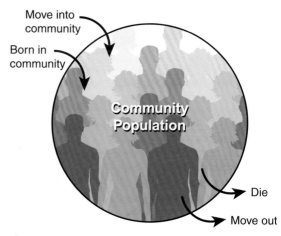

Figure 2.3 ■ A dynamic population.

in a study of 10,000 people exposed to a carcinogen and followed up for 20 years. However, a study of 100,000 people followed for 2 years would not show an increase, even though it involves the same number of person-years (200,000), because the follow-up time is too short.

BASIC ELEMENTS OF FREQUENCY STUDIES

To make sense of a study reporting prevalence, one needs careful definition of both the numerator and the denominator.

What Is a Case? Defining the Numerator

Cases might be people in the general population who develop a disease or patients in clinical settings with disease who develop an outcome event such as recurrence, complication of treatment, or death. In either situation, the way in which a case is defined affects rates.

Most clinical phenomena (serum cholesterol, serum calcium, thyroid hormone levels, etc.) exist on a continuum from low to high. The cutoff point defining a case can be placed at various points and this can have large effects on the resulting prevalence. We will discuss some of the reasons why one would place a cutoff at one or another point in Chapter 3 and the consequences for a diagnostic test performance in Chapter 8.

Example

The world is in an obesity epidemic. What is the prevalence of abnormal weight in the United States? It depends on how abnormal is defined. Figure 2.4 shows the distribution of body mass index (BMI, one way of measuring obesity that takes into account both weight and height) in U.S. men and women aged 40 to 59 years in 2007 through 2008 (9). The U.S. National Institutes of Health and World Health Organization have recommended a classification of BMI (Table 2.3). According to this classification, prevalence of obesity was 33.8%, whereas prevalence of overweight (which includes people with obesity and more) was 68%. A substantial proportion of the population, about 5%, was in the most extreme (Class III, "morbid obesity") weight class.

Rates may also be affected by how aggressively one looks for cases. For example, aspirin can induce asthma in some people. How often does this occur? It depends on the definition of a case. When people are simply asked whether they have a breathing problem after taking aspirin, rates are relatively low, about 3% in adults. When a case is defined more rigorously, by giving aspirin and measuring whether this was followed by bronchoconstriction, the prevalence of aspirin-induced asthma is much higher, about 21% in adults (10). The lower rate

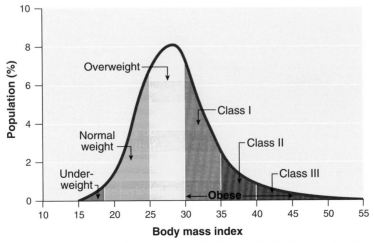

Figure 2.4 ■ The prevalence of overweight and obesity in men, 2007 to 2008. (Data from Flegal KM, Carroll MD, Ogden CL, et al. Prevalence and trends in obesity among US adults, 1999–2008. JAMA 2010;303(3):235–241.)

Table 2.3

Classification of Obesity According to the U.S. National Institutes of Health and World Health Organization

Classification	Body Mass Index (kg/m²)
Underweight	<18.5
Normal weight	18.5–24.9
Overweight	25.0–29.9
Obesity	≥30
Obesity Class I	30.0–34.9
Obesity Class II	35.0–39.9
Obesity Class III ("severe," "extreme," or "morbid")	≥40

Data from Flegal KM, Carroll MD, Ogden CL et al. Prevalence and trends in obesity among US adults, 1999–2008. JAMA 2010;303:235–241.

pertains to clinical situations, whereas the higher rate tells us something about the biology of this disease.

Incidence can also change if a more sensitive ways of detecting disease is introduced.

Example

Many cases of prostate cancer remain indolent and are not detected during life. With use of prostate-specific antigen (PSA), a blood test for prostate cancer, more of these indolent cases are now found. The test is relatively sensitive and leads to prostate biopsies that discover otherwise undetected cancers. The result of widespread PSA testing in the United States has been a rapid rise in the reported incidence of prostate cancer, more than double in a few years (11) (Fig. 2.5). The rise in incidence probably does not reflect an increase in the true incidence in the population because it has occurred so fast and because similar increases have not been seen in countries where PSA testing is less common. Incidence has subsequently fallen somewhat, presumably because the reservoir of prevalent cases, brought to attention by this new test, has been exhausted. However, incidence has not fallen to pre-PSA levels and seems to have reached a higher plateau, suggesting that new (incident) cases are being diagnosed more frequently since PSA testing was introduced.

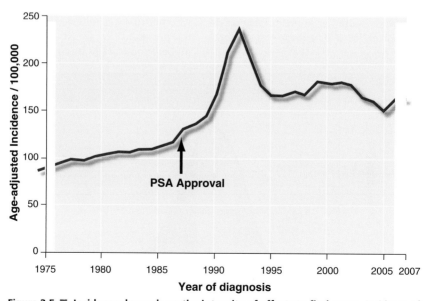

Figure 2.5 ■ Incidence depends on the intensity of efforts to find cases. Incidence of prostate cancer in the United States during the widespread use of screening with prostate-specific antigen (PSA). (Redrawn with permission from Wolf AMD, Wender RC, Etzioni RB et al. American Cancer Society guideline for the early detection of prostate cancer: Update 2010. CA Cancer Journal for Clinicians 2010;60:70–98.)

What Is the Population? Defining the Denominator

A rate is useful only to the extent that the population in which it is measured—the denominator of the rate—is clearly defined and right for the question. Three characteristics of the denominator are especially important.

First, all members of the population should be susceptible to the outcome of interest; that is, they should comprise a population at risk. If members of the population cannot experience the event or condition counted in the numerator, they do not belong in the denominator. For example, rates of cervical cancer should be assessed in women who still have a cervix; to the extent that cervical cancer rates are based on populations that include women who have had hysterectomies (or for that matter, men), true rates will be underestimated.

Second, the population should be relevant to the question being asked. For example, if we wanted to know the prevalence of HIV infection in the community, we would study a random sample of all people in a region. But if we wanted to know the prevalence of HIV infection among people who use street drugs, we would study them.

Third, the population should be described in sufficient detail so that it is a useful basis for judging to whom the results of the prevalence study applies. What is at issue here is the generalizability of rates—deciding whether a reported rate applies to the kind of patients that you are interested in. A huge gradient in rates of disease (e.g., for HIV infection) exists across practice settings from the general population to primary care practice to referral centers. Clinicians need to locate the reported rates on that spectrum if they are to use the information effectively.

Does the Study Sample Represent the Population?

As mentioned in Chapter 1, it is rarely possible to study all the people who have or might develop the condition of interest. Usually, one takes a sample so that the number studied is of manageable size. This leads to a central question: Does the sample accurately represent the parent population?

Random samples are intended to produce representative samples of the population. In a simple random sample, every individual in the population has an equal probability of being selected. A more general term, probability sample, is used when every person has a known (not necessarily equal) probability of being selected. Probability samples are useful because it is often more informative to include in the sample a sufficient number of people in particular subgroups of interest, such as ethnic minorities or the elderly. If members of these subgroups comprise only a small proportion of the population, a simple random sample of the entire population might not include enough of them. To remedy this, investigators can vary the sampling fraction, the fraction of all members of each subgroup included in the sample. Investigators can oversample low-frequency groups relative to the rest, that is, randomly select a larger fraction of them. The final sample will still be representative of the entire population if the different sampling fractions are taken into account in the analysis.

On average, the characteristics of people in probability samples are similar to those of the population from which they were selected, particularly when the sample is large. To the extent that the sample differs from the parent population, it is by chance and not because of systematic error.

Non-random samples are common in clinical research for practical reasons. They are called convenience samples (because their main virtue is that they were convenient to obtain, such as samples of patients who are visiting a medical facility, are cooperative, and are articulate) or grab samples (because the investigators just grabbed patients wherever they could find them).

Most patients described in the medical literature and encountered by clinicians are biased samples of their parent population. Typically, patients are included in research because they are under care in an academic institution, are available, are willing to be studied, are not afflicted with diseases other than the one under study, and perhaps also are particularly interesting, severely affected, or both. There is nothing wrong with this practice as long as it is understood to whom the results do (or do not) apply. However, because of biased samples, the results of clinical research often leave thoughtful clinicians with a large generalizability problem, from the research setting to their practice.

DISTRIBUTION OF DISEASE BY TIME, PLACE, AND PERSON

Epidemiology has been described as the study of the determinants of the distribution of disease in populations. Major determinants are time, place, and person. Distribution according to these factors can provide strong clues to the causes and control of disease, as well as to the need for health services.

Time

An epidemic is a concentration of new cases in time. The term pandemic is used when a disease is especially widespread, such as a global epidemic of particularly severe influenza (e.g., the one in 1918–1919) and the more slowly developing but worldwide rise in HIV infection/AIDS. The existence of an epidemic is recognized by an epidemic curve that shows the rise and fall of cases of a disease over time in a population.

Example

Figure 2.6 shows the epidemic curve for Severe Acute Respiratory Syndrome (SARS), in Beijing, People's Republic of China, during the spring of 2003 (12). In all, 2,521 probable cases were reported during the epidemic. Cases were called "probable" because, at the time, there were no hard and fast criteria for diagnosis. The working definition of a case included combinations of the following epidemiologic and clinical phenomena: contact with a patient with SARS or living or visiting an area where SARS was active, symptoms and signs of a febrile respiratory illness, chest radiograph changes, lack of response to antibiotics, and normal or decreased white blood cell count. Later, as more became known about this new disease, laboratory testing for the responsible coronavirus could be used to define a case. Cases were called "reported" to make clear that there was no assurance that all cases in the Beijing community were detected.

Figure 2.6 also indicates when major control measures were instituted. The epidemic declined in relation to aggressive quarantine measures involving the closing of public gathering places, identifying new cases early in their course, removing cases from the community, and isolating cases in facilities specifically for SARS. It is possible that the epidemic abated for reasons other than these control measures, but it is unlikely given that similar control measures in other places were also followed by a resolution of the epidemic. Whatever the cause, the decline in new cases allowed the World Health Organization to lift its advisory against travel to Beijing so that the city could reopen public places and resume normal international business and tourism.

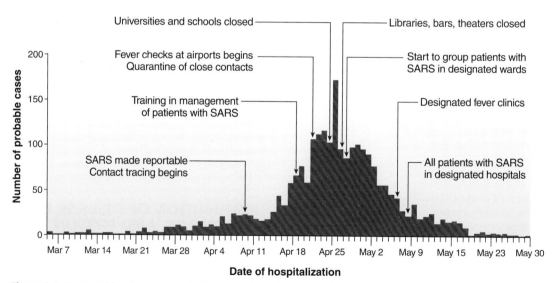

Figure 2.6 ■ An epidemic curve. Probable cases of severe acute respiratory syndrome in Beijing March 2003 through May 2003, in relation to control measures. (Adapted with permission from Pang X, Zhu Z, Xu F, et al. Evaluation of control measures implemented in the severe acute respiratory syndrome outbreak in Beijing, 2003. JAMA 2003;290: 3215–3221.)

Knowledge of a local epidemic helps clinicians get the right diagnosis. For example, while serving as a primary care physician on a military base in Germany, one author saw a child with a fever and rash on the hands and feet. With only a hospital-based clerkship in pediatrics to rely on, he was perplexed. But when he and his colleagues began seeing many such children in a short time span, they recognized (with the help of a pediatric consultant) that they were in the midst of an outbreak of coxsackievirus infection ("hand, foot, and mouth syndrome"), which is a distinctive but mild infectious disease of children.

Place

The geographic distribution of cases indicates where a disease causes a greater or less burden of suffering and provides clues to its causes.

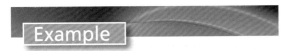

The incidence of colorectal cancer is very different in different parts of the world. Rates, even when adjusted for differences in age, are high in North America, Europe, and Australia and low in Africa and Asia (Fig. 2.7) (13). This observation has led to the hypothesis that environmental factors may play a large part in the development of this disease. This hypothesis has been supported by other studies showing that people moving from countries of low incidence to those of high incidence acquire higher rates of colorectal cancer during their lifetime.

When a disease such as iodine deficiency goiter or polio (after global efforts to eradicate it) is limited to certain places, the disease is called endemic.

Person

When disease affects certain kinds of persons at the same time and in the same places as other people who are not affected, this provides clues to causes and guidance on how health care efforts should be deployed. At the beginning of the AIDS pandemic, most cases were seen in homosexual men who had multiple sexual partners as well as among intravenous drug users. This led to the early hypothesis that the disease was caused

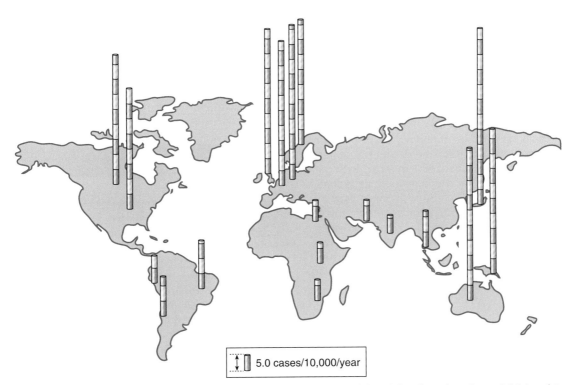

5.0 cases/10,000/year

Figure 2.7 ■ Colorectal cancer incidence for men according to area of the globe. (Data from Center MM, Jemal A, Smith RA, et al. Worldwide variations in colorectal cancer. CA Cancer J Clin 2009;59:366–378.)

by an infectious agent transmitted in semen and blood. Laboratory studies confirmed this hypothesis and discovered the human immunodeficiency virus. Identification of the kinds of people most affected also led to special efforts to prevent spread of the disease in them—for example, by targeting education about safe sex to those communities, closing public bathhouses, and instituting safe-needle programs.

USES OF PREVALENCE STUDIES

Properly performed prevalence studies are the very best ways of answering some important questions and are a weak way of answering others.

What Are Prevalence Studies Good For?

Prevalence studies provide valuable information about what to expect in different clinical situations.

Example

The approach to cervical lymphadenopathy depends on where and in whom it is seen. Children with persistent cervical adenopathy seen in primary care practice have only a 0.4% probability that the node represents cancer, mainly lymphoma. Clinicians should have a high threshold for biopsy, the definitive way of determining whether or not cancer is present. However, adults seen in primary care practice have a 4% chance of having an underlying cancer of the head and neck. For them, clinicians should have a lower threshold for lymph node biopsy. Rates of malignancy in referral centers are much higher, about 60% in adults with cervical adenopathy, and biopsies are usually done. The situation is different in different parts of the world. In resource-poor countries, mycobacterial infections are a more common cause of lymphadenopathy than cancer. Thus, knowledge of prevalence helps clinicians prioritize the diagnostic possibilities in their particular setting and for the particular patient at hand.

Prevalence of disease strongly affects the interpretation of diagnostic test results, as will be described in greater detail in Chapter 8.

Finally, prevalence is an important guide to planning health services. In primary care practice, being prepared for diabetes, obesity, hypertension, and lipid disorders should demand more attention than planning for

Hodgkin disease, aplastic anemia, or systemic lupus erythematosus. In contrast, some referral hospitals are well prepared for just these diseases, and appropriately so.

What Are Prevalence Studies Not Particularly Good For?

Prevalence studies provide only weak evidence of cause and effect. Causal questions are inherently about new events arising over time; that is, they are about incidence. One of the other limitations of prevalence studies, for this purpose, is that it may be difficult to know whether the purported cause actually preceded or followed the effect because the two are measured at the same point in time. For example, if inpatients with hyperglycemia are more often infected, is it because hyperglycemia impairs immune function leading to infection or has the infection caused the hyperglycemia? If a risk factor (e.g., family history or a genetic marker) is certain to have preceded the onset of disease or outcome, interpretation of the cause-and-effect sequence is less worrisome.

Another limitation is that prevalence may be the result of incidence of disease, the main consideration in causal questions, or it may be related to duration of disease, an altogether different issue. With only information about prevalence, one cannot determine how much each of the two, incidence and duration, contributes. Nevertheless, cross-sectional studies can provide compelling hypotheses about cause and effect to be tested by stronger studies.

The underlying message is that a well-performed cross-sectional study, or any other research design, is not inherently strong or weak but is only in relation to the question it is intended to answer.

Example

Children living on farms are less likely to have asthma than children who live in the same region but not on farms. Farm and urban environments differ in exposure to microbes, suggesting that exposure to microbes may protect against asthma. But the environments differ in many other ways. To strengthen this hypothesis, investigators in Germany examined mattress dust and also settled dust from children's bedrooms and found that greater microbial diversity was inversely related to asthma, independent of farming (14). Together, these observations suggest that exposure to a wider range of microbes may protect against asthma, a causal hypothesis to be tested by stronger research.

Review Questions

Read the following statements and mark the best answer.

2.1. Cancer registries report 40 new cases of bladder cancer per 100,000 men per year. Cases were from a complete count of all patients who developed bladder cancer in several regions of the United States, and the number of men at risk was estimated from the census data in those regions. Which rate is this an example of?

   A. Point prevalence
   B. Period prevalence
   C. Incidence density
   D. Cumulative incidence
   E. Complication rate

2.2. Sixty percent of adults in the U.S. population have a serum cholesterol >200mg/dL (5.2 mmol/L). Which rate is this an example of?

   A. Point prevalence
   B. Complication rate
   C. Incidence density
   D. Cumulative Incidence
   E. Period prevalence

2.3. You are reading a study of the prevalence of uterine cervix infections and want to decide if the study is scientifically sound. Which of the following is *not* important?

   A. Participants are followed up for a sufficient period of time for anemia to occur.
   B. The study is done on a representative sample of the population.
   C. All members of the population are women.
   D. Cervical infection is clearly defined.
   E. The study is done on a sample from a defined population.

2.4. A probability sample of a defined population:

   A. Is invalidated by oversampling.
   B. Is inferior to a random sample.
   C. Is not representative of the population.
   D. Results in a representative sample of the population only if there are enough people in the sample.

2.5. The incidence of rheumatoid arthritis is about 40/100,000/year and the prevalence is

about 1/100 persons. On average, how many years does the disease persist?

   A. 10
   B. 25
   C. 33
   D. 40
   E. 50

2.6. Which of the following studies is *not* a cohort study?

   A. The proportion of patients with stomach cancer who survive 5 years
   B. The risk of developing diabetes mellitus in children according to their weight
   C. Complications of influenza vaccine among children vaccinated in 2011
   D. The earlier course of disease in a group of patients now under care in a clinic
   E. Patients admitted to an intensive care unit and followed up for whether they are still alive at the time of hospital discharge

2.7. A sample for a study of incidence of medication errors is obtained by enrolling every 10th patient admitted to a hospital. What kind of sample is this?

   A. Stratified sample
   B. Probability sample
   C. Convenience sample
   D. Random sample
   E. Oversample

2.8. Cohort studies of children with a first febrile seizure have shown that they have a one in three chance of having another seizure during childhood. What kind of rate is this?

   A. Point prevalence
   B. Complication rate
   C. Cumulative Incidence
   D. Period prevalence
   E. Incidence density

2.9. Which of the following would not increase the observed incidence of disease?

   A. More aggressive efforts to detect the disease
   B. A true increase in incidence
   C. A more sensitive way of detecting the disease
   D. A lowering of the threshold for diagnosis of disease
   E. Studying a larger sample of the population

2.10. Infection with a fungus, coccidioidomycosis, is common in the deserts of the southwestern United States and in Mexico, but uncommon elsewhere. Which of the following best describes this infection?

A. Endemic
B. Pandemic
C. Incident
D. Epidemic
E. Prevalent

2.11. Twenty-six percent of adults report having experienced back pain lasting at least a day in the prior 3 months. Which of the following best describes this rate?

A. Cumulative Incidence
B. Incidence density
C. Point prevalence
D. Complication rate
E. Period prevalence

2.12. Which of the following best describes a "dynamic population"?

A. It is rapidly increasing in size.
B. It is uniquely suited for cohort studies.
C. People are continually entering and leaving the population.
D. It is the basis for measuring cumulative incidence.
E. It is the best kind of population for a random sample.

2.13. For a study of the incidence of idiopathic scoliosis (a deformity of the spine that becomes apparent after birth, most often in adolescence), which would be an appropriate cohort?

A. Children born in North Carolina in 2012 and examined for scoliosis until they are adults
B. Children who were referred to an orthopedic surgeon for treatment
C. Children who were found to have scoliosis in a survey of children in North Carolina
D. Children who have scoliosis and are available for study
E. Children who were randomly sampled from the population of North Carolina in the spring of 2012

2.14. Which of the following are prevalence studies especially useful for?

A. Describing the incidence of disease
B. Studying diseases that resolve rapidly
C. Estimating the duration of disease
D. Describing the proportion of people in a defined population with the condition of interest
E. Establishing cause and effect

2.15. Last year, 800,000 Americans died of heart disease or stoke. Which of the following best describes this statistic?

A. Incidence density
B. Point prevalence
C. Cumulative Incidence
D. Period prevalence
E. None of the above

Answers are in Appendix A.

REFERENCES

1. Roberts DE, Gupta G. Letter to the editor. New Engl J Med 1987;316:550.
2. Bryant GD, Norman GR. Expressions of probability: words and numbers. N Engl J Med 1980;302:411.
3. Toogood JH. What do we mean by "usually"? Lancet 1980;1:1094
4. Loftus EV Jr. Clinical epidemiology of inflammatory bowel disease: Incidence, prevalence, and environmental influences. Gastroenterology 2004;126:1504–1517.
5. Loftus EV Jr, Silverstein MD, Sandborn WJ, et al. Ulcerative colitis in Olmstead County, Minnesota, 1940-1993: incidence, prevalence, and survival. Gut 2000;46:336–343.
6. Sands K, Vineyard G, Platt R. Surgical site infections occurring after hospital discharge. J Infect Dis 1996;173:963–970.
7. Andrade L, Caraveo-Anduaga JJ, Berglund P, et al. The epidemiology of major depressive episodes: results from the International Consortium of Psychiatric Epidemiology (ICPE) surveys. Int J Methods Psychiatr Res 2003;12:3–21.
8. Yawn BP, Saddier P, Wollan PC, et al. A population-based study of the incidence and complication rates of herpes zoster before zoster vaccine introduction. Mayo Clin Proc 2007;82:1341–1349.
9. Flegal KM, Carroll MD, Ogden CL, et al. Prevalence and trends in obesity among US adults, 1999-2008. JAMA 2010;303:235–241.
10. Jenkins C, Costello J, Hodge L. Systematic review of prevalence of aspirin induced asthma and its implications for clinical practice. BMJ 2004;328:434–437.
11. Wolf AMD, Wender RC, Etzioni RB, et al. American Cancer Society Guideline for the early detection of prostate cancer: update 2010. CA Cancer J Clin 2010;60:70–98.
12. Pang X, Zhu Z, Xu F, et al. Evaluation of control measures implemented in the severe acute respiratory syndrome outbreak in Beijing, 2003. JAMA 2003;290:3215–3221.
13. Center MM, Jemal A, Smith RA, et al. Worldwide variations in colorectal cancer. CA Cancer J Clin 2009;59:366–378.
14. Ege MJ, Mayer M, Normand AC, et al. Exposure to environmental microorganisms in childhood asthma. N Engl J Med 2011;364:701–709.

Chapter 3

Abnormality

. . . the medical meaning of "normal" has been lost in the shuffle of statistics.

—Alvan Feinstein
1977

KEY WORDS

Nominal data
Dichotomous data
Ordinal data
Interval data
Continuous data
Discrete data
Validity
Accuracy
Items
Constructs
Scales
Content validity
Criterion validity
Construct validity

Reliability
Reproducibility
Precision
Range
Responsiveness
Interpretability
Sampling fraction
Frequency distribution
Central tendency
Dispersion
Skewed distribution
Normal distribution
Regression to the
    mean

Clinicians spend a great deal of time distinguishing "normal" from "abnormal." Is the thyroid normal or slightly enlarged? Is the heart murmur "innocent" (of no health importance) or a sign of valvular disease? Is a slightly elevated serum alkaline phosphatase evidence of liver disease, unrecognized Paget disease, or nothing important?

When confronted with something grossly different from the usual, there is little difficulty telling the two apart. We are all familiar with pictures in textbooks of physical diagnoses showing massive hepatosplenomegaly, huge goiters, or hands severely deformed by rheumatoid arthritis. It takes no great skill to recognize this degree of abnormality, but clinicians are rarely faced with this situation. Most often, clinicians must make subtler distinctions between normal and

abnormal. That is when skill and a conceptual basis for deciding become important.

Decisions about what is abnormal are most difficult among relatively unselected patients, usually found outside of hospitals. When patients have already been selected for special attention, as is the case in most referral centers, it is usually clear that something is wrong. The tasks are then to refine the diagnosis and to treat the problem. In primary care settings and emergency departments, however, patients with subtle manifestations of disease are mixed with those with the everyday complaints of basically healthy people. It is not possible to pursue all of these complaints aggressively. Which of many patients with abdominal pain have self-limited gastroenteritis and which have early appendicitis? Which patients with sore throat and hoarseness have a viral pharyngitis and which have the rare but potentially lethal *Haemophilus* epiglottitis? These are examples of how difficult and important distinguishing various kinds of abnormalities can be.

The point of distinguishing normal from abnormal is to separate those clinical observations that should be the basis for action from those that can be simply noted. Observations that are thought to be normal are usually described as "within normal limits," "unremarkable," or "non-contributory" and remain buried in the body of a medical record. The abnormal findings are set out in a problem list or under the heading "impressions" or "diagnoses" and are the basis for action.

Simply calling clinical findings normal or abnormal is undoubtedly crude and results in some misclassification. The justification for taking this approach is that it is often impractical or unnecessary to consider

Table 3.1

Summary of Clinical Data: A Patient's Problem List and the Data on Which It Is Based

Problem List	Raw Data
Acute myocardial infarction	Chest pain, troponin 40 µg/L (>99th percentile of upper reference limit), new ST elevation in leads II, III, and AVF
Hypertension	Several blood pressure measurements (mm Hg): 145/92, 149/93, 142/91
Diabetes mellitus	Several fasting plasma sugar measurements (mg/dL): 138, 135, 129
Renal failure	Serum creatinine 2.7 mg/dL
Obstructive pulmonary disease	Forced expiratory volume at 1 second (FEV1)/forced vital capacity (FVC) < 0.70

the raw data in all their detail. As Bertrand Russell pointed out, to be perfectly intelligible one must be at least somewhat inaccurate, and to be perfectly accurate, one is too often unintelligible. Physicians usually choose to err on the side of being intelligible—to themselves and others—even at the expense of some accuracy. Another reason for simplifying data is that each aspect of a clinician's work ends in a decision—to pursue evaluation or to wait, to begin a treatment or to reassure. Under these circumstances, some sort of "present/absent" classification is necessary.

Table 3.1 is an example of how relatively simple expressions of abnormality are derived from more complex clinical data. On the left is a typical problem list, a statement of the patient's important medical problems. On the right are some of the data on which the decisions to call them problems are based. Conclusions from the data, represented by the problem list, are by no means uncontroversial. For example, the mean of the four diastolic blood pressure measurements is 92 mm Hg. Some might argue that this level of blood pressure does not justify the label "hypertension" because it is not particularly high and there are some disadvantages to telling patients they are sick and recommending drugs. Others might consider the label appropriate, considering that this level of blood pressure is associated with an increased risk of cardiovascular disease and that the risk can be reduced by treatment, and the label is consistent with guidelines. Although crude, the problem list serves as a basis for decisions—about diagnosis, prognosis, and treatment—and clinical decisions must be made,

whether actively (by additional diagnostic tests and treatment) or passively (by no intervention).

This chapter describes some of the ways clinicians distinguish normal from abnormal. First, we consider how biologic phenomena are measured, how they vary, and how they are summarized. Then, we discuss how these data are used as a basis for value judgments about what is worth calling abnormal.

TYPES OF DATA

Measurements of clinical phenomena yield three kinds of data: nominal, ordinal, and interval.

Nominal Data

Nominal data occur in categories without any inherent order. Examples of nominal data are characteristics that are determined by a small set of genes (e.g., ABO blood type and sex) or are dramatic, discrete events (e.g., death, dialysis, or surgery). These data can be placed in categories without much concern about misclassification. Nominal data that are divided into two categories (e.g., present/absent, yes/no, alive/dead) are called dichotomous.

Ordinal Data

Ordinal data possess some inherent ordering or rank such as small to large or good to bad, but the size of the intervals between categories is not specified. Some clinical examples include 1+ to 4+ leg edema, heart murmurs grades I (heard only with special effort) to VI (audible with the stethoscope off the chest), and muscle strength grades 0 (no movement) to 5 (normal strength). Some ordinal scales are complex. The risk of birth defects from drugs during pregnancy is graded by the U.S. Food and Drug Administration on a five-category scale ranging from A, "no adverse effects in humans"; through B, an adverse effect in animal studies not confirmed in controlled studies in women or "no effect in animals without human data"; C, "adverse effect in animals without human data or no available data from animals or humans"; and D, "adverse effects in humans, or likely in humans because of adverse effects in animals"; to X, "adverse effects in humans or animals without indication for use during pregnancy" (1).

Interval Data

For interval data, there is inherent order and the interval between successive values is equal, no matter where one is on the scale. There are two types of interval data. Continuous data can take on any value in a continuum, regardless of whether they are reported that way. Examples include most serum chemistries, weight, blood pressure, and partial pressure of oxygen in arterial blood. The measurement and description of continuous variables may in practice be confined to a limited number of points on the continuum, often integers, because the precision of the measurement, or its use, does not warrant greater detail. For example, a particular blood glucose reading may in fact be 193.2846573 . . . mg/dL but is simply reported as 193 mg/dL. Discrete data can take on only specific values and are expressed as counts. Examples of discrete data are the number of a woman's pregnancies and live births and the number of migraine attacks a patient has in a month.

It is for ordinal and interval data that the question arises, "Where does normal leave off and abnormal begin?" When, for example, does a large normal prostate become too large to be considered normal? Clinicians are free to choose any cutoff point. Some of the reasons for the choices are considered later in this chapter.

PERFORMANCE OF MEASUREMENTS

Whatever the type of measurement, its performance can be described in several ways.

Validity

Validity is the degree to which the data measure what they were intended to measure—that is, the degree to which the results of a measurement correspond to the true state of the phenomenon being measured. Another word for validity is accuracy.

For clinical observations that can be measured by physical means, it is relatively easy to establish validity. The observed measurement is compared with some accepted standard. For example, serum sodium can be measured on an instrument recently calibrated against solutions made up with known concentrations of sodium. Laboratory measurements are commonly subjected to extensive and repeated validity checks. For example, it is common practice for blood glucose measurements to be monitored for accuracy by comparing readings against high and low standards at the beginning of each day, before each technician begins a day, and after any changes in the techniques, such as a new bottle of reagent or a new battery for the instrument. Similarly, accuracy of a lung scan for pulmonary embolus can be measured against pulmonary angiography, in which the pulmonary artery anatomy is directly visualized. The validity of a physical examination finding can be established by comparing it to the results of surgery or radiologic examinations.

Table 3.2

The CAGE Test for Detecting Alcohol Abuse and Dependence[a]
Have you ever felt you needed to **C**ut down on your drinking?
Have people **A**nnoyed you by criticizing your drinking?
Have you ever felt **G**uilty about your drinking?
Have you ever felt you needed a drink first thing in the morning (**E**ye opener) to steady your nerves or to get rid of a hangover?
One "yes" response suggests the need for closer assessment.
Two or more "yes" responses is strongly related to alcohol abuse, dependence, or both.

[a]Other tests, such as AUDIT, are useful for detecting less severe drinking patterns that can respond to simple counseling. Adapted from Ewing JA. Detecting alcoholism: the CAGE questionnaire. JAMA 1984;252:1905–1907.

Some other clinical measurements such as pain, nausea, dyspnea, depression, and fear cannot be verified physically. In patient care, information about these phenomena is usually obtained informally by "taking a history." More formal and standardized approaches, used in research, are structured interviews and questionnaires. Individual questions (items) are designed to measure specific phenomena (e.g., symptoms, feelings, attitudes, knowledge, beliefs) called constructs, and these items are grouped together to form scales. Table 3.2 shows one such scale, a brief questionnaire used to detect alcohol abuse and dependence.

Three general strategies are used to establish the validity of measurements that cannot be directly verified physically.

Content Validity

Content validity is the extent to which a particular method of measurement includes all of the dimensions of the construct one intends to measure and nothing more. For example, a scale for measuring pain would have content validity if it included questions about aching, throbbing, pressure, burning, and stinging, but not about itching, nausea, and tingling.

Criterion Validity

Criterion validity is present to the extent that the measurements predict a directly observable phenomenon. For example, one might see whether responses on a scale measuring pain bear a predictable relationship to pain of known severity: mild pain from minor abrasion, moderate pain from ordinary headache and peptic ulcer, and severe pain from renal colic. One might also show that responses to a scale measuring pain are related to other, observable manifestations of the severity of pain such as sweating, moaning, writhing, and asking for pain medications.

Construct Validity

Construct validity is present to the extent that the measurement is related in a coherent way to other measures, also not physically verifiable, that are believed to be part of the same phenomenon. Thus, one might be more confident in the construct validity of a scale for depression to the extent that it is related to fatigue and headache—constructs thought to be different from but related to depression.

Validity of a scale is not, as is often asserted, either present or absent. Rather, with these strategies, one can build a case for or against its validity under the conditions in which it is used, so as to convince others that the scale is more or less valid.

Because of their selection and training, physicians tend to prefer the kind of precise measurements that the physical and biologic sciences afford and may avoid or discount others, especially for research. Yet relief of symptoms and promoting satisfaction and a feeling of well-being are among the most important outcomes of patient care and are central concerns of patients and doctors alike. To guide clinical decisions, research must include them, lest the picture of medicine painted by the research be distorted.

As Feinstein (2) put it:

> The term "hard" is usually applied to data that are reliable and preferably dimensional (e.g., laboratory data, demographic data, and financial costs). But clinical performance, convenience, anticipation, and familial data are "soft." They depend on subjective statements, usually expressed in words rather than numbers, by the people who are the observers and the observed.
>
> To avoid such soft data, the results of treatment are commonly restricted to laboratory information that can be objective, dimensional, and reliable—but it is also dehumanized. If we are told that the serum cholesterol is 230 mg/dL, that the chest x-ray shows cardiac enlargement, and that the electrocardiogram has Q waves, we would not know whether the treated object was a dog or a person. If we were told that capacity at work was restored, that the medicine tasted good and was easy to take, and that the family was happy about the results, we would recognize a human set of responses.

Reliability

Reliability is the extent to which repeated measurements of a stable phenomenon by different people and instruments at different times and places get similar results. Reproducibility and precision are other words for this property.

The reliability of laboratory measurements is established by repeated measures—for example, of the same serum or tissue specimen—sometimes by different people and with different instruments. The reliability of symptoms can be established by showing that they are similarly described to different observers under different conditions.

The relationships between reliability and validity are shown in simple form in Figure 3.1. Measurements can be both accurate (valid) and reliable (precise), as shown in Figure 3.1A. Measurements can be very reliable but inaccurate if they are systematically off the mark, as in Figure 3.1B. On the other hand, measurements can be valid on the average but not be reliable, because they are widely scattered about the true value, as shown in Figure 3.1C. Finally, measurements can be both invalid and imprecise, as shown in Figure 3.1D. Small numbers of measurements with poor reliability are at risk of low validity because they are likely to be off the mark by chance alone. Therefore, reliability and validity are not altogether independent concepts. In general, an unreliable measurement cannot be valid and a valid measurement must be reliable.

Range

An instrument may not register very low or high values of the phenomenon being measured; that is, it has limited range, which limits the information it conveys. For example, the Basic Activities of Daily Living scale that measures patients' ability in dressing, eating, walking, toileting, maintaining hygiene, and transferring from bed or chair does not measure ability to read, write, or play the piano (activities that might be very important to individual patients).

Responsiveness

An instrument demonstrates responsiveness to the extent that its results change as conditions change. For example, the New York Heart Association scale—Classes I to IV (no symptoms of heart failure and no limitations of ordinary physical activity, mild symptoms and slight limitation of ordinary physical activity, marked limitation of ordinary physical activity because of fatigue, palpitation or dyspnea,

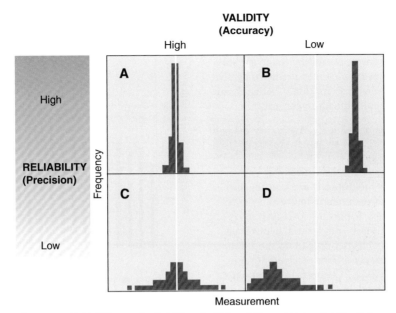

VALIDITY
(Accuracy)

Figure 3.1 ■ **Validity and reliability. A.** High validity and high reliability. **B.** Low validity and high reliability. **C.** High validity and low reliability. **D.** Low validity and low reliability. The white lines represent the true values.

and inability to carry out any physical activity, even at rest, because of symptoms)—is not sensitive to subtle changes in congestive heart failure, ones that might matter to patients. However, measurements of ejection fraction by echocardiography can detect changes so subtle that patients do not notice them.

Interpretability

Clinicians learn to interpret the significance of a PCO_2 of 50 or a blood sugar of 460 through experience, in which they repeatedly calibrate patients' current conditions and clinical courses against such test results. However, scales based on questionnaires may have little intuitive meaning to clinicians and patients who do not use them regularly. To overcome this interpretability disadvantage, researchers can "anchor" scale values to familiar states. To help clinicians interpret scale values, the numbers are anchored to descriptions of everyday performance. For example, values of the Karnofsky Performance Status Scale, a measure of functional capacity commonly used in studies of cancer patients receiving chemotherapy, range from 100 (normal) to 0 (dead). Just how bad is it to have a value of 60? At a scale value of 60, patients require occasional assistance but are able to care for most of their personal needs.

VARIATION

Overall variation is the sum of variation related to the act of measurement, biologic differences *within* individuals from time to time, and biologic differences *among* individuals (Table 3.3).

Variation Resulting from Measurement

All observations are subject to variation because of the performance of the instruments and observers involved in making the measurements. The conditions

Table 3.3

Sources of Variation	
Source of Variation	**Definition**
Measurement Variation	
Instrument	The means of making the measurement
Observer	The person making the measurement
Biologic Variation	
Within individuals	Changes in a person at different times and situations
Between individuals	Biologic differences from person to person

of measurement can lead to a biased result (lack of validity) or simply random error (lack of reliability). It is possible to reduce this source of variation by making measurements with great care and by following standard protocols. However, when measurements involve human judgment, rather than machines, variation can be particularly large and difficult to control.

Example

Findings on chest radiographs are used as part of the diagnosis of Acute Lung Injury and Acute Respiratory Distress Syndrome (ALI-ARDS), severe pulmonary disease with arterial hypoxemia that often requires intubation. But do specialists in these respiratory conditions read radiographs similarly? In one study, 21 experts in pulmonary critical care examined 28 chest x-rays from critically ill hypoxemic patients and decided whether the x-rays fulfilled radiographic criteria for the diagnosis of ALI-ARDS. The percentage of radiographs read as positive for the diagnosis ranged from 36% to 71% among the experts (Fig. 3.2), with more than a two-fold difference between the readers with the lowest positive and highest positive percentages. Radiographs with the greatest agreement among the experts showed abnormalities in all lung quadrants, whereas those with abnormalities only in the lower lung fields accounted for most variability (3).

Variations in measurements also arise because they are made on only a sample of the phenomenon being described, which may misrepresent the whole. Often, the sampling fraction (the fraction of the whole that is included in the sample) is very small. For example, a liver biopsy represents only about 1/100,000 of the liver. Because such a small part of the whole is examined, there is room for considerable variation from one sample to another.

If measurements are made by several different methods, such as different laboratories, technicians, or instruments, some of the measurements may be unreliable or may produce results that are systematically different from the correct value, which could contribute to the spread of values obtained.

Variation Resulting from Biologic Differences

Variation also arises because of biologic changes within individuals over time. Most biologic phenomena

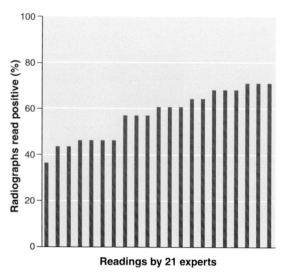

Figure 3.2 ■ **Observer variability.** Variability among 21 specialists reading chest x-rays for acute lung injury and acute respiratory distress syndrome. The percentage of radiographs read as positive for the diagnosis varied from 36% to 71% among the experts. (Data from Rubenfeld GD, Caldwell E, Granton J, et al. Interobserver variability in applying a radiographic definition for ARDS. Chest 1999;116: 1347–1353.)

change from moment to moment. A measurement at a point in time may not represent the usual value of these measurements.

Example

Clinicians estimate the frequency of ventricular premature beats (VPBs) to help determine the need for and effectiveness of treatment. For practical reasons, they may do so by making relatively brief observations—perhaps feeling a pulse for 1 minute or reviewing an electrocardiogram recording lasting several seconds. However, the frequency of VPBs in a given patient varies over time. To obtain a larger sample to estimate the VPB rate, a portable monitor was developed that tracks ventricular premature depolarizations (VPDs) electrocardiographically. Early studies found monitoring even for extended periods of time can be misleading. Figure 3.3 shows observations on one patient with VPDs, similar to other patients studied (4). VPDs per hour varied from <20 to 380 during a 3-day period, according to day and time of day. The

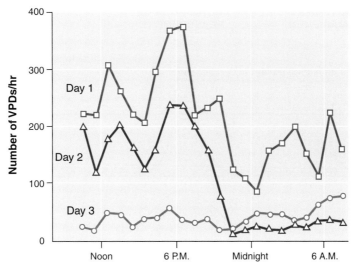

Figure 3.3 ■ **Biologic variability.** The number of ventricular premature beats (VPBs) per hour for one untreated patient on 3 consecutive days. (Data from Morganroth J, Michelson EL, Horowitz LN, et al. Limitations of routine long-term electrocardiographic monitoring to assess ventricular ectopic frequency. Circulation 1978;58:408–414.)

authors concluded, "To distinguish a reduction in VPB frequency attributable to therapeutic intervention rather than biologic or spontaneous variation alone required a greater than 83% reduction in VPB frequency if only two 24-hour monitoring periods were compared." Much shorter periods of observation could be even more misleading because of biologic variation. To deal with this biologic variability, modern devices are now able to monitor cardiac rhythm for extended periods of time.

Total Variation

The several sources of variation are cumulative. Figure 3.4 illustrates this for the measurement of blood pressure. When looking at a population distribution, variation in measurement for individual patients is added to variation for those individuals from time to time, which in turn is added to variation among different patients. Measurement variation contributes relatively little, although it accounts for as much as a 12 mm Hg among various observers. However, each patient's blood pressure varies a great deal from moment to moment throughout the day, so any single blood pressure reading might not represent the usual for that patient. Much of this variation is not random: Blood pressure is generally higher when people are awake, excited, visiting phy-

sicians, or taking over-the-counter cold medications. Of course, we are most interested in knowing how an individual's blood pressure compares with that of his or her peers, especially if the blood pressure level is related to complications of hypertension and the effectiveness of treatment.

Despite all these sources of variation that can distort the measurement of blood pressure, biologic differences among individuals is a predominant cause of variation in the case of blood pressure, so much so that several studies have found even a single casual blood pressure measurement can predict subsequent cardiovascular disease among a population.

Effects of Variation

Another way of thinking about variation is in terms of its net effect on the validity and reliability of a measurement and what can be done about it.

Random variation, for example, by unstable instruments or many observers with various biases that tend to balance each other out, results on average in no net misrepresentation of the true state of a phenomenon, even though individual measurements may be misleading. Inaccuracy resulting from random variation can be reduced by taking the average of a larger sample of what is being measured, for example, by counting more cells on a blood smear, examining a larger area of a urine sediment, or studying more patients. Also, the extent of random variation can be estimated by statistical methods (see Chapter 11).

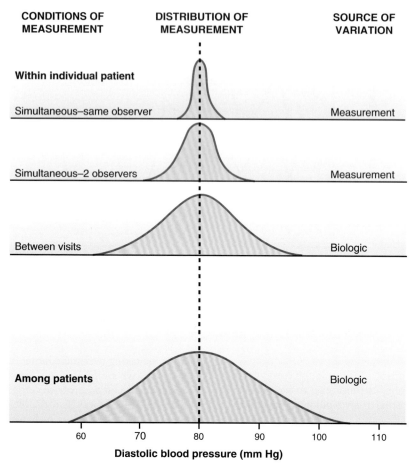

Figure 3.4 ■ **Sources of variation in the measurement of diastolic (phase V) blood pressure.** The dashed line indicates the true blood pressure. Multiple sources of variation, including within and among patients as well as intra- and inter-observer variation, all contribute to blood pressure measurement results.

On the other hand, biased results are systematically different from the true value, no matter how many times they are repeated. For example, all of the high values for VPDs shown in Figure 3.3 were recorded on the first day, and most of the low values on the third day. The days were biased estimates of each other because of variation in VPD rate from day to day.

DISTRIBUTIONS

Data that are measured on interval scales are often presented as a figure, called a frequency distribution, showing the number (or proportion) of a defined group of people possessing the different values of the measurement. Figure 3.5 shows the distribution of

blood neutrophil counts in normal black men and women.

Describing Distributions

Presenting interval data as a frequency distribution conveys the information in relatively fine detail, but it is often convenient to summarize distributions. Indeed, summarization is imperative when a large number of distributions are presented and compared.

Two basic properties of distributions are used to summarize them: central tendency, the middle of the distribution, and dispersion, how spread out the values are. Several ways of expressing central tendency and dispersion, along with their advantages and disadvantages, are illustrated in Figure 3.5 and summarized in Table 3.4.

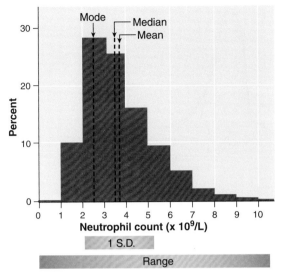

Figure 3.5 ■ Measures of central tendency and dispersion. The distribution of blood neutrophil counts in a national sample of blacks age 18 years and older. (The authors found that neutrophil counts were lower and neutropenia was more common in blacks compared to whites.) (Data from Hsieh MM, Everhart JE, Byrd-Holt DD, et al. Prevalence of neutropenia in the U.S. population: Age, sex, smoking status and ethnic differences. Ann Intern Med 2007;146:486–492.)

Actual Distributions

Distributions of clinical phenomena have many different shapes. The frequency distributions of four common blood tests (for potassium, alkaline phosphatase, glucose, and hemoglobin) are shown in Figure 3.6. In general, most of the values appear near the middle of the distribution, and except for the central part of the curves, there are no "humps" or irregularities. The high and low ends of the distributions stretch out into tails, with the tail at one end often being more elongated than the tail at the other (i.e., the curves are skewed toward the longer end). Whereas some of the distributions are skewed toward higher values, others are skewed toward lower values. In other words, all of these distributions are unimodal (have only one hump), and are roughly bell shaped, though not necessarily symmetrical. Otherwise, they do not resemble one another.

The distribution of values for many laboratory tests changes with characteristics of the patients such as age, sex, race, and nutrition. For example, the distribution of one such test, blood urea nitrogen (BUN, a test of kidney function), changes with age. A BUN of 25 mg/dL would be unusually high for a young person in her 20s, but not particularly remarkable for an 80-year-old.

Table 3.4

Expressions of Central Tendency and Dispersion

Expression	Definition	Advantages	Disadvantages
Central Tendency			
Mean	$\dfrac{\text{Sum of values for observations}}{\text{Number of observations}}$	Well suited for mathematical manipulation	Affected by extreme values
Median	The point where the number of observations above equals the number below	Not easily influenced by extreme values	Not well suited for mathematical manipulation
Mode	Most frequently occurring value	Simplicity of meaning	Sometimes there are no, or many, most frequent values
Dispersion			
Range	From lowest to highest value in a distribution	Includes all values	Greatly affected by extreme values
Standard Deviation[a]	The absolute value of the average difference of individual values from the mean[a]	Well suited for mathematical manipulation	For non-Gaussian distributions, does not describe a known proportion of the observations
Percentile, decile, quartile, etc.	The proportion of all observations falling between specified values	Describes "unusualness" of a value Does not make assumptions about the shape of a distribution	Not well suited for statistical manipulation

[a] $\sqrt{\dfrac{\Sigma(X - \bar{X})^2}{N - 1}}$, where X = each observation; $\bar{X}$ = mean of all observations; and N = number of observations.

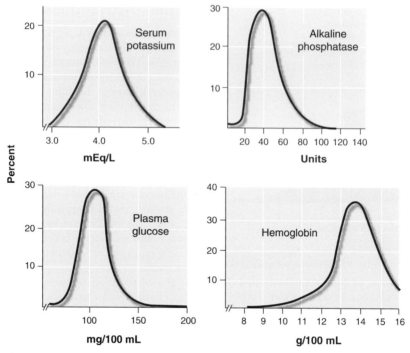

Figure 3.6 ■ Actual clinical distributions. (Data from Martin HF, Gudzinowicz BJ, Fanger H. Normal Values in Clinical Chemistry. New York: Marcel Dekker; 1975.)

The Normal Distribution

Another kind of distribution is called the normal distribution (or "Gaussian," after the mathematician who first described it). The normal distribution, based in statistical theory, describes the frequency distribution of repeated measurements of the same physical object by the same instrument. Dispersion of values represents random variation alone. A normal curve is shown in Figure 3.7. The curve is symmetrical and bell shaped. It has the mathematical property that about two-thirds of the observations fall within

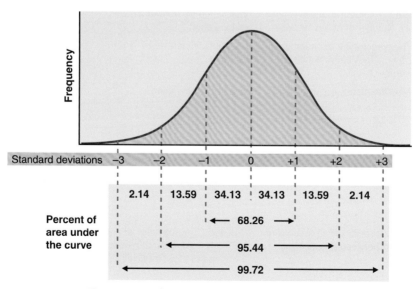

Figure 3.7 ■ The normal (Gaussian) distribution.

1 standard deviation of the mean, and about 95%, within 2 standard deviations.

Although clinical distributions often resemble a normal distribution the resemblance is superficial. As summarized in a perspective, "The experimental fact is that for most physiologic variables the distribution is smooth, unimodal, and skewed, and that mean ±2 standard deviations does not cut off the desired 95%. We have no mathematical, statistical, or other theorems that enable us to predict the shape of the distributions of physiologic measurements" (5).

The shapes of clinical distributions differ from one another because many differences among people, other than random variation, contribute to distributions of clinical measurements. Therefore, if distributions of clinical measurements resemble normal curves, it is largely by accident. Even so, it is often assumed, as a matter of convenience (because means and standard deviations are relatively easy to calculate and manipulate mathematically) that clinical measurements are "normally" distributed.

CRITERIA FOR ABNORMALITY

It would be convenient if the frequency distributions of clinical measurements for normal and abnormal people were so different that these distributions could be used to distinguish two distinct populations. This is actually the case for some abnormal genes. Sequences (genetic abnormalities coding) for the autosomal dominant condition familial adenomatous polyposis are either present or absent. People with the abnormal gene develop hundreds of polyps in their colon, whereas people without the gene rarely have more than a few, but this is the exception that proves the rule. Far more often, the various genetic abnormalities coding for the same disease produce a range of expressions. Even the expression of a specific genetic abnormality (such as substitution of a single base pair) differs substantially from one person to another, presumably related to differences in the rest of the genetic endowment as well as exposure to external causes of the disease.

Therefore, most distributions of clinical variables are not easily divided into "normal" and "abnormal." They are not inherently dichotomous and do not display sharp breaks or two peaks that characterize normal and abnormal results. This is because disease is usually acquired by degrees, so there is a smooth transition from low to high values with increasing degrees of dysfunction. Laboratory tests reflecting organ failure, such as serum creatinine for kidney failure or ejection fraction for heart failure, behave in this way.

Another reason why normals and abnormals are not seen as separate distributions is that even when people with and without a disease have substantially different frequency distributions, the distributions almost always overlap. When the two distributions are mixed together, as they are in naturally occurring populations, the abnormals are usually not seen as separate because they comprise such a small proportion of the whole. The curve for people with disease is "swallowed up" by the larger curve for healthy, normal people.

Example

Phenylketonuria (PKU) is an inherited disease characterized by progressive mental retardation in childhood. A variety of mutant alleles coding for phenylalanine hydroxylase results in dysfunction of the enzyme and, with a normal diet, accumulation of phenylalanine that results in symptoms. The genes are in principle either abnormal or not (Fig. 3.8A). The diagnosis, which becomes apparent in the first year of life, is confirmed by persistently high phenylalanine levels (several times the usual range) and low tyrosine levels in the blood.

It is common practice to screen newborns for PKU with a blood test for phenylalanine a few days after birth, in time to treat before there is irreversible damage. However, even though the abnormal genes are present or absent (Fig. 3.8A), the test misclassifies some infants because at that age there is an overlap in the distributions of serum phenylalanine concentrations in infants with and without PKU and because infants with PKU make up only a small proportion of those screened, <1/10,000 (Fig. 3.8B). Some newborns with PKU are in the normal range either because they have not yet ingested enough phenylalanine-containing protein or because they have a combination of alleles associated with mild disease. Some children who are not destined to develop PKU have relatively high levels—for example, because their mothers have abnormal phenylalanine metabolism. The test is set to be positive at the lower end of the overlap between normal and abnormal levels, to detect most infants with the disease, even though only about 1 out of 10 infants with an abnormal screening test turns out to have PKU.

A

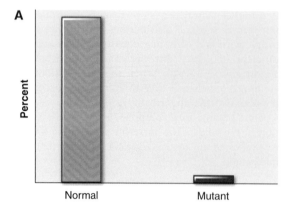

Alleles for phenylalanine hydroxylase

B

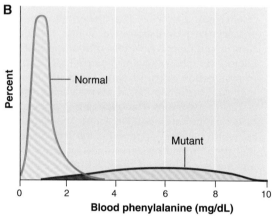

Figure 3.8 ■ Screening for phenylketonuria (PKU) in infants: dichotomous and overlapping distributions of normal and abnormal. A. Alleles coding for phenylalanine hydroxylase are either normal or mutant. **B.** The distributions of blood phenylalanine levels in newborns with and without PKU overlap and are of greatly different magnitude. (The prevalence of PKU, which is <1/10,000, is exaggerated so that its distribution can be seen in the figure.)

If there is no sharp dividing line between normal and abnormal, and the clinician can choose where the line is placed, what ground rules should be used to decide? Three criteria have proven useful: being unusual, being sick, and being treatable. For a given measurement, the results of these approaches bear no necessary relation to one another, so what is considered abnormal by one criterion might be normal by another.

Abnormal = Unusual

Normal often refers to the frequently occurring or usual condition. Whatever occurs often is considered normal, and what occurs infrequently is abnormal.

This is a statistical definition, based on the frequency of a characteristic in a defined population. Commonly, the reference population is made up of people without disease, but this need not be the case. For example, we may say that it is normal to have pain after surgery or itching with eczema.

It is tempting to be more specific by defining what is unusual in mathematical terms. One commonly used way of establishing a cutoff point between normal and abnormal is to agree, somewhat arbitrarily, that all values beyond 2 standard deviations from the mean are abnormal. On the assumption that the distribution in question approximates a normal distribution, 2.5% of observations would then appear in each tail of the distribution and be considered abnormally high or abnormally low.

Of course, as already pointed out, most biologic measurements are not normally distributed. Therefore, it is better to describe unusual values, whatever the proportion chosen, as a fraction (or percentile) of the actual distribution. In this way, it is possible to make a direct statement about how infrequent a value is without making assumptions about the shape of the distribution from which it came.

Despite this, the statistical definition of normality, with the cutoff point at 2 standard deviations from the mean, is most commonly used. However, it can be ambiguous or misleading for several reasons:

■ If all values beyond an arbitrary statistical limit, say the 95th percentile, were considered abnormal, then the frequency of all diseases would be the same (if one assumed the distribution was normal, 2.5% if we consider just the extreme high or low ends of the distribution). Yet, it is common knowledge that diseases vary in frequency; diabetes and osteoarthritis are far more common than ovalocytosis and hairy cell leukemia.

■ There is no general relationship between the degree of statistical unusualness and clinical disease. The relationship is specific to the disease in question and the setting. Thus, obesity is quite common in the United States but uncommon in many developing countries. For some measurements, deviations from usual are associated with disease to an important degree only at quite extreme values, well beyond the 95th or even the 99th percentile. Failure of organs such as the liver and kidneys becomes symptomatic only when most of usual function is lost.

■ Sometimes extreme values are actually beneficial. For example, people with unusually low blood pressure are, on average, at lower risk of cardiovascular disease than people with more usual blood pressures. People with unusually high bone density are at lower than average risk of fractures.

■ Many measurements are related to risk of disease over a broad range of values, with no threshold dividing normal from increased risk. Blood pressure is an example.

Example

Figure 3.9 shows that usual systolic blood pressure is related to ischemic heart disease mortality throughout a broad range of blood pressures, from 115 to 185 mm Hg. The Figure shows that even a systolic blood pressure of 120 mm Hg is riskier than 115 mm Hg, but patients are rarely prescribed medicines for hypertension at that level. For every 20 mm Hg higher systolic blood pressure, there is about a two-fold higher ischemic heart disease death rate, with no evidence of a threshold down to 115 mm Hg systolic pressure, the lowest level for which there are adequate data (6). Examining the slope of the curve, it seems unlikely that even a systolic blood pressure of 115 mm Hg is absolutely "safe." At what point, then, should normal and abnormal systolic blood pressure be defined? In terms of pharmacologic treatment for most patients, the goal is currently, somewhat arbitrarily, set at 140 mm Hg.

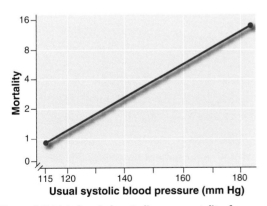

Figure 3.9 ■ Ischemic heart disease mortality for people ages 40 to 49 years is related to systolic blood pressure throughout the range of values occurring in most people. There is no threshold between normal and abnormal. "Mortality" is presented as a multiple of the baseline rate. (Data from Prospective Studies Collaboration. Age-specific relevance of usual blood pressure to vascular mortality: a meta-analysis of individual data for one million adults in 61 prospective studies. Lancet 2002;360:1903–1913.)

Abnormal = Associated with Disease

As the above example demonstrates, a sounder approach to distinguishing normal from abnormal is to call abnormal those observations that are clinically meaningful departures from good health—that is, associated with a meaningful risk of having or developing disease, disability, or death. Using this approach to defining abnormality can sometimes lead to different levels of a condition being abnormal.

Example

At what point does higher than average weight for height become a health problem in older individuals? Figure 3.10A shows the relationship between body mass index (BMI, weight in kilograms divided by height in meters squared) and the risk of death from all causes over 14 years in U.S. men aged 65 years of older on Medicare (7). The risk was high for men with the lowest BMI (probably because of weight loss associated with illness), and then was stable over a broad range of BMIs. Among the heavier men, only those with a markedly elevated BMI of 35 or above had increased mortality. Contrast this result with the risk for functional decline (in the ability to do light and heavy housework, make meals, shop, use the telephone, and manage money) over a 2-year period (Fig. 3.10B). The percentage of men declining functionally was related to weight across the BMI range, almost doubling from 21% to 38% as BMI increased. The cutoff point between normal and abnormal BMI depends on the health outcome in question.

Abnormal = Treating the Condition Leads to a Better Clinical Outcome

It makes intuitive sense to define a clinical condition or finding as "abnormal" if treatment of it leads to a better outcome. This approach makes particularly good sense for asymptomatic conditions. If a condition is causing no trouble, and treatment makes no difference, why try to treat it? However, even for symptomatic patients, it is sometimes difficult to

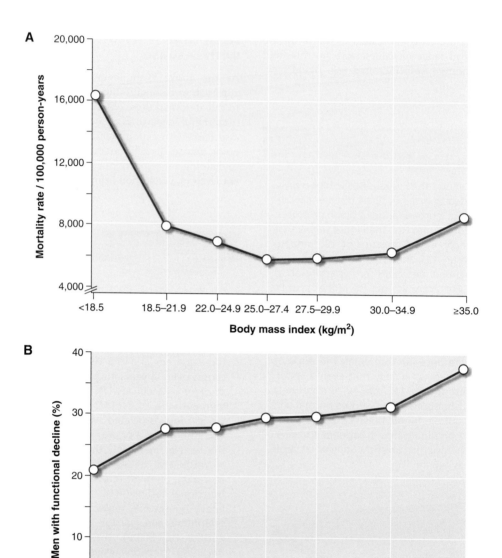

Figure 3.10 ■ Abnormal as associated with disease and other patient outcomes. The relationship between body mass index and **(A)** total mortality and **(B)** functional decline in men age 65 and older on Medicare. Body mass index is weight in kilograms divided by height in meters squared. Mortality rates are adjusted for age and smoking. (Redrawn with permission from Wee CC, Huskey KW, Ngo LH, et al. Obesity, race and risk for death or functional decline among Medicare beneficiaries. A cohort study. Ann Intern Med 2011;154:645–655.)

distinguish between clinical findings that will and will not improve with treatment. Modern technology, especially newer imaging techniques, are now able to detect abnormalities in patients so well that it is not always clear what is found is related to the patient's complaint. The result is an increasingly common dilemma for both patients and clinicians.

Example

Magnetic resonance imaging (MRI) of the knee is frequently performed in middle-aged and elderly patients presenting with knee pain; if a meniscal tear is found, the symptoms are usually attributed to the tear and arthroscopic meniscectomy may be performed. Nevertheless, the prevalence of meniscal tears and their relationship to knee symptoms is not clear, especially in older people. A study was undertaken in which 991 randomly selected middle-aged and elderly adults without prior knee surgery underwent MRI scans of their knees and were asked (independently) about knee-joint symptoms (8). Among people with radiographic evidence of osteoarthritis, 63% of those with frequent knee pain, aching, or stiffness had at least one meniscal tear show on the MRI, a result that might be suspected. Surprisingly, the result was almost the same (60%) among people without these symptoms. Among participants without evidence of osteoarthritis, the comparable percentages were 32% and 23%. The authors concluded that meniscal tears are common irrespective of knee symptoms, and often accompany knee osteoarthritis. Ironically, surgical treatment of meniscal repairs increases the risk of osteoarthritis, raising the stakes for determining if a meniscal tear is indeed the cause of a patient's knee pain.

Another reason to limit the definition of "abnormal" to a condition that is treatable is that not every condition conferring an increased risk can be successfully treated: The removal of the condition may not remove risk, either because the condition itself is not a cause of disease but is only related to a cause or because irreversible damage has already occurred. To label people abnormal can cause worry and a sense of vulnerability that may not be justified for some health problems if treatment cannot improve the outlook.

What is considered treatable changes with time. At their best, therapeutic decisions are grounded on evidence from well-conducted clinical trials (Chapter 9). As new knowledge is acquired from the results of clinical trials, the level at which treatment is considered useful may change.

Example

Folic acid, a vitamin that occurs mainly in green leafy vegetables, was discovered early in the 20th century. Diets low in folic acid were found to cause a vitamin deficiency syndrome with anemia. For many years, adequate intake of folic acid was defined in the "recommended dietary allowance" as the amount necessary to prevent anemia. More recently, however, reasons for a new and higher level of "normal" intake have emerged. Low folic acid levels in early pregnancy were linked to neural tube defects in infants, even though the folic acid levels were well above those needed to prevent anemia. Subsequent studies showed that folic acid supplementation in high-risk women prevented about three-quarters of the malformations. Thus, a higher level for "normal" folic acid intake during childbearing years has emerged because of new information about the levels needed to prevent disease. The optimal level is at least two times (and some suggest eight times) higher than the older criterion for normal intake. As a practical matter, these levels of intake are feasible in most people only by vitamin supplements, not by diet alone.

REGRESSION TO THE MEAN

When clinicians encounter an unexpectedly abnormal test result, they tend to repeat the test. Often, the second test result is closer to normal. Why does this happen? Should it be reassuring?

Patients selected because they represent an extreme value in a distribution can be expected, on average, to have less extreme values on subsequent measurements. This phenomenon, called regression to the mean, occurs for purely statistical reasons, not because the patients have necessarily improved.

Regression to the mean arises in the following way (Fig. 3.11): People are selected for inclusion in

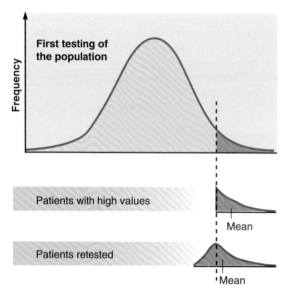

Figure 3.11 ■ Regression to the mean.

a study or for further diagnosis or treatment because their initial measurement for a trait falls beyond an arbitrarily selected cutoff point in the tail of a distribution of values for all the patients examined. Some of these people will remain above the cutoff point on subsequent measurements because their true values are usually higher than average, but others who were found to have values above the cutoff point during the initial screening usually have lower values on

retesting. They were selected only because they happened, through random variation, to have a high value at the time they were first measured. When the measurement is made again, these people have lower values than they had during the first screening. This phenomenon tends to drag down the mean value of the subgroup originally found to have values above the cutoff point.

Thus, patients who are singled out from others because of a laboratory test result that is unusually high or low can be expected, on average, to be closer to the center of the distribution if the test is repeated. Moreover, subsequent values are likely to be more accurate estimates of the true value, which could be obtained if measurements were repeated for a particular patient many times. Therefore, the time-honored practice of repeating laboratory tests that are found to be abnormal and of considering the second one the correct result is not merely wishful thinking. It has a sound theoretical basis. It also has an empirical basis. For example, in a study of liver function tests (aspartate aminotransferase, alanine aminotransferase, alkaline phosphatase, gamma-glutamyltransferase, and bilirubin) in a cross-section of the U.S. population, 12% to 38% of participants who had abnormally high values on initial testing had normal values on retesting (9). However, the more extreme the initial reading was—more than two times the normal range—the more likely the repeat test would remain abnormal. For participants with normal initial testing, values on retesting remained normal in more than 95%.

Review Questions

For each of the numbered clinical scenarios below (3.1–3.5), select from the lettered options the most appropriate term for the type of data.

3.1. Deep tendon reflex grade 0 (no response), 1+ (somewhat diminished), 2+ (normal), 3+ (brisker than average), and 4+ (very brisk).

   A. Interval—Continuous
   B. Dichotomous
   C. Nominal
   D. Ordinal
   E. Interval—Discrete

3.2. Cancer recurrent/not recurrent 5 years after initial treatment.

   A. Interval—Continuous
   B. Dichotomous
   C. Nominal
   D. Ordinal
   E. Interval—Discrete

3.3. Serum sodium 139 mg/dL.

   A. Interval—Continuous
   B. Dichotomous
   C. Nominal
   D. Ordinal
   E. Interval—Discrete

3.4. Three seizures per month.

   A. Interval—Continuous
   B. Dichotomous
   C. Nominal
   D. Ordinal
   E. Interval—Discrete

3.5. Causes of upper gastrointestinal bleeding: duodenal ulcer, gastritis, esophageal, or other varices.

   A. Interval—Continuous
   B. Dichotomous
   C. Nominal
   D. Ordinal
   E. Interval—Discrete

For questions 3.6–3.10, choose the best answer.

3.6. When it is not possible to verify measurement of a phenomenon, such as itching, by the physical senses, which of the following can be said about its validity?

   A. It is questionable, and one should rely on "hard" measures such as laboratory tests.
   B. It can be established by showing that the same value is obtained when the measurement is repeated by many different observers at different times.
   C. It can be supported by showing that the measurement is related to other measures of phenomena such as the presence of diseases that are known to cause itching.
   D. It can be established by showing that measurement results in a broad range of values.
   E. It cannot be established.

3.7. A physician or nurse measures a patient's heart rate by feeling the pulse for 10 seconds each time she comes to clinic. The rates might differ from visit to visit because of all the following *except:*

   A. The patient has a different pulse rate at different times.
   B. The measurement may misrepresent the true pulse by chance because of the brief period of observation.
   C. The physician and nurse use different techniques (e.g., different degrees of pressure on the pulse).
   D. The pulse rate varies among patients.
   E. An effective treatment was begun between visits.

3.8. "Abnormal" is commonly defined by all of the following *except:*

   A. The level at which treatment has been shown to be effective
   B. The level at which death rate is increased
   C. Statistically unusual values
   D. Values that do not correspond to a normal distribution
   E. The level at which there is an increased risk of symptoms

3.9. All of the following statements are true *except:*

   A. The normal distribution describes the distribution of most naturally occurring phenomena.
   B. The normal distribution includes 2.5% of people in each tail of the distribution (beyond 2 standard deviations from the mean).
   C. The normal distribution is unimodal and symmetrical.
   D. The normal distribution is the most common basis for defining abnormal laboratory tests measured on interval scales.

3.10. You see a new patient who is a 71-year-old woman on no medicines and without history of heart disease in herself or her family. She has never smoked and is not diabetic. Her blood pressure is 115/75 mm Hg, she is about 15 pounds overweight. A total cholesterol test done 2 days ago was high at as 250 mg/dL and the HDL cholesterol was 59 mg/dL. The Framingham risk calculator estimates that the patient's risk of developing general cardiovascular disease in the next 10 years is 9%. You know that treating cholesterol at the level found reduces cardiovascular risk. The patient wants to know if she should start taking a statin. Which of the following statements is *least correct*?

   A. The patient is likely to have a lower serum cholesterol the next time it is measured.
   B. The estimation of a 9% probability of cardiovascular disease in the next 10 years could be influenced by chance.
   C. The patient should be given a prescription for a statin to lower her risk of coronary heart disease.

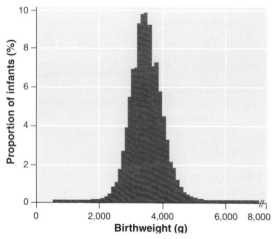

Figure 3.12 ■ **The distribution of birth weights of full-term babies born to non-diabetic mothers.** (Redrawn with permission from Ludwig DS, Currie J. The association between pregnancy weight gain and birthweight: a within-family comparison. Lancet 2010;376:984–990.)

Figure 3.12 shows the distribution of birthweight of more than a million full-term babies born to mothers without diabetes. Questions 3.11–3.13 relate to the figure. For each question, choose the best answer.

3.11. Which statement about the central tendency is *incorrect*?

  A. The mean birthweight is below 4,000 g.
  B. There is more than one mode birth weight.
  C. Mean and median birth weights are similar.

3.12. Which statement about dispersion is most correct?

  A. The range is the best way to describe the babies' birth weights.
  B. Standard deviations should not be calculated because the distribution is skewed.
  C. Ninety-five percent of the birth weights will fall within about 2 standard deviations of the mean.

3.13. One standard deviation of babies' birth weights encompasses approximately:

  A. Weights from 2,000 to 4,000 g
  B. Weights from 3,000 to 4,000 g
  C. Weights from 2,000 to 6,000 g

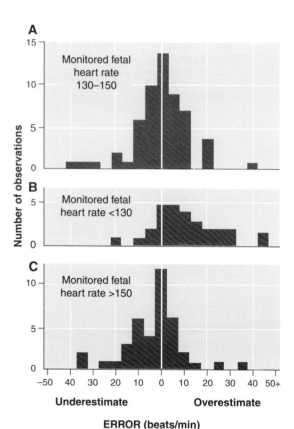

Figure 3.13 ■ **Observer variability.** Comparing fetal heart auscultation to electronic monitoring of fetal heart rate. (Redrawn with permission from Day E, Maddem L, Wood C. Auscultation of foetal heart rate: an assessment of its error and significance. Br Med J 1968;4:422–424.)

Figure 3.13 compares fetal heart rates measured by electronic monitoring (white middle bar), to measurements by hospital staff in three different circumstances: when fetal heart rate of beats per minute by electronic monitoring was normal (130–150), low (<130), and high (>150). Questions 3.14–3.16 relate to the figure. For each question, choose the best answer.

3.14. The distribution of hospital staff measurements around the electronic monitor measurement in Panel A of Figure 3.13 could be due to:

  A. Chance
  B. Inter-observer variability
  C. Biased preference for normal results
  D. A and B
  E. A and C
  F. B and C
  G. A, B, and C

3.15. The distribution of hospital staff measurements around the electronic monitor measurement in Panel B of Figure 3.13 could be due to:

A. Chance
B. Inter-observer variability
C. Biased preference for normal results
D. A and B
E. A and C
F. B and C
G. A, B, and C

3.16. The distribution of hospital staff measurements around the electronic monitor measurement in Panel C of Figure 3.13 could be due to:

A. Chance
B. Inter-observer variability
C. Biased preference for normal results
D. A and B
E. A and C
F. B and C
G. A, B, and C

Answers are in Appendix A.

REFERENCES

1. Sharma P, Parekh A, Uhl K. An innovative approach to determine fetal risk: the FDA Office of Women's Health pregnancy exposure registry web listing. Womens Health Issues 2008;18:226–228.
2. Feinstein AR. The need for humanized science in evaluating medication. Lancet 1972;2:421–423.
3. Rubenfeld GD, Caldwell E, Granton J, et al. Interobserver variability in applying a radiographic definition for ARDS. Chest 1999;116:1347–1353.
4. Morganroth J, Michelson EL, Horowitz LN, et al. Limitations of routine long-term electrocardiographic monitoring to assess ventricular ectopic frequency. Circulation 1978;58:408–414.
5. Elveback LR, Guillier CL, Keating FR. Health, normality, and the ghost of Gauss. JAMA 1970;211:69–75.
6. Prospective Studies Collaboration. Age-specific relevance of usual blood pressure to vascular mortality: a meta-analysis of individual data for one million adults in 61 prospective studies. Lancet 2002;360:1903–1913.
7. Wee CC, Huskey KW, Ngo LH, et al. Obesity, race and risk for death or functional decline among Medicare beneficiaries. A cohort study. Ann Intern Med 2011;154:645–655.
8. Englund M, Guermazi A, Gale D. Incidental meniscal findings on knee MRI in middle-aged and elderly persons. N Engl J Med 2008;359:1108–1115.
9. Lazo M, Selvin E, Clark JM. Brief communication: clinical implications of short-term variability in liver function test results. Ann Intern Med 2008;148:348–352.

Chapter 4

Risk: Basic Principles

The lesson . . . is that a large number of people at a small risk may give rise to more cases of disease than the small number who are at a high risk.

—Geoffrey Rose
1985

KEY WORDS

Risk	Calibration
Risk factor	Discrimination
Exposure	Concordance
Latency period	statistic
Immediate causes	C-statistic
Distant causes	Sensitivity
Marker	Specificity
Risk prediction model	Receiver operating
Risk prediction tool	characteristic (ROC)
Risk stratification	curve

Risk generally refers to the probability of some untoward event. In medicine, clinicians deal with probabilities in virtually every patient encounter. They work with basic principles of risk whether they are diagnosing a complaint, describing prognosis, deciding on treatment, or discussing prevention with the patient. Patient encounters no longer deal only with the patient's complaints, but increasingly involve checking for risk factors that might lead to poor health in the future. In medical research, more and more effort is devoted to elucidating risk factors for diseases. A major rationale for the Human Genome Project is to predict diseases that will become manifest over a person's lifetime. Clinical journals publish epidemiologic studies investigating possible health risks. All this effort has improved our understanding about risks to health and how to study them, and has helped improve the health of patients and populations, sometimes in dramatic ways. For example, research that led to the understanding that smoking, hypertension, and hyperlipidemia increase

the risk of cardiovascular disease (CVD) has helped decrease cardiovascular mortality in the United States by half over the past several decades.

People have a strong interest in their risk of disease, a concern reflected in television and newspaper headlines, and the many Web sites and popular books about risk reduction. The risk of breast and prostate cancer, heart disease and stroke, Alzheimer disease, autism, and osteoporosis are examples of topics in which the public has developed a strong interest. Discerning patients want to know their individual risks and how to reduce them.

In this chapter, we will concentrate on the underlying principles about risk, important regardless of where risk confronts the clinician and patient along the spectrum of care. As much as possible, we will deal with concepts rather than terminology and methods, covering those important details in later chapters. Chapters 5 and 6 deal with risks for adverse health effects in the distant future, often years or even decades away; they describe scientific methods used to indicate the probability that people who are exposed to certain "risk factors" will subsequently develop a particular disease or bad health outcome more often than similar people who are not exposed. In acute care settings such as intensive care units, emergency rooms, and hospital wards, the concern is about risks patients with known disease might or might not experience, termed prognosis (Chapter 7); the time horizon of prognosis spans from minutes and hours to months and years, depending on the study. Chapters 8, 9, and 10 revisit risk as it relates to diagnosis, treatment, and prevention. In each case, the approach to assessing risk is somewhat different. However, the fundamental principles of determining risks to health are similar.

RISK FACTORS

Characteristics associated with an increased risk of becoming diseased are called risk factors. Some risk factors are inherited. For example, having the haplotype HLA-B27 greatly increases one's risk of acquiring the spondyloarthropathies. Work on the Human Genome Project has identified many other diseases for which specific genes are risk factors, including colon and breast cancer, osteoporosis, and amyotrophic lateral sclerosis. Other risk factors, such as infectious agents, drugs, and toxins, are found in the physical environment. Still others are part of the social environment. For example, bereavement after the loss of a spouse, change in daily routines, and crowding all have been shown to increase rates of disease—not only for emotional illness but physical illness as well. Some of the most powerful risk factors are behavioral; examples include smoking, drinking alcohol to excess, driving without seat belts, engaging in unsafe sex, eating too much, and exercising too little.

Exposure to a risk factor means that a person, before becoming ill, has come in contact with or has manifested the factor in question. Exposure can take place at a single point in time, as when a community is exposed to radiation during a nuclear accident. More often, however, contact with risk factors for chronic disease takes place over a period of time. Cigarette smoking, hypertension, sexual promiscuity, and sun exposure are examples of risk factors, with the risk of disease being more likely to occur with prolonged exposure.

There are several different ways of characterizing the amount of exposure or contact with a putative risk factor: ever been exposed, current dose, largest dose taken, total cumulative dose, years of exposure, years since first exposure, and so on. Although the various measures of dose tend to be related to one another, some may show an exposure–disease relationship, whereas others may not. For example, cumulative doses of sun exposure constitute a risk factor for non-melanoma skin cancer, whereas episodes of severe sunburn are a better predictor of melanoma. If the correct measure is not chosen, an association between a risk factor and disease may not be evident. Choice of an appropriate measure of exposure to a risk factor is usually based on all that is known about the clinical and biologic effects of the exposure, the pathophysiology of the disease, and epidemiologic studies.

RECOGNIZING RISK

Risk factors associated with large effects that occur rapidly after exposure are easy for anyone to recognize. It is not difficult to appreciate the relationship between exposure and medical conditions such as sunburn and aspirin overdose, or the poor prognosis of hypotension at the onset of myocardial infarction, because the deleterious effect follows exposure relatively rapidly and is easy to see.

The sudden increase of a rare disease, or the dramatic clinical presentation of a new disease is also easy to recognize, and invites efforts to find a cause. AIDS was such an unusual syndrome that the appearance of just a few cases raised suspicion that some new agent (as it turned out, a retrovirus) might be responsible, a suspicion confirmed relatively quickly after the first cases of the disease. A previously unidentified coronavirus was confirmed as the cause of severe adult respiratory syndrome (SARS) in a matter of weeks after the first reported cases of the highly lethal infection in 2003. Similarly, decades ago, physicians quickly noticed when several cases of carcinoma of the vagina, a very rare condition, began appearing. A careful search for an explanation was undertaken, and maternal exposure to diethylstilbestrol (a hormone used to stabilize pregnancies in women with a history of miscarriage) was found.

Most morbidity or mortality, however, is caused by chronic diseases for which the relationship between exposure and disease is far less obvious. It is usually impossible for individual clinicians, however astute, to recognize risk factors for chronic disease based on their own experiences with patients. This is true for several reasons, which are discussed in the following pages.

Long Latency

Many chronic diseases have a long latency period between exposure to a risk factor and the first manifestations of disease. Radiation exposure in childhood, for example, increases the risk for thyroid cancer in adults decades later. Similarly, hypertension precedes heart disease by decades, and calcium intake in young and middle-aged women affects osteoporosis and fracture rates in old age. When patients experience the consequence of exposure to a risk factor years later, the original exposure may be all but forgotten and the link between exposure and disease obscured.

Immediate Versus Distant Causes

The search for risk factors usually is a search for causes of disease. In clinical medicine, physicians are more interested in immediate causes of disease—infectious, physiologic, or anatomic changes leading to sickness such as a coronavirus causing SARS or hypocalcemia leading to seizures. But distant causes, more remote causes, may be important in the causal pathway. For example, lack of maternal education is a risk factor for low-birth-weight infants. Other factors related to education, such as poor nutrition, less prenatal care, cigarette smoking, and the like are more direct causes of low birth weight. Nevertheless, studies in India have shown that improving maternal education lowers infant mortality.

Common Exposure to Risk Factors

Many risk factors, such as cigarette smoking or eating a diet high in sugar, salt, and fat, have become so common in Western societies that for many years their dangers went unrecognized. Only by comparing patterns of disease among people with and without these risk factors, using cross-national studies or investigating special subgroups—Mormons, for example, who do not smoke, or vegetarians who eat diets low in cholesterol—were risks recognized that were, in fact, large. It is now clear that about half of lifetime users of tobacco will die because of their habit; if current smoking patterns persist, it is predicted that in the 21st century, more than 1 billion deaths globally will be attributed to smoking (1).

A relationship between the sleeping position of babies and the occurrence of sudden infant death syndrome (SIDS) is another example of a common exposure to a risk factor and the dramatic effect associated with its frequency, an association that went unrecognized until relatively recently.

Example

SIDS, the sudden, unexplained death of an infant younger than 1 year of age, is a leading cause of infant mortality. Studies suggest that there are many contributing factors. In the late 1980s and 1990s, several investigations found that babies who were placed face down in their cribs were three to nine times more likely to die of SIDS than those placed on their backs. In 1992, the American Academy of Pediatrics issued a recommendation to place infants on their backs to sleep but indicated that side positioning for sleep was an acceptable alternative. The percentage of babies placed in the prone position for sleep fell from 70% in 1992 to 24% in 1996, with a concomitant 40% drop in the number of SIDS cases (2). Ongoing research led to evidence that side positioning of babies also increased the risk of SIDS (3), and the American Academy of Pediatrics updated its recommendations in 2005 to make it clear that side sleeping was no longer recommended.

Low Incidence of Disease

The incidence of most diseases, even ones thought to be "common," is actually uncommon. Thus, although lung cancer is the most common cause of cancer deaths in Americans, and people who smoke are as much as 20 times more likely to develop lung cancer than those that do not smoke, the yearly incidence of lung cancer in people who have smoked heavily for 30 years, is 2 to 3 per 1,000. In the average physician's practice, years may pass between new cases of lung cancer. It is difficult for the average clinician to draw conclusions about risks from such infrequent events.

Small Risk

The effects of many risk factors for chronic disease are small. To detect a small risk, a large number of people must be studied to observe a difference in disease rates between exposed and unexposed persons. For example, drinking alcohol has been known to increase the risk of breast cancer, but it was less clear whether low levels of consumption, such as drinking just one glass of wine or its equivalent a day, conferred risk. A study of 2,400,000 women-years was needed to find that women who averaged a glass a day increased their risk of developing breast cancer 15% (4). Because of the large numbers of woman-years in the study, chance is an unlikely explanation for the result, but even so, such a small effect could be due to bias. In contrast, it is not controversial that hepatitis B infection is a risk factor for hepatoma, because people with certain types of serologic evidence of hepatitis B infection are up to 60 times (not just 1.15 times) more likely to develop liver cancer than those without it.

Multiple Causes and Multiple Effects

There is usually not a close, one-to-one relationship between a risk factor and a particular disease.

RISK FACTORS

Hypercholesterolemia

Positive family history

Thiamine deficiency

Valvular disease

Viral infection

Smoking

Diabetes

Alcohol

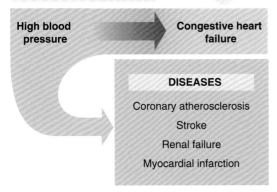

DISEASES

Coronary atherosclerosis

Stroke

Renal failure

Myocardial infarction

Figure 4.1 ■ **Relationship between risk factors and disease: hypertension and congestive heart failure.** Hypertension causes many diseases, including congestive heart failure, and congestive heart failure has many causes, including hypertension.

A given risk factor may contribute to many diseases, and a disease may have multiple causes. The relationship between hypertension and congestive failure is an example (Fig. 4.1). Some people with hypertension develop congestive heart failure, and many do not. Also, many people who do not have hypertension develop congestive heart failure because there are other causes. The relationship is also difficult to recognize because hypertension causes several diseases other than congestive heart failure. Thus, although hypertension is the third leading cause of congestive heart failure, physicians were not aware of this relationship until the 1970s, when adequate evidence became available after careful study of large numbers of people over many years.

Risk Factors May or May Not Be Causal

Just because risk factors predict disease, it does not necessarily follow that they cause disease. A risk factor may predict a disease outcome indirectly, by virtue of an association with some other variable that actually is a determinant of disease. That is, the risk factor is confounded with a truly causal factor.

A risk factor that is not a cause of disease is called a marker of disease, because it "marks" the increased probability of disease. Not being a cause does not diminish the value of a risk factor as a way of predicting the probability of disease, but it does imply that removing the risk factor might not remove the excess risk associated with it.

Example

Homocystinuria, a rare pediatric disease caused by autosomal recessive genes and very high levels of the amino acid homocysteine, is associated with severe premature atherosclerosis. The possibility that slightly elevated homocysteine levels also could be a risk factor for coronary heart disease in adults has been investigated. Multiple studies have found that there is a relationship; each increase of 5 μmol/L in homocysteine level increases the risk of CVD by 20% (5). Because of this relationship, clinical studies were undertaken to determine if lowering homocysteine levels with folic acid as well as vitamins B_6 and B_{12} would reduce the risk of major cardiovascular events among people with known CVD or diabetes. Surprisingly, several large studies found that even though homocysteine levels were lowered, the vitamin supplementation did not protect against future cardiovascular events in these patients (6). Thus, although elevated homocysteine levels was a marker for future CVD in adults, it does not appear to be a causal factor, at least among patients with known CVD or diabetes.

There are several ways of deciding whether a risk factor is a cause or merely a marker for disease. These are covered in Chapter 5.

For all these reasons, individual clinicians are rarely in a position to recognize, let alone confirm, associations between exposure and chronic diseases. They may notice an association when a dramatic disease occurs quickly after an unusual exposure, but most diseases and most exposures do not conform to such a pattern. For accurate information about risk, clinicians must turn to the medical literature, particularly to carefully constructed studies that involve a large number of patients.

PREDICTING RISK

A single powerful risk factor, as in the case of hepatitis B and hepatocellular cancer, can be very helpful clinically, but most risk factors are not strong. If drinking a glass of wine a day increases the risk of breast cancer by 15%, and the average 10-year risk of developing breast cancer for women in their 40s is 1 in 69 (or 1.45%), having a glass of wine with dinner would increase the 10-year risk to about 1 in 60 (or 1.67%). Some women might not think such a difference in the risk of breast cancer is meaningful.

Combining Multiple Risk Factors to Predict Risk

Because most chronic diseases are caused by several relatively weak risk factors acting together, statistically combining their effects can produce a more powerful prediction of risk than considering one risk factor at a time. Statistically combining risk factors produces a **risk prediction model** or a **risk prediction tool** (also sometimes called a clinical prediction tool or a risk assessment tool). Risk prediction tools are increasingly common in clinical medicine; well-known models used for long-term predictions include the Framingham Risk Score for predicting cardiovascular events and the National Cancer Institute's Breast Cancer Risk Assessment Tool for predicting breast cancer occurrence. Shorter-term hospital risk prediction tools include the Patient At Risk of Re-admission Scores (PARR) and the Critical Care Early Warning Scores. Prediction tools have also combined diagnostic test results, for example, to diagnose acute myocardial infarction when a patient presents with chest pain, or for diagnosing the occurrence of pulmonary embolism. The statistical methods used to combine multiple risk factors are discussed in Chapter 11.

Risk prediction models help with two important clinical activities. First, a good risk prediction model aids **risk stratification**, dividing groups of people into subgroups with different risk levels (e.g., low, medium, and high). Using the risk stratification approach can also help determine whether adding a newly proposed

risk factor for a disease improves the ability to predict disease, that is, improves risk stratification.

Example

CVD is the most common cause of death globally. In the United States, despite decreasing incidence, CVD accounts for a third of all deaths. Over the past 50 years, several risk factors, including hypertension, hypercholesterolemia, cigarette smoking, diabetes mellitus, marked obesity, physical inactivity, and family history have been identified. When used in risk prediction tools, these risk factors help to predict risk of CVD. In clinical practice, risk prediction is most useful when people are stratified into either high or low risk—so that patients and doctors feel comfortable either watching or intervening. It is less clear what to do with people calculated by a risk prediction tool to be at moderate risk of CVD. Efforts have been made to improve risk prediction tools for CVD by adding risk factors that reclassifies persons initially classified at moderate risk to either high- or low-risk categories. One such risk factor is a plasma marker for inflammation—C-reactive protein (CRP). A synthesis of studies of CRP found that adding it to risk prediction models improves risk stratification for CVD (7). Figure 4.2 illustrates how adding the results of the test for CRP improved the risk stratification of a risk prediction tool for CVD in women by reclassifying women into higher or lower risk categories that more accurately matched rates of CVD over a 10-year period (8).

Even if a risk factor improves a risk prediction model, a clinical trial is necessary that demonstrates lowering or removing the risk factor protects patients. In the case of CRP, such a trial has not yet been reported, so it is possible that it is a marker rather than a causal factor for CVD.

Risk Prediction in Individual Patients and Groups

Risk prediction tools are often used to predict the future for individuals, with the hope that each person will know his or her risks, a hope summarized by the term "personalized medicine." As an example, Table 4.1 summarizes the information used in

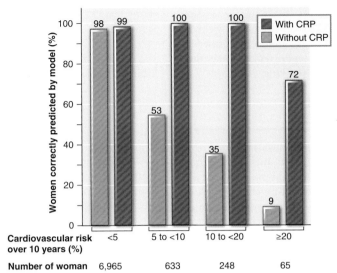

Figure 4.2 ■ Effect of adding a new risk factor to a risk prediction model. Comparison of risk prediction models for CVD over 10 years among 7,911 non-diabetic women, with and without CRP as a risk factor. Adding CRP into the risk model improved risk stratification of the women, especially to strata at higher risk by the model without CRP. (Data from Ridker PM, Buring JE, Rifal N et al. Development and validation of improved algorithms for the assessment of global cardiovascular risk in women. JAMA 2007;297:611–619.)

Table 4.1

Example of a Risk Prediction Tool: The NCI Breast Cancer Risk Assessment Tool[a]

Risk Factors Included in the Model[b]

1. What is the woman's age?
2. What was the woman's age at the time of her first menstrual period?
3. What was the woman's age at the time of her first live birth of a child?
4. How many of the woman's first-degree relatives—mother, sisters, daughters—have had breast cancer?
5. Has the woman ever had a breast biopsy?
   5a. How many breast biopsies (positive or negative) has the woman had?
   5b. Has the woman had at least one breast biopsy with atypical hyperplasia?
6. What is the woman's race/ethnicity?
   6a. What is the sub race/ethnicity?

[a]The risk assessment tool is not for women with a history of breast cancer, ductal carcinoma in situ (DCIS), or lobular carcinoma in situ (LCIS).
[b]A woman (or her clinician) chooses answers to each question from a drop-down menu.
Available at http://www.cancer.gov/bcrisktool/.

The National Cancer Institute (NCI) Breast Cancer Risk Assessment Tool. A woman or her clinician enters information, and the tool calculates a 5-year and lifetime (to age 90) risk of developing breast cancer. However, it turns out that predicting what will happen in a single individual is much more difficult than prediction in a group of similar people.

First, because predictions are expressed as probabilities of future events, there is a basic incompatibility between the incidence of a disease over 5 years (say, 15%) in a group of people and the chance that an individual in the group will develop the disease. A single person will either develop the disease or not. (You cannot be "somewhat pregnant.") So, in a sense, the average of the group is always wrong for an individual because the two are expressed in different terms, a probability determined by what happened to a group in the past versus the prospective prediction of presence or absence of disease in an individual.

Second, the presence of even a strong risk factor does not necessarily mean that an individual is very likely to get the disease. As pointed out earlier in this chapter, many years of smoking can increase a smoker's risk of lung cancer approximately 20-fold compared with non-smokers. Even so, the smoker has about a 1 in 10 chance of developing lung cancer in the next 10 years. Most risk factors (and risk prediction tools) for most diseases are much weaker than the risk of lung cancer with smoking.

EVALUATING RISK PREDICTION TOOLS

Determining how well a particular risk prediction tool works is done by asking two questions: (i) how accurately does the tool predict the *proportion* of different groups of people who will develop the disease (calibration), and (ii) how accurately does it identify *individuals* who will and will not develop the disease (discrimination)? To answer these questions, the tool is tested on a large group of people who have been followed for several years (sometimes, decades) with known outcomes of disease for each person in the group.

Calibration

Calibration, determining how well a prediction tool correctly predicts the proportion of a group who will develop disease, is conceptually and operationally simple. It is measured by comparing the number of people in a group predicted or estimated (E) by the prediction tool to develop disease to the number who are observed (O) to develop the disease. Ratios of E/O close to 1.0 mean the risk tool is well calibrated—it predicts a proportion of people that is very close to the actual proportion that develops the disease. Evaluations of the NCI breast cancer risk assessment tool have found it is highly accurate in predicting the proportion of women in a group who will develop breast cancer in the next 5 years, with E/O ratios close to 1.0.

Discrimination

Discriminating among individuals in a group who will and will not develop disease is difficult, even for well-calibrated risk tools. The most common method used to measure discrimination accuracy is to calculate a concordance statistic (often shortened to c-statistic). It estimates how often in pairs of randomly selected individuals, one of whom went on to develop the disease of interest and one of whom did not, the risk prediction score was higher for the one who developed disease. If the risk prediction tool did not improve prediction at all, the resulting estimate would be like a coin toss and the c-statistic would be 0.50. If the risk prediction tool worked perfectly, so that in every pair the diseased individual had a higher score than the non-diseased individual, the c-statistic would be 1.0. In one study assessing discrimination of the NCI breast cancer risk tool, the c-statistic was calculated as 0.58 (9). It is clear that this is not a high c-statistic, but just what the meaning of values between 0.5 and 1.0 is difficult to understand clinically.

The clearest (although rarest) method to understand how well a risk prediction model discriminates is to compare visually the predictions for individuals to the observed results for all individuals in the study. Figure 4.3A illustrates perfect discrimination by a hypothetical risk prediction tool; the tool completely separates people destined to develop disease from those destined not to develop disease. Figure 4.3B illustrates the ability of the NCI breast cancer risk prediction tool to discriminate between women who subsequently did and did not develop breast cancer over a 5-year period and visually shows what a c-statistic of 0.58 means. Although the average risk scores are slightly higher for the women who developed breast cancer, and the their curve on the graph is slightly to the right of those who did not develop breast cancer, the individual risk prediction scores of the two groups overlap substantially; there is no place along the *x*-axis of risk that separates women into groups who did and did not develop breast cancer. This is so even though the calibration of the model was very good.

Sensitivity and Specificity of a Risk Prediction Tool

Yet another way to assess a risk prediction tool's ability to distinguish who will and will not develop disease is to determine its sensitivity and specificity (a topic that will be discussed more thoroughly in Chapters 8 and 10). Sensitivity of a risk prediction tool is the ability of the tool to identify those individuals destined to develop a disease and is expressed as the percentage of people who the tool correctly identifies will develop the disease. A tool's specificity is the ability to identify individuals who will not develop the disease, expressed as percentage of people the tool correctly identifies who will not develop the disease. Looking at Figure 4.3, a 5-year risk of 1.67% was chosen as a cut point between "low" and "high" risk. Using that cut point, the sensitivity was estimated as 44% (44% of women who developed breast cancer had a risk score ≥1.67%) and specificity was estimated as 66% (66% of women who did not develop breast cancer had a risk score <1.67%). In other words, the risk prediction tool missed more than half the women who developed breast cancer over a 5-year period,

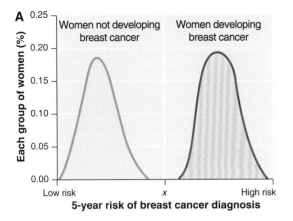

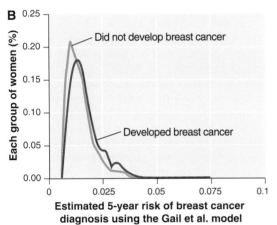

Figure 4.3 ■ A. The ability of a hypothetically perfect breast cancer risk prediction tool to discriminate between women who did and did not develop breast cancer. The group on the left have low risk scores and did not develop breast cancer, whereas the group on the right have higher scores and did develop breast cancer. There is no overlap of the two groups and the c-statistic would be 1.0. (Redrawn with permission from Elmore JA, Fletcher SW. The risk of cancer risk prediction: "What is my risk of getting breast cancer?" J Natl Cancer Inst 2006;98:1673–1675.) **B. The ability of an actual risk prediction tool to discriminate between women who did and did not develop breast cancer over a 5-year period.** The risk scores of the two groups overlap substantially, with no place along the x-axis that separates women who did and did not develop breast cancer. (Redrawn with permission from Rockhill Levine B.)

while assigning about a third of women not destined to develop the disease to the high-risk group. Studies of prediction tools that include information about sensitivity and specificity often also display a receiver operating characteristic (ROC) curve, a method of analysis that combines the results of sensitivity and specificity and can be used to compare different tools. ROCs are discussed in detail in Chapter 8.

Risk Stratification

As already mentioned, and as shown in Figure 4.2, risk stratification can be used to assess how well a risk prediction tool works and to determine whether adding a new risk factor improves the tool's ability to classify people correctly into clinically meaningful risk groups. Better risk stratification improves a tool's calibration. Risk stratification may not dramatically affect the tool's discrimination ability. For example, examining Figure 4.2, the risk tool that included CRP correctly assigned 99% of 6,965 women to the lowest risk stratum (<5% CVD events over 10 years). The study found that CVD events occurred in 101 (1.4%) women assigned to the lowest risk stratum, a result consistent with <5%, but because the vast majority (88%) of women were assigned to the lowest risk stratum, more women in that group developed CVD (101) than in all the other risk groups combined (97). This result, similar to what happened with the breast cancer risk tool (Fig. 4.3B), is a common, frustrating occurrence with risk prediction.

Why Risk Prediction Tools Do Not Discriminate Well Among Individuals

Why is it that a risk prediction tool that predicts so well the proportion of a group of people who will develop disease does so poorly at discriminating between those individuals who will and will not develop disease? A major problem is the strength (or more correctly, the weakness) of the prediction tool. Discrimination requires a very strong risk factor (or combination of risk factors) to separate a group of people into those who will and will not develop a disease, with even moderate success. If people who will develop the disease are just two or three or even five times more likely to develop the disease, risk prediction tools will not discriminate well. They need to be many times (some authors suggested at least 200 times [10]) more likely to develop the disease. Few risk prediction rules are that powerful.

Another problem is that for most chronic diseases, risk factors are widely spread throughout the population. Thus, even people at low risk can develop the disease. Figure 4.3B shows that some women with the lowest risk score developed breast cancer. In fact, in absolute numbers more women with low scores developed breast cancer than those with high scores because (thank goodness), in most groups of women, there are relatively few with high scores.

In summary, risk prediction models are an important way of combining individual risk factors to achieve better stratification of people into groups of graded risk, as illustrated in Figure 4.2. It is helpful for an individual patient and clinician to understand to which risk group a well-constructed risk model assigns the patient, but the limitations of the assignment should also be understood. In addition, it is important to keep in mind the counterintuitive fact that for most diseases, most of the people destined to develop a disease are not at high risk.

CLINICAL USES OF RISK FACTORS AND RISK PREDICTION TOOLS

Risk Factors and Pretest Probability for Diagnostic Testing

Knowledge of risk can be used in the diagnostic process because the presence of a risk factor increases the probability of disease. However, most risk factors (and even risk prediction tools) are limited in their ability to predict disease in symptomatic patients because they usually are not as strong a predictor of disease as are clinical findings of early disease. As stated by Geoffrey Rose (11):

> Often the best predictor of future major diseases is the presence of existing minor disease. A low ventilatory function today is the best predictor of its future rate of decline. A high blood pressure today is the best predictor of its future rate of rise. Early coronary heart disease is better than all of the conventional risk factors as a predictor of future fatal disease.

As an example of Rose's dictum, although age, male gender, smoking, hypertension, hyperlipidemia, and diabetes are important predictors for future coronary artery disease, they are far less important when evaluating a patient presenting to the emergency department with chest pain (12). The specifics of the clinical situation, such as presence and type of chest pain and results of an electrocardiogram, are the most powerful first steps in determining whether the patient is experiencing an acute myocardial infarction (13).

The absence of a very strong risk factor may help to rule out disease. Thus, it is reasonable to consider mesothelioma in the differential diagnosis of a pleural mass in a patient who is an asbestos worker. However, mesothelioma is a much less likely diagnosis for the patient who has never been exposed to asbestos.

Using Risk Factors to Choose Treatment

Risk factors have long been used in choosing (and developing) treatments. Patients with CVD who also have elevated lipids are treated with statins or other lipid lowering drugs. Specific treatments for hyperlipidemia and hypertension are highly effective treatments for diabetic patients with those conditions. In oncology, "targeted" therapies have been developed for certain cancers.

Example

The HER2 receptor is an epidermal growth factor receptor that is overexpressed in approximately 20% of breast cancers. HER2-positive breast cancer is associated with a worse prognosis than HER2-negative cancers. A monoclonal antibody to the HER2 protein was developed and tested in several clinical trials involving women with HER2-positive breast cancer. Women who received both standard therapy and the monoclonal antibody treatment had half as many breast cancer events as those receiving only standard treatment (14,15). Testing for the HER2 protein is now a standard procedure to help determine optimal breast cancer treatment.

Risk Stratification for Screening Programs

Knowledge of risk factors occasionally can be used to improve the efficiency of screening programs by selecting subgroups of patients at substantially increased risk. Although the risk for breast cancer associated with deleterious genetic mutations is very low in the general population, it is much higher in women with multiple close relatives who developed the disease at a relatively early age; blood tests screening for gene mutations are usually reserved for women whose family history indicates they are at substantially increased risk. Similarly, screening for colorectal cancer is recommended for the general population starting at age 50. However, people with a first-degree relative with a history of colorectal cancer are at increased risk for the disease, and expert groups suggest that screening these people should begin at age 40.

Removing Risk Factors to Prevent Disease

If a risk factor is also a cause of disease, removing it can prevent disease. Prevention can occur regardless of whether the mechanism by which the disease develops is known. Some of the classic successes in the history of epidemiology illustrate this point. Before bacteria were identified, John Snow noted in 1854 that an increase rate of cholera occurred among people drinking water supplied by a particular company, and the epidemic subsided after he cut off that supply. In the process, he established that cholera was spread by contaminated water supplies. In modern times, the same approach is used to investigate outbreaks of food-borne illnesses, to identify the source and take remedial action to stop the outbreak. Today, the biologic cause is quickly determined as well and helps to pinpoint the epidemic source. The concept of cause and its relationship to prevention is discussed in Chapter 12.

Review Questions

For questions 4.1–4.10, select the best answer.

4.1. In the mid-20th century, chest surgeons in Britain were impressed that they were operating on more men with lung cancer, most of whom were smoking. How might the surgeons' impression that smoking was a risk factor for developing lung cancer have been wrong?

  A. Smoking had become so common that more men would have a history of smoking, regardless of whether they were undergoing operations for lung cancer.
  B. Lung cancer is an uncommon cancer, even among smokers.
  C. Smoking confers a low risk of lung cancer.
  D. There are other risk factors for lung cancer.

4.2. Risk factors are easier to recognize:

  A. When exposure to a risk factor occurs a long time before the disease.
  B. When exposure to the risk factor is associated with a new disease.
  C. When the risk factor is a marker rather than a cause of disease.

4.3. Risk prediction models are useful for:

  A. Predicting onset of disease
  B. Diagnosing disease
  C. Predicting prognosis
  D. All of the above

4.4. Figure 4.2 shows:

  A. The risk model incorporating CRP results assigned too many women to the intermediate risk strata.
  B. The risk model incorporating CRP results predicts which individual women will develop CVD better than the risk model without CRP results.
  C. The number of women developing CVD over 10 years is likely highest in the group with a risk of <5%.

4.5. A risk model for colon cancer estimates that one of your patients has a 2% chance of developing colorectal cancer in the next 5 years. In explaining this to your patient, which of the following statements is most correct?

  A. Because colorectal cancer is the second most common non-skin cancer in men, he should be concerned about it.
  B. The model shows that your patient will not develop colorectal cancer in the next 5 years.
  C. The model shows that your patient is a member of a group of people in whom a very small number will develop colorectal cancer in the next 5 years.

4.6. In general, risk prediction tools are best at:

  A. Predicting future disease in a given patient.
  B. Predicting future disease in a group of patients.
  C. Predicting which individuals will and will not develop disease.

4.7. When a risk factor is a marker for future disease:

A. The risk factor can help identify people at increased risk of developing the disease.
B. Removing the risk factor can help prevent the disease.
C. The risk factor is not confounding a true causal relationship.

4.8. A risk factor is generally least useful in:

A. The risk stratification process
B. Diagnosing a patient's complaint
C. Preventing disease

4.9. Figure 4.3B shows that:

A. The risk model is well calibrated.
B. The risk model works well at stratifying women into different risk groups.

C. Most women developing breast cancer over 5 years are at higher risk.
D. The risk model does not discriminate very well.

4.10. It is difficult for risk models to determine which individuals will and will not develop disease for all of the following reasons *except:*

A. The combination of risk factors is not strongly related to disease.
B. The risk factors are common throughout a population.
C. The model is well calibrated.
D. Most people destined to develop the disease are not at high risk.

Answers are in Appendix A.

REFERENCES

1. Vineis P, Alavanja M, Buffler P, et al. Tobacco and cancer: recent epidemiological evidence. J Natl Cancer Inst 2004;96:99–106.
2. Willinger M, Hoffman HJ, Wu KT, et al. Factors associated with the transition to nonprone sleep positions of infants in the United States: The National Infant Sleep Position Study. JAMA 1998;280:329–335.
3. Li DK, Petitti DB, Willinger M, et al. Infant sleeping position and the risk of sudden infant death syndrome in California, 1997–2000. Am J Epidemiol 2003;157:446–455.
4. Chen WY, Rosner B, Hankinson SE, et al. Moderate alcohol consumption during adult life, drinking patterns and breast cancer risk. JAMA 2011;306:1884–1890.
5. Humphrey LL, Rongwei F, Rogers K, et al. Homocysteine level and coronary heart disease incidence: a systematic review and meta-analysis. Mayo Clin Proc 2008;83:1203–1212.
6. Martí-Carvajal AJ, Solà I, Lathyris D, et al. Homocysteine lowering interventions for preventing cardiovascular events. Cochrane Database Syst Rev 2009;4:CD006612.
7. Buckley DI, Fu R, Freeman M, et al. C-reactive protein as a risk factor for coronary heart disease: a systematic review and meta-analyses for the U.S. Preventive Services Task Force. Ann Intern Med 2009;151:483–495.
8. Ridker PM, Hennekens CH, Buring JE, et al. C-reactive protein and other markers of inflammation in the prediction of cardiovascular disease in women. N Engl J Med 2000;342:836–843.
9. Rockhill B, Speigelman D, Byrne C, et al. Validation of the Gail et al. model of breast cancer risk prediction and implications for chemoprevention. J Natl Cancer Inst 2001;93:358–366.
10. Wald NJ, Hackshaw AK, Frost CD. When can a risk factor be used as a worthwhile screening test? BMJ 1999;319:1562–1565.
11. Rose G. Sick individuals and sick populations. Int J Epidemiol 1985;14:32–38.
12. Han JH, Lindsell CJ, Storrow AB, et al. The role of cardiac risk factor burden in diagnosing acute coronary syndromes in the emergency department setting. Ann Emerg Med 2007;49:145–152.
13. Panju AA, Hemmelgarn BR, Guyatt GH, et al. Is this patient having a myocardial infarction? The rational clinical examination. JAMA 1998;280:1256–1263.
14. Piccart-Gebhart MJ, Procter M, Leyland-Jones B, et al. Trastuzumab after adjuvant chemotherapy in HER2-positive breast cancer. N Engl J Med 2005;353:1659–1672.
15. Romond EH, Perez EA, Bryant J, et al. Trastuzumab plus adjuvant chemotherapy for operable HER2-positive breast cancer. N Engl J Med 2005;353:1673–1684.

Chapter 5

Risk: Exposure to Disease

From the study of the characteristics of persons who later develop coronary heart disease (CHD) and comparison with the characteristics of those who remain free of this disease, it is possible many years before any overt symptoms or signs become manifest . . . to put together a profile of those persons in whom there is a high risk of developing CHD . . . It has seldom been possible in noninfectious disease to identify such highly susceptible individuals years before the development of disease.

—Thomas Dawber and William Kannel
1961

KEY WORDS

Observational study	Extraneous variable
Cohort study	Covariate
Cohort	Crude measure of effect
Exposed group	Confounding
Unexposed group	Intermediate outcome
Incidence study	Confounding variable/
Prospective cohort	Confounder
study	Controlling
Retrospective/historical	Restriction
cohort study	Matching
Case-cohort design	Stratification
Measure of effect	Standardization
Absolute risk	Multivariable analysis
Attributable risk	Logistic regression
Risk difference	Cox proportional
Relative risk	hazard
Risk ratio	Unmeasured
Population-	confounder
attributable risk	Residual confounding
Population-	Effect modification
attributable fraction	Interaction

STUDIES OF RISK

This chapter describes how investigators obtain estimates of risk by observing the relationship between exposure to possible risk factors and the subsequent incidence of disease. It describes methods used to determine risk by following groups into the future and also discusses several ways of comparing risks as they affect individuals and populations. Chapter 6 describes methods of studying risk by looking backward in time.

The most powerful way to determine whether exposure to a potential risk factor results in an increased risk of disease is to conduct an experiment in which the researcher determines who is exposed. People currently without disease are divided into groups of equal susceptibility to the disease in question. One group is exposed to the purported risk factor and the other is not, but the groups otherwise are treated the same. Later, any difference in observed rates of disease in the groups can be attributed to the risk factor. Experiments are discussed in Chapter 9.

When Experiments Are Not Possible or Ethical

The effects of most risk factors in humans cannot be studied with experimental studies. Consider some of the risk questions that concern us today: Are inactive people at increased risk for cardiovascular disease, everything else being equal? Do cellular phones cause brain cancer? Does obesity increase the risk of cancer? For such questions, it is usually not possible to conduct an experiment. First, it would be unethical to impose possible risk factors on a group of healthy people for the purposes of scientific research. Second, most people would balk at having their diets and behaviors constrained by others for long periods of time. Finally, the experiment would have to go on for many years, which is difficult and expensive. As a result, it is usually necessary to study risk in less obtrusive ways.

Clinical studies in which the researcher gathers data by simply observing events as they happen, without playing an active part in what takes place, are called observational studies. Most studies of risk are observational studies and are either cohort studies, described in the rest of this chapter, or case-control studies, described in Chapter 6.

Cohorts

As defined in Chapter 2, the term cohort is used to describe a group of people who have something in common when they are first assembled and who are then observed for a period of time to see what happens to them. Table 5.1 lists some of the ways in which cohorts are used in clinical research. Whatever members of a cohort have in common, observations of them should fulfill three criteria if the observations are to provide sound information about risk of disease.

Table 5.1

Cohorts and Their Purposes		
Characteristic in Common	**To Assess Effect of**	**Example**
Age	Age	Life expectancy for people age 70 (regardless of birth date)
Date of birth	Calendar time	Tuberculosis rates for people born in 1930
Exposure	Risk factor	Lung cancer in people who smoke
Disease	Prognosis	Survival rate for patients with brain cancer
Therapeutic intervention	Treatment	Improvement in survival for patients with Hodgkin lymphoma given combination chemotherapy
Preventive intervention	Prevention	Reduction in incidence of pneumonia after pneumococcal vaccination

1. They do not have the disease (or outcome) in question at the time they are assembled.
2. They should be observed over a meaningful period of time in the natural history of the disease in question so that there will be sufficient time for the risk to be expressed. For example, if one wanted to learn whether neck irradiation during childhood results in thyroid neoplasms, a 5-year follow-up would not be a fair test of this hypothesis, because the usual time period between radiation exposure and the onset of disease is considerably longer.
3. All members of the cohort should be observed over the full period of follow-up or methods must be used to account for dropouts. To the extent that people drop out of the study and their reasons for dropping out are related in some way to the outcome, the information provided by an incomplete cohort can misrepresent the true state of affairs.

Cohort Studies

The basic design of a cohort study is illustrated in Figure 5.1. A group of people (a cohort) is assembled, none of whom has experienced the outcome of interest, but all of whom could experience it. (For example, in a study of risk factors for endometrial cancer, each member of the cohort should have an intact uterus.) Upon entry into the study, people in the cohort are classified according to those characteristics (possible risk factors) that might be related to outcome. For each possible risk factor, members of the cohort are classified either as exposed (i.e., possessing the factor in question, such as hypertension) or unexposed. All the members of the cohort are then observed over time to see which of them experience the outcome, say, cardiovascular disease, and the rates of the outcome events are compared in the exposed and unexposed groups. It is then possible to see whether potential risk factors are related to subsequent outcome events. Other names for cohort studies are incidence studies, which emphasize that patients are followed over time; prospective studies, which imply the forward direction in which the patients are pursued; and longitudinal studies, which call attention to the basic measure of new disease events over time.

The following is a description of a classic cohort study that has made important contributions to our understanding of cardiovascular disease risk factors and to modern methods of conducting cohort studies.

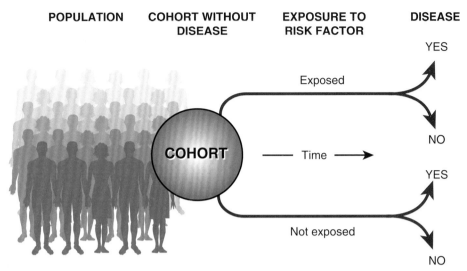

Figure 5.1 ■ **Design of a cohort study of risk.** Persons without disease are divided into two groups—those exposed to a risk factor and those not exposed. Both groups are followed over time to determine what proportion of each group develops disease.

Example

The Framingham Study (1) was begun in 1949 to identify factors associated with an increased risk of coronary heart disease (CHD). A representative sample of 5,209 men and women, aged 30 to 59 years, was selected from approximately 10,000 persons of that age living in Framingham, a small town near Boston. Of these, 5,127 were free of CHD when first examined and, therefore, were at risk of developing CHD. These people were re-examined biennially for evidence of coronary disease. The study ran for 30 years and now continues as the Framingham Offspring Study (2). It demonstrated that the risk of developing CHD is associated with elevated blood pressure, high serum cholesterol, cigarette smoking, glucose intolerance, and left ventricular hypertrophy. There was a large difference in risk of CHD between those with none and those with all of these risk factors. Combining the risk factors identified in this study gave rise to one of the most often used risk prediction tools in clinical medicine—the Framingham Risk Score for cardiovascular disease.

Prospective and Historical Cohort Studies

Cohort studies can be conducted in two ways (Fig. 5.2). The cohort can be assembled in the present and followed into the future (a prospective cohort study), or it can be identified from past records and followed forward from that time up to the present (a retrospective cohort study or a historical cohort study). The Framingham Study an example of a prospective cohort study. Useful retrospective cohort studies are appearing increasingly in the medical literature because of the availability of large computerized medical databases.

Prospective Cohort Studies

Prospective cohort studies can assess purported risk factors not usually captured in medical records, including many health behaviors, educational level, and socioeconomic status, which have been found to have important health effects. When the study is planned before data are collected, researchers can be sure to collect information about possible confounders. Finally, all the information in a prospective cohort study can be collected in a standardized manner that decreases measurement bias.

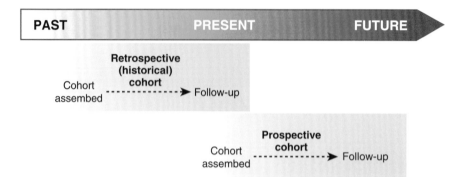

Figure 5.2 ■ Retrospective and prospective cohort studies. Prospective cohorts are assembled in the present and followed forward into the future. In contrast, retrospective cohorts are made by going back into the past and assembling the cohort, for example, from medical records, then following the group forward to the present.

Example

How much leisure time physical activity is needed to achieve health benefits? Several guidelines suggest a minimum of 30 minutes a day for 5 days a week, but most people do not follow the recommendation. Can less physical activity achieve health benefits? A prospective cohort study was undertaken among more than 415,000 adults who answered a standard questionnaire about their physical activity and were followed for an average of 8 years (3). Results showed that increasing amounts of leisure activity were correlated with reduced all-cause mortality and longer life expectancy compared to those who reported no activity. As little as 15 minutes of activity per day correlated with a decreased mortality of 14% and an increased life expectancy of 3 years, even when accounting for education level, physical labor at work, and other health conditions.

Historical Cohort Studies Using Medical Databases

Historical cohort studies can take advantage of computerized medical databases and population registries that are used primarily for patient care or to track population health. The major advantages of historical cohort studies over classical prospective cohort studies are that they take less time, are less expensive, and are much easier to do. However, they cannot undertake studies of factors not recorded in computerized databases, so patients' lifestyle, social standing, education, and other important health determinants usually cannot be included in the studies. Also, information in many databases, especially medical care information, is not collected in a standardized manner, leading to the possibility of bias in results. Large computerized databases are particularly useful for studying possible risk factors and health outcomes that are likely to be recorded in medical databases in somewhat standard ways, such as diagnoses and treatments.

Example

The incidence of autism increased sharply in the 1990s, coinciding with an increasing vaccination of young children for measles, mumps, and rubella (MMR). A report linking MMR vaccination and autism in several children caused widespread alarm that vaccination (or the vaccine preservative, thimerosal) was responsible for the increasing incidence of autism. In some countries, MMR vaccination rates among young children dropped, resulting in new outbreaks and even deaths from measles. Because of the seriousness of the situation, several studies were undertaken to evaluate MMR vaccine as a possible risk factor. In Denmark, a retrospective cohort study included all children (537,303) born from January 1991 through December 1998 (4). The investigators reviewed the children's countrywide health records and determined that 82% received the MMR vaccine (physicians must report vaccinations to the government in order to receive payment); 316 children were diagnosed with autism, and another 422 with autistic-spectrum disorders. The frequency of autism among children who had been vaccinated was similar (in fact, slightly less) to that among children not receiving MMR vaccine. This, along with other studies, provided strong evidence against the suggestion that MMR vaccine causes autism. Subsequently, the original study leading to alarm was investigated for fraud and conflict of interest and was retracted by *The Lancet* in 2010 (5).

Case-Cohort Studies

Another method using computerized medical databases in cohort studies is the case-cohort design. Conceptually, it is a modification of the retrospective cohort design that takes advantage of the ability to determine the frequency of a given medical condition in a large group of people. In a case-cohort study, all exposed people in a cohort, but only a small random sample of unexposed people are included in the study and followed for some outcome of interest. For efficiency, the group of unexposed people is "enriched" with all those who subsequently suffer the outcome of interest (i.e., become cases). The results are then adjusted to reflect the sampling fractions used to obtain the sample. This efficient approach to a cohort study requires that frequencies of outcomes be determined in the entire group of unexposed people; thus, the need for a large, computerized, medical database.

Example

Does prophylactic mastectomy protect women who are at increased risk for breast cancer? A case-cohort study was done to examine this question in six health maintenance organizations, all of which had computerized databases of diagnoses and surgical procedures on their members. Investigators identified all 276 women who underwent bilateral prophylactic mastectomy over a number of years and followed them forward over time to determine if they developed breast cancer. For the com-

parison group, the investigators randomly sampled a similar group of women not undergoing the procedure and enriched the sample with women who subsequently developed breast cancer. "Enrichment" was accomplished by knowing who among 666,800 eligible women developed breast cancer—through examination of the computerized database. The investigators randomly sampled about 1% of comparison women of a certain age who developed breast cancer,[†] but only about .01% of women who did not. Adjustments for the sampling fractions were then made during the analysis. The results showed that bilateral prophylactic mastectomy was associated with a 99% reduction in breast cancer among women at higher risk (6).

Advantages and Disadvantages of Cohort Studies

Well-conducted cohort studies of risk, regardless of type, are the best available substitutes for a true experiment when experimentation is not possible. They follow the same logic as a clinical trial and allow measurement of exposure to a possible risk factor while avoiding any possibility of bias that might occur if exposure were determined after the outcome was already known. The most important scientific disadvantage of cohort studies (in fact, all observational studies) is that they are subject to a great many more potential biases than are experiments. People who are exposed to a certain risk factor in the natural course of events are likely to differ in a great many ways from a comparison group of people not exposed to the factor. If some of these other differences are also related to the disease in question, they could confound any association observed between the putative risk factor and the disease.

The uses, strengths, and limitations of the different types of cohort studies are summarized in Table 5.2. Several of the advantages and disadvantages apply regardless of type. However, the potential

---

[†]Strictly speaking, the study was a modification of a standard case-cohort design that would have included all cases, not just 1%, of 26,800 breast cancers that developed in the comparison group of women not undergoing prophylactic mastectomy. However, because breast cancer occurs commonly, a random sample of the group sufficed.

Table 5.2

Advantages and Disadvantages of Cohort Studies

Advantages	Disadvantages
All Cohort Study Types	
The only way of establishing incidence (i.e., absolute risk) directly	Susceptible to confounding and other biases
Follows the same logic as the clinical question: If persons are exposed, do they get the disease?	
Exposure can be elicited without the bias that might occur if outcome were known before documentation of exposure	
Can assess the relationship between exposure and many diseases	
Prospective Cohort Studies	
Can study a wide range of possible risk factors	Inefficient because many more subjects must be enrolled than experience the event of interest; therefore, cannot be used for rare diseases
Can collect lifestyle and demographic data not available in most medical records	Expensive because of resources necessary to study many people over time
Can set up standardized ways of measuring exposure and degree of exposure to risk factors	Results not available for a long time
	Assesses the relationship between disease and exposure to only relatively few factors (i.e., those recorded at the outset of the study)
Retrospective (Historical) Cohort Studies	
More efficient than prospective cohort studies because data have already been collected for another purpose (i.e., during patient care or for a registry)	Range of possible risk factors that can be studied is narrower than that possible with prospective cohort studies
Cheaper than prospective cohort studies because resources not necessary to follow many people over time	Cannot examine patient characteristics not available in the data set used
Faster than prospective cohort studies because patient outcomes have already occurred	Measurement of exposure and degree of exposure may not be standardized
Case-cohort Studies	
All advantages of retrospective cohort studies apply	All disadvantages of retrospective cohort studies apply
Even more efficient than retrospective cohort studies because only a sample of unexposed group is analyzed	Difficult for readers to understand weighting procedures used in the analysis

for difficulties with the quality of data is different for the three. In prospective studies, data can be collected specifically for the purposes of the study and with full anticipation of what is needed. It is thereby possible to avoid measurement biases and some of the confounders that might undermine the accuracy of the results. However, data for historical cohorts are usually gathered for other purposes—often as part of medical records for patient care. Except for carefully selected questions, such as the relationship between vaccination and autism, the data in historical cohort studies may not be of sufficient quality for rigorous research.

Prospective cohort studies can also collect data on lifestyle and other characteristics that might influence the results, and they can do so in standard ways. Many of these characteristics are not routinely available in retrospective and case-cohort studies, and those that are usually are not collected in standard ways.

The principal disadvantage of prospective cohort studies is that when the outcome is infrequent, which is usually so in studies of risk, a large number of people must be entered in a study and remain under observation for a long time before results are available. Having to measure exposure in many people and then follow them for years is inefficient when few ultimately develop the disease. For example, the Framingham Study of cardiovascular disease (the most common cause of death in America) was the largest study of its kind when it began. Nevertheless, more than 5,000 people had to be followed for several years before the first, preliminary conclusions could be published. Only 5% of the people had experienced a coronary event during the first 8 years. Retrospective and case-cohort studies get around the problem of time but often sacrifice access to important and standardized data.

Another problem with prospective cohort studies results from the people under study usually being "free living" and not under the control of researchers. A great deal of effort and money must be expended to keep track of them. Prospective cohort studies of risk, therefore, are expensive, usually costing many millions, sometimes hundreds of millions, of dollars.

Because of the time and money required for prospective cohort studies, this approach cannot be used for all clinical questions about risk, which was a major reason for efforts to find more efficient, yet dependable, ways of assessing risk, such as retrospective and case-cohort designs. Another method, case-control studies, is discussed in Chapter 6.

WAYS TO EXPRESS AND COMPARE RISK

The basic expression of risk is incidence, which is defined in Chapter 2 as the number of new cases of disease arising during a given period of time in a defined population that is initially free of the condition. In cohort studies, the incidence of disease is compared in two or more groups that differ in exposure to a possible risk factor. To compare risks, several measures of the association between exposure and disease, called measures of effect, are commonly used. These measures represent different concepts of risk, elicit different impressions of the magnitude of a risk, and are used for different purposes. Four measures of effect are discussed in the following text. Table 5.3 summarizes the four, along with absolute risk, and Table 5.4 demonstrates their use with the risk of lung cancer among smokers and non-smokers.

Absolute Risk

Absolute risk is the probability of an event in a population under study. Its value is the same as that for incidence, and the terms are often used interchangeably. Absolute risk is the best way for individual patients and clinicians to understand how risk factors may affect their lives. Thus, as Table 5.4 shows, although smoking greatly increases the chances of dying from lung cancer, among smokers the absolute risk of dying from lung cancer each year in the population studied was 341.3 per

Table 5.3

Measures of Effect		
Expression	**Question**	**Definition[a]**
Absolute risk	What is the incidence of disease in a group initially free of the condition?	$I = \dfrac{\text{\# new cases over a given period of time}}{\text{\# people in the group}}$
Attributable risk (risk difference)	What is the incidence of disease attributable to exposure?	$AR = I_E - I_{\bar{E}}$
Relative risk (risk ratio)	How many times more likely are exposed persons to become diseased, relative to non-exposed persons?	$RR = \dfrac{I_E}{I_{\bar{E}}}$
Population-attributable risk	What is the incidence of disease in a population, associated with the prevalence of a risk factor?	$AR_P = AR \times P$
Population-attributable fraction	What fraction of the disease in a population is attributable to exposure to a risk factor?	$AF_P = \dfrac{AR_P}{I_T}$

[a]Where I_E = incidence in exposed persons; $I_{\bar{E}}$ = incidence in non-exposed persons; P = prevalence of exposure to a risk factor; and I_T = total incidence of disease in a population.

Table 5.4

Calculating Measures of Effect: Cigarette Smoking and Death from Lung Cancer in Men[a]	
Simple Risks	
Death rate (absolute risk or incidence) from lung cancer in smokers	341.3/100,000/yr
Death rate (absolute risk or incidence) from lung cancer in non-smokers	14.7/100,000/yr
Prevalence of cigarette smoking	32.1%
Lung cancer mortality rate in population	119.4/100,000/yr
Compared Risks	
Attributable risk	= 341.3/100,000/yr − 14.7/100,000/yr = 326.6/100,000/yr
Relative risk	= 341.3/100,000/yr ÷ 14.7/100,000/yr = 23.2
Population-attributable risk	= 326.6/100,000/yr × 0.321 = 104.8/100,000/yr
Population-attributable fraction	= 104.8 /100,000/yr ÷ 119.4/100,000/yr = 0.88

[a]Data from Thun MJ, Day-Lally CA, Calle EE, et al. Excess mortality among cigarette smokers: Changes in a 20-year interval. Am J Public Health 1995;85:1223–1230.

100,000 (3 to 4 lung cancer deaths per 1,000 smokers per year).

Attributable Risk

One might ask, "What is the additional risk (incidence) of disease following exposure, over and above that experienced by people who are not exposed?" The answer is expressed as attributable risk, the absolute risk (or incidence) of disease in exposed persons minus the absolute risk in non-exposed persons. In Table 5.4, the attributable risk of lung cancer death in smokers is calculated as 326.6 per 100,000 per year. Attributable risk is the additional incidence of disease related to exposure, taking into account the background incidence of disease from other causes. Note that this way of comparing rates implies that the risk factor is a cause and not just a marker. Because of the way it is calculated, attributable risk is also called risk difference, the differences between two absolute risks.

Relative Risk

On the other hand, one might ask, "How many times more likely are exposed persons to get the disease relative to non-exposed persons?" To answer this question, relative risk or risk ratio, is the ratio of incidence in exposed persons to incidence in non-exposed persons, estimated in Table 5.4 as 23.2. Relative risk (or an estimate of relative risk, odds

ratios, discussed in Chapter 6) is the most commonly reported result in studies of risk, not only because of its computational convenience but also because it is a common metric in studies with similar risk factors but with different baseline incidence rates. Because relative risk indicates the strength of the association between exposure and disease, it is a useful measure of effect for studies of disease etiology.

Interpreting Attributable and Relative Risk

Although attributable and relative risk are calculated from the same two components—the incidence (or absolute risk) of an outcome from an exposed and unexposed group—the resulting size of the risk may appear to be quite different depending on whether attributable or relative risk is used.

Example

Suppose a risk factor doubles the chance of dying of a certain disease (i.e., the relative risk is 2). Then suppose that the frequency of the risk factor varies in four groups of unexposed people, from 1 in 10 in one group, all the way to 1 in 10,000 in another group, as illustrated below. The resulting calculations for relative risk and attributable risk would be:

Incidence			
Unexposed Group	**Exposed Group**	**Relative Risk**	**Attributable Risk**
1/10,000	2/10,000	2.0	0.2/1,000
1/1,000	2/1,000	2.0	2/1,000
1/100	2/100	2.0	20/1,000
1/10	2/10	2.0	200/1,000

Because the calculation of relative risk cancels out incidence, it does not clarify the size of risk in discussions with patients or help much in the decision to try to alter a risk in a patient. The patient and clinician will probably be much more concerned when the doubling of a death rate goes from 100 to 200 in 1,000 than from 1 to 2 in 10,000. A real-life example of how absolute risk changes even though relative risk is stable is illustrated in a study of fracture risk in postmenopausal women according to baseline measurements of bone mineral density (BMD) and age (7). The relative risk of low BMD changed little over several decades (ranging from 1.97 to 2.78), whereas attributable risk almost doubled (from 14.4 to 23.8 per 1,000 women-years) because the risk of fractures increased with age regardless of BMD (Table 5.5).

In most clinical situations, it is best simply to concentrate on the attributable risk by comparing the absolute risks in exposed and unexposed people. Ironically, because most medical research presents results as relative risk, clinicians often emphasize relative risks when advising patients.

Population Risk

Another way of looking at risk is to ask, "How much does a risk factor contribute to the overall rates of disease in groups of people, rather than individuals?" This information is useful for determining which risk factors are particularly important and which are trivial to the overall health of a community, and can inform those who must prioritize the deployment of health care resources.

To estimate population risk, it is necessary to take into account the frequency with which members of a community are exposed to a risk factor. **Population-attributable risk** is the product of the attributable risk and the prevalence of exposure to the risk factor in a population. It measures the excess incidence of disease in a community that is associated with a risk factor. One can also describe the fraction of disease occurrence in a population associated with a particular risk factor, the **population-attributable fraction**. It is obtained by dividing the population-attributable risk by the total incidence of disease in the population. In the case of cigarette smoking and lung cancer (Table 5.4), smoking annually contributes about 105 lung cancer deaths for every 100,000 men in the population (population-attributable risk), and accounts for 88% of all lung cancer deaths

Table 5.5

Comparing Relative Risk and Attributable Risk in the Relationship of Bone Mineral Density (BMD) T-scores, Fractures, and Age

	Fracture Incidence (Absolute Risk per 1,000 Person-years)			
Age	**BMD T-score >−1.0**	**BMD T-score <−2.0**	**Relative Risk[a]**	**Attributable Risk[b] per 1,000 Person-years**
50–59	4.5	19.0	2.63	14.4
60–69	50.0	22.0	2.78	16.4
70–79	7.5	30.5	2.37	20.3
80–99	16.5	42.0	1.97	23.8

[a]Adjusted.
[b]Estimated from Figure 2 of reference.
Data from Siris ES, Brenneman SK, Barrett-Connor E, et al. The effect of age and bone mineral density on the absolute, excess, and relative risk of fracture in postmenopausal women aged 55-99: results from the National Osteoporosis Risk Assessment (NORA). Osteoporosis Int 2006;17:565–574.

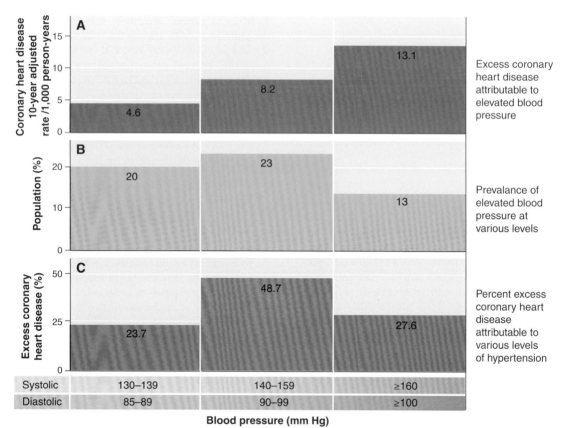

Figure 5.3 ■ Relationships among attributable risk, prevalence of risk factor, and population risk for coronary heart disease (CHD) death due to hypertension. Panel A shows that the attributable risk for CHD increases as blood pressure levels increase. However, because mild and moderate hypertension are more prevalent than severe hypertension (Panel B), most excess CHD deaths caused by hypertension are not due to the highest levels of blood pressure (Panel C). (Data from Wilson PWF, Agostino RB, Levy D, et al. Prediction of coronary heart disease using risk factor categories. Circulation 1998;97:1837–1847.)

in the population (population-attributable fraction). Note how important the prevalence of the risk factor (smoking) is to these calculations. As smoking rates fall, the fraction of lung cancer due to smoking also falls.

As discussed in Chapter 4, if a relatively weak risk factor is very prevalent in a community, it could account for more disease than a very strong, but rare, risk factor. Figure 5.3 illustrates this for hypertension and the development of coronary heart disease. Figure 5.3A shows the attributable (excess) risk of coronary heart disease according to various levels of hypertension among a group of about 2,500 men followed for 10 years. Risk increased with increasing blood pressure. However, few men had very high blood pressure (Fig. 5.3B). As a result, the highest level of hypertension contributed only about a quarter of excess coronary heart disease in the population (Fig. 5.3C).

Paradoxically, then, physicians could save more lives with effective treatment of lower, rather than higher, levels of hypertension. This fact, so counterintuitive to clinical thinking, has been termed "the prevention paradox" (8).

Measures of population risk are less frequently encountered in the clinical literature than are measures of absolute, attributable, and relative risks, but a particular clinical practice is as much a population for the doctor as is a community for health policymakers. In addition, how the prevalence of exposure affects community risk can be important in the care of individual patients. For instance, when patients cannot give a history or when exposure is difficult for them to recognize, physicians depend on the usual prevalence of exposure to estimate the likelihood of various diseases. When considering treatable causes of cirrhosis in a North American patient, for example, it would be more useful to consider alcohol than schistosomes, inasmuch as few North Americans are exposed to schistosomes. Of course, one might take a very different stance in the Nile Delta, where schistosomiasis is prevalent, and the people, who are mostly Muslims, rarely drink alcohol.

TAKING OTHER VARIABLES INTO ACCOUNT

Thus far, we mainly have been discussing exposure and disease in isolation as if they were the only two variables that matter. But, in fact, many other variables are part of the phenomenon being studied; these other variables can have one of two important effects on the results. They can cause an unwanted, artificial change in the observed relationship between exposure and disease (confounding), leading to incorrect conclusions about the relationship; or they can modify the magnitude of the exposure–disease relationship (effect modification), which is valuable information for clinicians. This section discusses these two effects, which are so important to the interpretation of research results, especially in observational studies.

Extraneous Variables

Extraneous variables is a general term for variables that are part of the system being studied but are not (i.e., are "extraneous" to) the exposure and disease of primary interest. For example, in a study of exercise and sudden death, the other variables that are relevant to that study include age, body mass index, coexisting diseases, all of the cardiovascular risk factors, and everything having to do with the ability to exercise. Another term favored by statisticians is covariates. Neither term is particularly apt. Extraneous variables are not at all "extraneous" because they can have important effects of the exposure–disease relationship. Also, covariates may or may not "covary" (change in relation to each other, exposure, or disease), but these are the terms that are used.

Simple Descriptions of Risk

Observational studies can disregard these other variables and simply compare the course of disease in two naturally occurring groups, one exposed to a risk or prognostic factor and the other not, without implying that exposure itself was responsible for whatever differences in outcome are observed. Crude measures of effect (not adjusted for other variables) can be useful in predicting events, without regard to causes.

Example

British investigators followed up a cohort of 17,981 children who had been diagnosed with childhood cancer before 15 years of age (9). After follow-up of up to 66 years, there were 11 times as many deaths as would have occurred in the general population. The excess death rate declined with age, but 45 years after the cancer diagnosis, the death rate was still three times the expected rate. Deaths were mainly from second primary cancers and circulatory diseases. The investigators did not gather evidence for or against the several possible reasons for the excess death rates such as the effects of treatment with radiation and chemotherapy, genetic risk, or environmental risk factors. Nevertheless, knowing that death rates are substantially higher, as well as the causes of death, is useful in planning for the care of adults who have survived childhood cancer.

Usually, investigators want to report more than crude measures of effect. They want to demonstrate how exposure is related to disease *independently* of all the other variables that might affect the relationship. That is, they want to come as close as possible to describing cause and effect.

CONFOUNDING

The validity of observational studies is threatened above all by confounding. We have already described confounding in conceptual terms in Chapter 1, noting that confounding occurs when exposure is associated or "travels together" with another variable, which is itself related to the outcome, so that the effect of exposure can be confused with or distorted by the effect of the other variable. Confounding causes a systematic error—a bias—in inference, whereby the effects of one variable are attributed to another. For example, in a study of whether vitamins protect against cardiovascular events, if people who choose to take vitamins are also more likely to follow a healthy lifestyle (e.g., not smoke cigarettes, exercise, eat a prudent diet, and avoid obesity), taking vitamins will be associated with lower cardiovascular disease rates regardless of whether vitamins protect against cardiovascular disease. Confounding can increase or decrease an observed association between exposure and disease.

Working Definition

A confounding variable is one that is:

- Associated with exposure
- Associated with disease
- Not part of the causal chain from exposure to disease

A confounding variable cannot be in the causal chain between exposure and disease; although variables that are in the chain are necessarily related to both exposure and disease, they are not initiating events. (Such variables are sometimes referred to as intermediate outcomes.) If their effects were removed, this would also remove any association that might exist between exposure and disease. For example, in a study of diet and cardiovascular disease, serum cholesterol is a consequence of diet; if the effect of cholesterol were removed, it would incorrectly diminish the association between diet and cardiovascular disease.

In practice, while confounding variables (colloquially called confounders) may be examined one at a time, usually many variables can confound the exposure–disease relationship and all are examined and controlled for concurrently.

Potential Confounders

How does one decide which variables should be considered *potential* confounders? One approach is to identify all the variables that are known, from other studies, to be associated with either exposure or disease. Age is almost always a candidate, as are known risk factors for the disease in question. Another approach is to screen variables in the study data for statistical associations with exposure and disease, using liberal criteria for "association" so as to err on the side of not missing potential confounding. Investigators may also consider variables that just make sense according to their clinical experience or the biology of disease, regardless of whether there are strong research studies linking them to exposure or disease. The intention is to cast a broad net so as not to miss possible confounders. This is because of the possibility that a variable may confound the exposure–disease relationship by chance, because of the particular data at hand, even though it is not a confounder in nature.

Confirming Confounding

How does one decide whether a variable that might confound the relationship between exposure and disease actually does so? One approach is to simply show that the variable is associated with exposure and (separately) to show that it is associated with disease.

Another approach is to see if the crude relationship between exposure and disease is different when taking the potential confounder into account. The following example illustrates both approaches.

Example

As pointed out in an example in Chapter 4, several observational studies have shown that high levels of homocysteine in the blood are related to cardiovascular disease and that the vitamin folate lowers homocysteine levels. A cohort study examined the relation between intake of folate and the incidence of stroke (10). A total of 83,272 female nurses aged 34 to 59 years at the beginning of the study were followed up for 18 years with biennial questionnaires to assess diet and stroke. The relative risk of stroke, comparing highest to lowest quintile of folate intake and adjusted for age, was 0.83, suggesting that folate protected against stroke. However, folate intake was inversely associated with intake of saturated and trans-fatty acids and smoking (all cardiovascular risk factors) and positively associated with likelihood of exercising (a protective factor) (Fig. 5.4). When these other factors were taken into account, folate was no longer protective; the relative risk was 0.99. The authors concluded that their study did not show an independent effect of folate on stroke incidence; the crude relationship between exposure and disease had been confounded by other cardiovascular risk and protective factors.

CONTROL OF CONFOUNDING

To determine whether a factor is independently related to risk or prognosis, it is ideal to compare cohorts with and without the factor, everything else being equal. But in real life, "everything else" is usually not equal in observational studies.

What can be done about this problem? There are several possible ways of controlling[†] for differences

---

[†]Unfortunately, the term "control" also has several other meanings: the non-exposed people in a cohort study, the patients in a clinical trial who do not receive the experimental treatment, and non-diseased people (non-cases) in a case-control study.

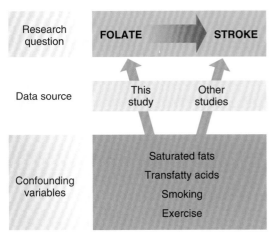

Figure 5.4 ■ Example of confounding. The relationship between folate intake and incidence of stroke was confounded by several cardiovascular risk and protective factors.

between groups. Controlling is a general term for any process aimed at removing the effects of extraneous variables while examining the independent effects of individual variables. A variety of methods can be applied during the design or analysis of research (summarized in Table 5.6 and described in the following text). One or more of these strategies should be applied in any observational study that attempts to describe the effect of one variable independent of other variables that might affect the outcome. The

basic question is, "Are the differences between groups in risk or prognosis related to the particular factor under study or to some other factor(s)?"

Randomization

The best way to balance all extraneous variables between groups is to randomly assign patients to groups so that each patient has an equal chance of falling into the exposed or unexposed group (see Chapter 9). A special feature of randomization is that it balances not only variables known to affect outcome and included in the study, but also unknown or unmeasured confounders. Unfortunately, it is usually not possible to study risk or prognostic factors with randomized trials.

Restriction

Patients who are enrolled in a study can be confined to only those possessing a narrow range of characteristics, a strategy called restriction. When this is done, certain characteristics can be made similar in the groups being compared. For example, the effect of prior cardiovascular disease on prognosis after acute myocardial infarction could be studied in patients who had no history of cigarette smoking or hypertension. However, this approach is limiting. Although restriction on entry to a study can certainly produce homogeneous groups of patients, it does so at the expense of generalizability. In the course of excluding

Table 5.6

Methods for Controlling Confounding

Method	Description	Phase of Study Design	Phase of Study Analysis
Randomization	Assign patients to groups in a way that gives each patient an equal chance of falling into one or the other group.	+	
Restriction	Limit the range of characteristics of patients in the study	+	
Matching	For each patient in one group, select one or more patients with the same characteristics (except for the one under study) for a comparison group.	+	+
Stratification	Compare rates within subgroups (strata) with otherwise similar probability of the outcome.		+
Simple adjustment	Mathematically adjust crude rates for one or a few characteristics so that equal weight is given to strata of similar risk.		+
Multivariable adjustment	Adjust for differences in a large number of factors related to outcome, using mathematical modeling techniques.		+
Best-case/Worst-case analysis	Describe how different the results could be under the most extreme (or simply very unlikely) assumption about selection bias.		+

Table 5.7

Example of Stratification: Hypothetical Death Rates after Coronary Bypass Surgery in Two Hospitals, Stratified by Preoperative Risk

Preoperative Risk	Hospital A			Hospital B		
	Patients	Deaths	Rate (%)	Patients	Deaths	Rate (%)
High	500	30	6	400	24	6
Medium	400	16	4	800	32	4
Low	300	2	0.67	1,200	8	0.67
Total	1,200	48	4	2,400	64	2.7

potential subjects, cohorts may no longer be representative of most patients with the condition. Also, after restriction, it is no longer possible, in that study, to learn anything more about the effects of excluded variables.

Matching

Matching is another way of making patients in two groups similar. In its simplest form, for each patient in the exposure group, one or more patients with the same characteristics (except for the factor of interest) would be selected for a comparison group. Matching is typically done for variables that are so strongly related to outcome that investigators want to be sure they are not different in the groups being compared. Often, patients are matched for age and sex because these variables are strongly related to risk or prognosis for many diseases, but matching for other variables, such as stage or severity of disease and prior treatments, may also be useful.

Although matching is commonly done and can be very useful, it has limitations. Matching controls bias only for those variables involved in the match. Also, it is usually not possible to match for more than a few variables because of practical difficulties in finding patients who meet all of the matching criteria. Moreover, if categories for matching are relatively crude, there may be room for substantial differences between matched groups. For example, if women in a study of risk for birth of a child with Down syndrome were matched for maternal age within 10 years, there could be a nearly 10-fold difference in frequency related to age if most of the women in one group were 30 years old and most in the other 39 years old. Finally, as with restriction, once one matches on a variable, its effects on outcomes can no longer be evaluated in the study. For these reasons, although matching may be done for a few characteristics that

are especially strongly related to outcome, investigators rely on other ways of controlling for bias as well.

Stratification

With stratification, data are analyzed and results presented according to subgroups of patients, or strata, of similar risk or prognosis (other than the exposure of interest). An example of this approach is the analysis of differences in hospital morality for a common surgical procedure, coronary bypass surgery (Table 5.7). This is especially relevant today because of several high-profile examples of "report cards" for doctors and hospitals, and the concern that the reported differences may be related to patient rather than surgeon or hospital characteristics.

Suppose we want to compare the operative mortality rates for coronary bypass surgery at Hospitals A and B. Overall, Hospital A noted 48 deaths in 1,200 bypass operations (4%), and Hospital B experienced 64 deaths in 2,400 operations (2.6%).

The crude rates suggest that Hospital B is superior. But is it really superior if everything else is equal? Perhaps the preoperative risk among patients in Hospital A was higher than in Hospital B and that, rather than hospital care, accounted for the difference in death rates. To see if this possibility accounts for the observed difference in death rates, patients in each of these hospitals are grouped into strata of similar underlying preoperative risk based on age, prior myocardial function, extent of occlusive disease, and other characteristics. Then the operative mortality rates within each stratum of risk are compared.

Table 5.7 shows that when patients are divided by preoperative risk, the operative mortality rates in each risk stratum are identical in two hospitals: 6% in high-risk patients, 4% in medium-risk patients, and 0.67% in low-risk patients. The crude rates were misleading because of important differences in the risk characteristics of the patients treated at the two hospitals: 42% of Hospital A's patients and only 17% of Hospital B's patients were high risk.

An advantage of stratification is that it is a relatively transparent way of recognizing and controlling for bias.

Standardization

If an extraneous variable is especially strongly related to outcomes, two rates can be compared without bias related to this variable if they are adjusted to equalize the weight given to that variable. This process, called standardization (or adjustment), shows what the overall rate would be for each group if strata-specific rates were applied to a population made up of similar proportions of people in each stratum.

To illustrate this process, suppose the operative mortality in Hospitals A and B can be adjusted to a common distribution of risk groups by giving each risk stratum the same weight in the two hospitals. Without adjustment, the risk strata receive different weights in the two hospitals. The mortality rate of 6% for high-risk patients receives a weight of 500/1,200 in Hospital A and a much lower weight of 400/2,400 in Hospital B. The other risk strata were also weighted differently in the two hospitals. The result is a crude rate for Hospital A, which is the sum of the rate in each stratum times its weight: $(500/1,200 \times 0.06) + (400/1,200 \times 0.04) + (300/1,200 \times 0.0067) = 0.04$. Similarly, the crude rate for Hospital B is $(400/2,400 \times 0.06) + (800/2,400 \times 0.04) + (1,200/2,400 \times 0.0067) = 0.027$.

If equal weights were used when comparing the two hospitals, the comparison would be fair (free of the effect of different proportions in the various risk groups). The choice of weights does not matter as long as it is the same in the two hospitals. Weights could be based on those existing in either of the hospitals or any reference population. For example, if each stratum were weighted 1/3, then the standardized rate for Hospital A = $(1/3 \times 0.06) + (1/3 \times 0.04) + (1/3 \times 0.0067) = 0.035$, which is exactly the same as the standardized rate for Hospital B. The consequence of giving equal weight to strata in each hospital is to remove the apparent excess risk of Hospital A.

Standardization is commonly used in relatively crude comparisons to adjust for a single variable such as age that is obviously different in groups being compared. For example, the crude results of the folate/stroke example were adjusted for age, as discussed earlier. Standardization is less useful as a stand-alone

strategy to control for confounding when multiple variables need to be considered.

Multivariable Adjustment

In most clinical situations, many variables act together to produce effects. The relationships among these variables are complex. They may be related to one another as well as to the outcome of interest. The effect of one might be modified by the presence of others, and the joint effects of two or more might be greater than their individual effects taken together.

Multivariable analysis makes it possible to consider the effects of many variables simultaneously. Other terms for this approach include mathematical modeling and multivariable adjustment. Modeling is used to adjust (control) for the effects of many variables simultaneously to determine the independent effects of one. This method also can select, from a large set of variables, those that contribute independently to the overall variation in outcome. Modeling can also arrange variables in order of the strength of their contribution. There are several kinds of prototypic models, according to the design and data in the study. Cohort and case-control studies typically rely on logistic regression, which is used specifically for dichotomous outcomes. A Cox proportional hazard model is used when the outcome is the time to an event, as in survival analyses (see Chapter 7).

Multivariable analysis of observational studies is the only feasible way of controlling for many variables simultaneously during the analysis phase of a study. Randomization also controls for multiple variables, but during the design and conduct phases of a study. Matching can account for only a few variables at a time, and stratified analyses of many variables run the risk of having too few patients in some strata. The disadvantage of modeling is that for most of us it is a "black box," making it difficult to recognize where the method might be misleading. At its best, modeling is used in addition to, not in place of, matching and stratified analysis.

Overall Strategy for Control of Confounding

Except for randomization, all ways of dealing with extraneous differences between groups share a limitation: They are effective only for those variables that are singled out for consideration. They do not deal with risk or prognostic factors that are not known at the time of the study or those that are known but not taken into account.

For this reason and the complementary strengths and weakness of the various methods, one should not rely on only one or another method of controlling for bias but rather uses several methods together, layered one on another.

Example

In a study of whether ventricular premature contractions are associated with reduced survival in the years following acute myocardial infarction, one might deal with confounding as follows:

- *Restrict* the study to patients who are not very old or young and who do not have unusual causes, such as arteritis or dissecting aneurysm, for their infarction.
- *Match* for age, a factor strongly related to prognosis but extraneous to the main question.
- Using *stratified analysis*, examine the results separately for strata of differing clinical severity. This includes the presence or absence of congestive heart failure or other diseases, such as chronic obstructive pulmonary disease.
- Using *multivariable analysis*, adjust the crude results for the effects of all the variables other than the arrhythmia, taken together, that might be related to prognosis.

OBSERVATIONAL STUDIES AND CAUSE

The end result of a careful observational study, controlling for a rich array of extraneous variables, is to come as close as possible to describing a truly independent effect, one that is separate from all the other variables that confound the exposure–disease relationship. However, it is always possible that some important variables were not taken into account, either because their importance was not known or because they were not or could not be measured. The consequence of unmeasured confounders is residual confounding. For this reason, in single studies the results should be thought of (and investigators should describe their results) as "independent associations" and not necessarily as establishing cause. Chapter 12 describes how to build a case for a causal association.

EFFECT MODIFICATION

A very different issue from confounding is whether the presence or absence of a variable changes the effect of exposure on disease, called effect modification. As Rothman (11) puts it,

> The most central difference is that, whereas confounding is a bias that the investigator hopes to prevent or, if necessary, to remove from the data, effect modification is an elaborated description of the effect itself. Effect modification is thus a finding to be reported rather than a bias to be avoided. Epidemiologic analysis is generally aimed at eliminating confounding and discovering and describing effect modification.

Statisticians call effect modification interaction, and biologists call it synergy or antagonism, depending on whether the third factor increases or decreases the effect.

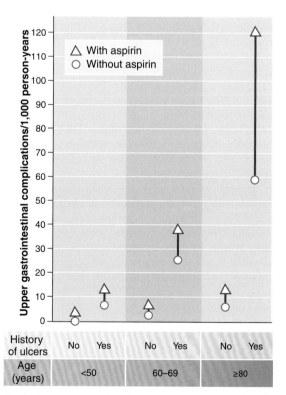

Figure 5.5 ■ Example of effect modification. The additional risk of gastrointestinal complications from aspirin is modified by age and history of peptic ulcer disease. (Data from Patrono C, Rodriguez LAG, Landolfi R, et al. Low-dose aspirin for the prevention of atherothrombosis. N Engl J Med 2005;353:2373–2383.)

Example

Aspirin has been shown to prevent cardiovascular events. Whether it should be recommended depends on a patient's risk of cardiovascular events and of complications of aspirin, mainly upper gastrointestinal bleeding. Figure 5.5 shows that the additional rate of gastrointestinal complications (the incidence attributable to aspirin) depends on two other factors, age and prior history of peptic ulcer disease (12). In men younger than 50 years old with no history of ulcers, the rate of complications is about 1/1,000 person-years, and there is virtually no additional risk related to aspirin. Risk increases a little with age among men without a history of ulcers. However, among men with a history of ulcer disease, the rate of complications rises sharply with age, and even much more with aspirin use. At the highest level of risk, in men older than age 80 and with an ulcer history, aspirin doubles risk from 60 to 120/1,000 person-years.

This example shows that age and history of peptic ulcer disease modify the effect of aspirin on gastrointestinal complications. The additional information provided by effect modification enables clinicians to tailor their recommendations about the use of aspirin more closely to the characteristics of an individual patient.

Confounding and effect modification are independent of each other. A given variable might be a confounder, effect modifier, both, or neither, depending on the research question and data.

Review Questions

For question 5.1, select the best answer.

5.1. Which of the following statements is not correct for *both* prospective and retrospective cohort studies?

A. They measure incidence of disease directly.
B. They allow assessment of possible associations between exposure and many diseases.
C. They allow investigators to decide beforehand what data to collect.
D. They avoid bias that might occur if measurement of exposure is made after the outcome of interest is known.

Questions 5.2–5.4 are based on the following example:

A study was done examining the relationship of smoking, stroke, and age (13). The 12-year incidence per 1,000 persons (absolute risk) of stroke according to age and smoking status was:

Age	Non-smokers	Smokers
45–49	7.4	29.7
65–69	80.2	110.4

5.2. What was the relative risk of stroke of smokers compared to non-smokers in their 40s?

A. 1.4
B. 4.0
C. 22.3
D. 30.2
E. 72.8
F. 80.7

5.3. What was the attributable risk per 1,000 people of stroke among smokers compared to non-smokers in their 60s?

A. 1.4
B. 4.0
C. 22.3
D. 30.2
E. 72.8
F. 80.7

5.4. Which of the following statements about the study results is incorrect?

A. To calculate population-attributable risk of smoking among people in their 60s, additional data are needed.

B. More cases of stroke due to smoking occurred in people in their 60s than in their 40s.

C. When relative risk is calculated, the results reflect information about the incidence in exposed and unexposed persons, whereas the results for attributable risk do not.

D. The calculated relative risk is a stronger argument for smoking as cause of stroke for persons in their 40s than the calculated risk for persons in their 60s.

E. Depending on the question asked, age could be considered either a confounding variable or an effect modifier in the study.

Questions 5.5–5.11 are based on the following example:

Deep venous thrombosis (DVT) is a serious condition that occasionally can lead to pulmonary embolism and death (14). The incidence of DVT is increased by several genetic and environmental factors, including oral contraceptives (OCs) and a genetic mutation, factor V Leiden. These two risk factors, OCs and factor V Leiden, interact. Heterozygotes for factor V Leiden have 4 to 10 times the risk of DVT of the general population. In women without the genetic mutation, incidence of DVT rises from about 0.8/10,000 women/yr among those not on OCs to 3.0/10,000 women/yr for those taking the pill. The baseline incidence of DVT in heterozygotes for factor V Leiden is 5.7/10,000 women/yr, rising to 28.5/10,000 women/yr among those taking OCs. Mutations for factor V Leiden occur in about 5% of whites but are absent in Africans and Asians.

For questions 5.5–5.10., select the one best answer.

5.5. What is the absolute risk of DVT in women who do not have the mutation and do not take OCs?

A. 0.8/10,000/yr
B. 1.3/10,000/yr
C. 2.2/10,000/yr
D. 9.5/10,000/yr
E. 25.5/10,000/yr

5.6. What is the attributable risk of DVT for women taking OCs who do not carry the mutation for factor V Leiden compared to those not taking OCs and not carrying the mutation?

A. 0.8/10,000/yr
B. 1.3/10,000/yr
C. 2.2/10,000/yr
D. 9.5/10,000/yr
E. 25.5/10,000/yr

5.7. What is the attributable risk of DVT for women taking OCs who carry factor V Leiden compared to women on OCs but not carrying the mutation?

A. 0.8/10,000/yr
B. 1.3/10,000/yr
C. 2.2/10,000/yr
D. 9.5/10,000/yr
E. 25.5/10,000/yr

5.8. In a population with 100,000 white women, all of whom take OCs, what is the population-attributable risk for DVT in women who are heterozygous for factor V Leiden?

A. 0.8/10,000/yr
B. 1.3/10,000/yr
C. 2.2/10,000/yr
D. 9.5/10,000/yr
E. 25.5/10,000/yr

5.9. What is the relative risk of DVT in women taking OCs and heterozygous for factor V Leiden compared to women who take OCs but do not carry the mutation?

A. 3.8
B. 7.1
C. 9.5
D. 28.5
E. 35.6

5.10. What is the relative risk of DVT in women taking OCs and without the mutation compared to women without the mutation who are not taking OCs?

A. 3.8
B. 7.1
C. 9.5
D. 28.5
E. 35.6

5.11. Given the information in this study and calculations for questions 5.5–5.10, which of the following statements about risk of developing DVT is incorrect?

A. Factor V Leiden modifies the effect of OCs on the annual risk of developing DVT by increasing risk from about 3 per 10,000 to about 30 per 10,000 women.
B. Being heterozygous for factor V Leiden confers about twice the risk for DVT as taking OCs.
C. Women heterozygous for factor V Leiden should be advised against taking OCs because of the high relative risk for DVT among such women.

For question 5.12, select the best answer

5.12. In a study to determine if regularly taking aspirin prevents cardiovascular death, aspirin users died as often as non-users. However, aspirin users were sicker and had illnesses more likely to be treated with aspirin. Which of the following methods is the best way to account for the propensity of people to take aspirin?

A. Calculate the absolute risk of cardiovascular death in the two groups and the risk difference attributable to using aspirin.
B. Create subgroups of aspirin users and non-users with similar indications for using the medication and compare death rates among the subgroups.
C. For each person using aspirin, match a non-user on age, sex, and comorbidity and compare death rates in the two groups.

REFERENCES

1. Dawber TR. The Framingham Study: The Epidemiology of Atherosclerotic Disease. Cambridge, MA: Harvard University Press; 1980.
2. Kannel WB, Feinleib M, McNamara PM, et al. An investigation of coronary heart disease in families. The Framingham Offspring Study. Am J Epidemiol 1979;110:281–290.
3. Wen CP, Wai J PM, Tsai MK, et al. Minimum amount of physical activity for reduced mortality and extended life expectancy: a prospective cohort study. Lancet 2011;378:1244–1253.
4. Madsen KM, Hviid A, Vestergaard M, et al. A population-based study of measles, mumps, and rubella vaccination and autism. N Engl J Med 2002;347:1477–1482.
5. The Editors of The Lancet. Retraction—ileal-lymphoid-nodular hyperplasia, non-specific colitis, and pervasive developmental disorder in children. Lancet 2010;375:445.
6. Geiger AM, Yu O, Herrinton LJ, et al. (on behalf of the CRN PROTECTS Group). A case-cohort study of bilateral prophylactic mastectomy efficacy in community practices. Am J Epidemiol 2004;159:S99.
7. Siris ES, Brenneman SK, Barrett-Connor E, et al. The effect of age and bone mineral density on the absolute, excess, and relative risk of fracture in postmenopausal women aged 55–99: results from the National Osteoporosis Risk Assessment (NORA), Osteoporosis Int 2006; 17:565–574.
8. Hofman A, Vandenbroucke JP. Geoffrey Rose's big idea. Br Med J 1992;305:1519–1520.
9. Reulen RC, Winter DL, Frobisher C, et al. long-term cause-specific mortality among survivors of childhood cancers. JAMA 2010;304:172–179.
10. Al-Delaimy WK, Rexrode KM, Hu FB, et al. Folate intake and risk of stroke among women. Stroke 2004;35: 1259–1263.
11. Rothman KJ. Modern Epidemiology. Boston: Little Brown and Co.; 1986.
12. Patrono C, Rodriguez LAG, Landolfi R, et al. Low-dose aspirin for the prevention of atherothrombosis. N Engl J Med 2005;353:2373–2383.
13. Psaty BM, Koepsell TD, Manolio TA, et al. Risk ratios and risk differences in estimating the effect of risk factors for cardiovascular disease in the elderly. J Clin Epidemiol 1990;43: 961–970.
14. Vandenbroucke JP, Rosing J, Bloemenkamp KW, et al. Oral contraceptives and the risk of venous thrombosis. N Engl J Med 2001;344:1527–1535.

Chapter 6

Risk: From Disease to Exposure

". . . take two groups presumed to be representative of persons who do and do not have the disease and determine the percentage of each group who have the characteristic. . . . This yields, not a true rate, but rather what is usually referred to as a relative frequency."
—Jerome Cornfield
1952

KEY WORDS

Latency period
Case-control study
Control
Population-based
  case-control study
Nested case-control
  study
Matching
Umbrella matching

Overmatching
Recall bias
Odds ratio
Estimated relative
  risk
Prevalence odds ratio
Crude odds ratio
Adjusted odds ratio
Epidemic curve

Cohort studies are a wonderfully logical and direct way of studying risk, but they have practical limitations. Most chronic diseases take a long time to develop. The latency period, the period of time between exposure to a risk factor and the expression of its pathologic effects, is measured in decades for most chronic diseases. For example, smoking precedes coronary disease, lung cancer, and chronic bronchitis by 20 years or more, and osteoporosis with fractures occurs in the elderly because of diet and exercise patterns throughout life. Also, relatively few people in a cohort develop the outcome of interest, even though it is necessary to measure exposure in, and to follow-up, all members of the cohort. The result is that cohort studies of risk require a lot of time and effort, not to mention money, to get an answer. The inefficiency is especially limiting for very rare diseases.

Some of these limitations can be overcome by modifications of cohort methods, such as retrospective cohort or case-cohort designs, described in the preceding chapter. This chapter describes another way of studying the relationship between a potential risk (or protective) factor and disease more efficiently: case-control studies. This approach has two main advantages over cohort studies. First, it bypasses the need to collect data on a large number of people, most of whom do not get the disease and so contribute little to the results. Second, it is faster because it is not necessary to wait from measurement of exposure until effects occur.

But efficiency and timeliness come at a cost: Managing bias is a more difficult and sometimes uncertain task in case-control studies. In addition, these studies produce only an estimate of relative risk and no direct information on other measures of effect such as absolute risk, attributable risk, and population risks, all described in the Chapter 5.

The respective advantages and disadvantages of cohort and case-control studies are summarized in Table 6.1.

Despite the drawbacks of case-control studies, the trade-off between scientific strength and feasibility is often worthwhile. Indeed, case-control studies are indispensable for studying risk for very uncommon diseases, as shown in the following example.

Table 6.1

Summary of Characteristics of Cohort and Case-Control Studies

Cohort Study	Case-Control Study
Begins with a defined cohort	Begins with sampled cases and controls
Exposure measured in members of the cohort	Exposure measured in cases and controls, sometimes after outcomes
Cases arise in the cohort during follow-up	Exposure occurs before samples became cases and controls
Incidence measured for exposed and non-exposed members of the cohort	Exposure measured for cases and controls
Can calculate absolute, relative, attributable, and population risks directly	Can estimate relative risk but there is no information on incidence

Example

In the mid 2000s, clinicians began reporting cases of an unusual form of femoral fracture in women. Bisphosphonates, drugs taken to prevent osteoporosis, were suspected because they had been introduced in the decades before and act by reducing bone remodeling. Case series reported an association between bisphosphonates and atypical fractures, but the women in these studies took other drugs and had other diseases that could also have been related to their risk of fractures. To provide a more definitive answer to whether bisphosphonates were independently associated with atypical fractures, investigators in Sweden did a case-control study (1). From the National Swedish Patient Register, they identified all 59 women age 55 years or older with atypical femoral fractures in 2008. They also identified 263 controls, women in the same registry who had had ordinary femoral fractures (to match for underlying vulnerability to fractures). Other variables that might be related to both bisphosphonate use and atypical fractures were recorded, including age, use of bone-modifying drugs such as corticosteroids or estrogens, and diseases such as osteoporosis and previous fractures. After taking these other factors into account, women taking bisphosphonates were 33 times more likely to develop atypical fractures.

By adding a comparison group and accounting for other variables that might be related to bisphosphonate use and atypical fractures, the investigators were able to take the inference that bisphosphonates might be a cause of atypical fractures well beyond what was possible with case series alone.

This chapter, the third about risk, is titled "From Disease to Exposure" because case-control studies involve looking backward from disease to exposure, in contrast to cohort studies, which look forward from exposure to disease.

CASE-CONTROL STUDIES

The basic design of a case-control study is diagrammed in Figure 6.1. Two samples are selected: patients who have developed the disease in question and an otherwise similar group of people who have not developed the disease. The researchers then look back in time to measure the frequency of exposure to a possible risk factor in the two groups. The resulting data can be used to estimate the relative risk of disease related to a risk factor.

Example

Head injuries are relatively common among alpine skiers and snowboarders. It seems plausible that helmets would prevent these injuries, but critics point out that helmets might also increase head injuries by reducing field of vision, impairing hearing, and giving athletes a false sense of security. To obtain more definitive evidence of helmets' actual effects, investigators in Norway did a case-control study (Fig. 6.2) (2). Cases and controls were chosen from visitors to eight major Norwegian alpine ski resorts during the 2002 winter season. Cases were all 578 people with head injuries reported by the ski patrol. Controls were a sample of people waiting in line at the bottom of the main ski lift at each of the eight resorts. For both cases and controls, investigators recorded other factors that might confound the relationship between helmet use and head injury, including age, sex, nationality, type of equipment, previous ski school attendance, rented or owned equipment, and skiing ability. After taking confounders into account, helmet use was associated with a 60% reduction in risk of head injury.

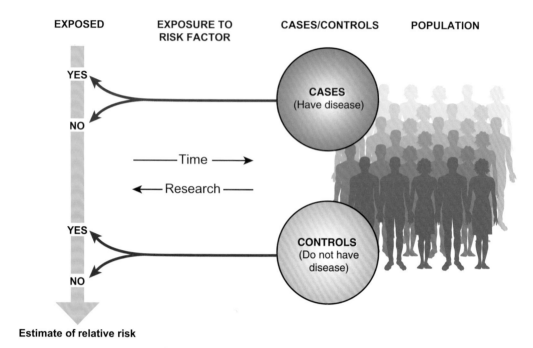

Figure 6.1 ■ Design of case-control studies.

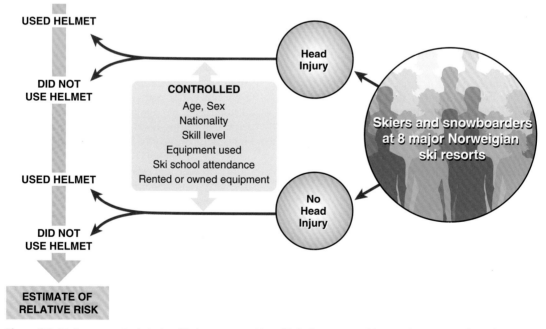

Figure 6.2 ■ A case-control study of helmet use and head injuries among skiers and snowboarders. (Summary of Sulheim S, Holme I, Ekeland A, et al. Helmet use and risk of head injuries in alpine skiers and snowboarders. JAMA 2006;295:919–924.)

The word control comes up in other situations, too. It is used in experimental studies to refer to people, animals, or biologic materials that have not been exposed to the study intervention. In diagnostic laboratories, "controls" refer to specimens that have a known amount of the material being tested for. As a verb, *control* is used to describe the process of taking into account, neutralizing, or subtracting the effects of variables that are extraneous to the main research question. Here, the term is used in the context of case-control studies to refer to people who do not have the disease or outcome under study.

DESIGN OF CASE-CONTROL STUDIES

The validity of case-control studies depends on the care with which cases and controls are selected, how well exposure is measured, and how completely potentially confounding variables are controlled.

Selecting Cases

The cases in case-control research should be new (incident) cases, not existing (prevalent) ones. The reasons are based on the concepts discussed in Chapter 2. The prevalence of a disease at a point in time is a function of both the incidence and duration of that disease. Duration is in turn determined by the rate at which patients leave the disease state (because of recovery or death) or persist in it (because of a slow course or successful palliation). It follows from these relationships that risk factors for prevalent disease may be risk factors for incidence, duration, or both; the relative contributions of the two cannot be determined. For example, if prevalent cases were studied, an exposure that caused a rapidly lethal form of the disease would result in fewer cases that were exposed, reducing relative risk and thereby suggesting that exposure is less harmful than it really is or even that it is protective.

At best, a case-control study should include all the cases or a representative sample of all cases that arise in a defined population. For example, the bisphosphonates study included all residents of Sweden in 2008 and the helmets study all skiers and snowboarders in eight major resorts in Norway (accounting for 55% of all ski runs in the country).

Some case-control studies, especially older ones, have identified cases in hospitals and referral centers where uncommon diseases are most likely to be found. This way of choosing cases is convenient, but it raises validity problems. These centers may attract particularly severe or atypical cases or those with unusual exposures—the wrong sample if the underly-

ing research question in case-control studies is about ordinary occurrences of disease and exposures.

Also, it is difficult in this situation to be confident that controls, however they are chosen, are truly similar to cases in all ways other than exposure, which is critical to the validity of this kind of study (see the Selecting Controls section). Fortunately, it is rarely necessary to take this scientific risk because there are many databases that make true population sampling possible.

However the cases might be identified, it should be possible for both them and controls to be exposed to the risk factor and to experience the outcome. For example, in a case-control study of exercise and sudden death, cases and control would have to be equally able to exercise (if they chose to) to be eligible.

It goes without saying that diagnosis should be rigorously confirmed for cases (and excluded for controls), and the criteria made explicit. In the bisphosphonates study, investigators agreed on explicit criteria for atypical fractures of the femur and reviewed all radiographs, not just reports of them, to classify fracture type. One investigator then reviewed a random sample of radiographs for a second time without knowing how each had been classified, and there was complete agreement between the original and the second classifications.

Selecting Controls

Above all, the validity of case-control studies depends on the comparability of cases and controls. To be comparable, cases and controls should be members of the same base population and have an equal opportunity of being exposed. The best approach to meeting these requirements is to ensure that controls are a random sample of all non-cases in the same population or cohort that produced the cases.

The Population Approach

Studies in which cases and controls are a complete or random sample of a defined population are called population-based case-control studies. In practice, most of these populations are dynamic—that is, continually changing, with people moving in and out of the population—as described in Chapter 2 (3). This might bias the result, especially if cases and controls are sampled over a long period of time and exposure is changing rapidly during this time. This concern can be laid to rest if there is evidence that population turnover is in fact so small as to have little effect on the study results or if cases and controls are matched on calendar time—that is, controls are selected on the same date as the onset of disease in the cases.

The Cohort Approach

Another way of ensuring that cases and controls are comparable is to draw them from the same cohort. In this situation, the study is said to be a **nested case-control study** (it is "nested" in the cohort).

In the era of large databases and powerful computers, why not just analyze cohort data as a cohort study rather than a case-control study? After all, the inefficiency of including many exposed members of the cohort, even though few of them will experience the outcome, could be overcome by computing power. The usual reason for case-control analyses of cohort data is that some of the study variables, especially some covariates, may not be available in the cohort database and, therefore, have to be gathered from other sources for each patient in the study. Obtaining the missing information from medical records, questionnaires, genetic analyses, and linkage to other databases can be very expensive and time-consuming. Therefore, there is a practical advantage to having to assemble this information only for cases and a sample of non-cases in the cohort, not every member of the cohort.

With nested case-control studies, there is an opportunity to obtain both a crude measures of incidence from a cohort analysis and a strong estimate of relative risk, that takes into account a rich set of covariates, from a case-control analysis. With this information one has the full set of risk described in Chapter 5—absolute risk for exposed and non-exposed people, relative risk, attributable risk, and population risks.

The bisphosphonate example illustrates the advantages of complementary cohort and case control analyses. A cohort analysis, taking only age into account, showed that the increase in absolute risk of atypical fractures related to bisphosphonate use was five cases per 10,000 patient-years. Collection of data on covariates was done by linking to other databases and was presumably too resource-intensive to be done on the entire national sample. With these data for cases and controls, a much more credible estimate of relative risk was possible in the case-control analysis. The estimate of relative risk of 33 from the case-control analysis was consistent with the crude relative risk from the cohort analysis (not accounting for potential confounders other than age), which was 47. Because of the two analyses, both cohort and case-control, the authors could point out that the relative risk of atypical fracture was large but the absolute risk was small.

Hospital and Community Controls

If population- or cohort-based sampling is not possible, a fallback position is to select controls in such a way that the selection *seems* to produce controls that are comparable to cases. For example, if cases are selected from a hospital ward, the controls might be selected from patients with different diseases, apparently unrelated to the exposure and disease of interest, in the same hospital. As pointed out earlier, for most risk factors and diseases, case-control studies in health care settings are more fallible than population- or cohort-based sampling because hospitalized patients are usually a biased sample of all people in the community, the people to whom the results should apply.

Another approach is to obtain controls from the community served by the hospital. However, many hospitals do not draw patients exclusively from the surrounding community; some people in the community go to other hospitals, and some people in other communities pass up their own neighborhood hospital to go to the study hospital. As a result, cases and controls may be systematically different in ways that distort the exposure-disease relationship.

Multiple Control Groups

If none of the available control groups seems ideal, one can see how choice of controls affects results by selecting several control groups with apparently complementary scientific strengths and weaknesses. Similar estimates of relative risk obtained using different control groups is evidence against bias because it is unlikely that the same biases would affect otherwise dissimilar groups in the same direction and to the same extent. If the estimates of relative risks are different, it is a signal that one or more are biased and the reasons need to be investigated.

Example

In the helmets and head injury example (2), the main control group was uninjured people skiing or snowboarding on the same hills on the same days, but one could imagine disadvantages to these controls, such as their not having similar risk-taking behavior to cases. To examine the effect of choice of control group on results, the investigators repeated the analyses with a different control group—skiers with other injuries. The estimated relative risk was similar—a reduction in risk of 55% rather than 60% with the original control group—suggesting that choice of control group did not substantially affect results.

Multiple Controls per Case

Having several control *groups* per case group should not be confused with having several controls for each case. If the number of cases is limited, as is often so with rare diseases, the study can provide more information if there is more than one control per case. More controls produce a gain in the ability to detect an increase or decrease in risk if it exists, a property of a study called "statistical power" (see Chapter 11). As a practical matter, the gain is worthwhile up to about three or four controls per case, after which little is gained by including even more controls.

Matching

If some characteristics seem especially strongly related to either exposure or disease, such that one would want to be sure that they occur similarly in cases and controls, they can be matched. With matching, for each case with a set of characteristics, the study includes one or more controls that possess the same characteristics. Researchers commonly match for age and sex, because these are often strongly related to both exposure and disease, but matching may extend beyond these demographic characteristics (e.g., to risk profile or disease severity) when other factors are known to be strongly associated with an exposure or outcome. Matching increases the useful information obtainable from a set of cases and controls by reducing differences between groups in determinants of disease other than the one being considered, thereby allowing a more powerful (sensitive) measure of association.

Sometimes, cases and controls are made comparable by umbrella matching, matching on a variable such as hospital or community that is a proxy for many other variables that could confound the exposure–disease relationship and would be difficult to measure one at a time, if that were possible at all. Examples of variables that might be captured under an umbrella include social disadvantage related to income, education, race, and ethnicity; propensity to seek health care or follow medical advice; and local patterns of health care.

Matching can be overdone, biasing study results. Overmatching can occur if investigators match on variables so closely related to exposure that exposure rates in cases and controls becomes more similar than they are in the population. The result is to make the observed estimate of relative risk closer to 1 (no effect). There are many reasons why the matching variable might be related to exposure. It may be part of the chain of events leading from exposure to disease. Other variables might be highly related to each other because they have similar root causes; education,

income, race, and ethnicity tend to be related to each other, so if one matches on one, it will obscure effects of the others. Matching on diseases with the same treatment would result in overmatching for studies of the effects of that treatment. For example, in a study of non-steroidal anti-inflammatory drugs (NSAIDs) and renal failure, if cases and controls were matched for the presence of arthritic symptoms, which are commonly treated with NSAIDs, matched pairs would have an artificially similar history of NSAID use.

A disadvantage of matching is that once a variable is matched for, and so made similar in cases and controls, it is no longer possible to learn how it affects the exposure–disease relationship. Also, for many studies it is not possible to find matched controls for more than a few case characteristics. This can be overcome, to some extent, if the number of potential controls is huge or if the matching criteria are relaxed (e.g., by matching age within a 5-year range rather than the same year). In summary, matching is a useful way of controlling for confounding, but it can limit the questions that can be asked in the study and can cause rather than remove bias.

Measuring Exposure

The validity of case-control studies also depends on avoiding misclassification when measuring exposure. The safest approach is to depend on complete, accurate records that were collected before disease developed. Examples include pharmacy records for studies of prescription drug risks, surgical records for studies of surgical complications, and stored blood specimens for studies of risk related to biomolecular abnormalities. With such records, knowledge of disease status cannot bias reporting of exposure.

However, many important exposures can only be measured by asking cases and controls or their proxies about them. Among these are exercise, diet, and over-the-counter and recreational drug use. The following example illustrates how investigators can "harden" data from interviews that are inherently vulnerable to bias.

Example

What are the risk factors for suicide in China? Investigators studied 519 people who had committed suicide and 536 people who had died from other injuries (4). Both groups came from 23 geographically representative sites in China. Exposure was measured by interviews with family members and close associates. The authors noted that as with other studies that depended on a "psychological autopsy" for measurement of exposure, "interviewers were aware of the cause of death of the deceased (suicide or other injury) so we could not completely eliminate potential interviewer bias." They went on to explain that they "tried to keep this bias to a minimum by using the same interview schedule for cases and controls, employing objective measures of potential risk factors, independently obtaining evidence from two sources (family members and close associates), and giving extensive training to interviewers." They also chose controls who died from injuries to match for one important characteristic that might affect responses in the interview, the recent death of a family member or associate.

The study identified eight predictors of suicide: high depression symptom score, previous suicide attempt, acute stress just prior to death, low quality of life, high chronic stress, severe interpersonal conflict in the 2 days before death, a blood relative with previous suicidal behavior, and a friend or associate with previous suicidal behavior.

When cases and controls are asked to recall their previous exposures, bias can occur for several reasons. Cases, knowing they have the disease under study, may be more likely to remember whether they were exposed, a problem called recall bias. For example, parents of a child with Reyes syndrome (an encephalopathy) may be more likely to recall aspirin use after widespread efforts to make parents aware of an association between aspirin use and Reyes syndrome in febrile children. A man with prostate cancer might be more likely to report a prior vasectomy after stories of an association were in the news. With all the publicity surrounding the possible risks of various environmental and drug exposures, it is entirely possible that victims of disease would remember their exposures more often than people without the disease.

Investigators can limit recall bias by not telling patients the specific purpose of the study. It would be unethical not to inform participants in research about the general nature of the study question, but to provide detailed information about specific questions and hypotheses could so bias the resulting information as to commit another breach of ethics—involving subjects in a flawed research project.

Physicians may be more likely to ask about an exposure and record that information in the medical record in cases than in controls if exposure is already suspected of being a cause. Thus, a physician may be more likely to record a family history of prostate cancer in a patient with prostate cancer or to record cell phone use in a patient with brain cancer. This bias should be understandable to all students of physical diagnosis. If a resident admitting a relatively young woman with acute myocardial infarction is aware of the reported association with use of birth control pills, he or she might question the patient more intensely about birth control pill use and to record this information more carefully. Protections against this kind of bias are the same as those mentioned earlier: multiple sources of information and "blinding" the data gatherers by keeping them in the dark about the specific hypothesis under study.

The existence of disease can also lead to exposure, especially when the exposure under study is a medical treatment. Early manifestations of the disease may lead to treatment, while the study question is just the other way around: whether treatment causes disease. If this problem is anticipated, it can be dealt with in the design of the study, as illustrated in the following example.

Example

Do beta-blocker drugs prevent first myocardial infarctions in patients being treated for hypertension? A case-control study addressed this question (5). Because angina is a major indication for use of beta-blockers, and also a symptom of coronary disease, the investigators carefully excluded any subjects with a history that suggested angina or other manifestation of coronary heart disease. They found that patients with hypertension treated with beta-blockers had a reduced risk of non-fatal myocardial infarctions, even after those with angina or other evidence of coronary disease were carefully excluded.

All that might be said about bias in measurement of exposure can also be said of confounders. Many important covariates (e.g., smoking, diet, exercise, as well as race and ethnicity) may be poorly recorded in medical records and databases and, therefore, must be obtained by interview if they are to be included in the study at all.

Multiple Exposures

Thus far, we have described case-control studies of a single, dichotomous exposure, but case-control studies are an efficient means of examining a far richer array of exposures: the effects of multiple exposures, various doses of the same exposure, and exposures that are early symptoms (not risk factors) of disease.

Example

Ovarian cancer is notoriously difficult to diagnose early in its course when treatment might be more effective. Investigators in England did a case-control study of symptoms of ovarian cancer in primary care (6). Cases were 212 women over 40 years of age diagnosed with primary ovarian cancer in 39 general practices in Devon, England, 2000–2007; 1,060 controls without ovarian cancer were matched to cases by age and practice. Symptoms were abstracted from medical records for the year before diagnosis. Seven symptoms were independently associated with ovarian cancer: abdominal distension, postmenopausal bleeding, loss of appetite, increased urinary frequency, abdominal pain, rectal bleeding, and abdominal bloating. After excluding symptoms reported in the 180 days before diagnosis (to get a better estimate of "early" symptoms), three remained independently associated with ovarian cancer: abdominal distension, urinary frequency, and abdominal pain.

THE ODDS RATIO: AN ESTIMATE OF RELATIVE RISK

Figure 6.3 shows the dichotomous classification of exposure and disease typical of both cohort and case-control studies and compares how risk is calculated differently for the two. These concepts are illustrated with the bisphosphonates study, which had both a cohort and a case-control component.

In the cohort study, participants were divided into two groups at the outset—exposed to bisphosphonates $(a + b)$ and not exposed to bisphosphonates $(c + d)$. Cases of atypical fracture emerged naturally over time in the exposed group (a) and the unexposed group (c). This provides appropriate numerators and denominators to calculate the incidence of atypical fracture in the exposed

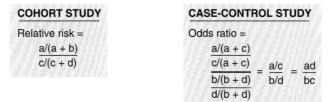

	Cases	Noncases	
Exposed	a	b	a + b
Not exposed	c	d	c + d
	a + c	b + d	

COHORT STUDY

Relative risk =
$$\frac{a/(a + b)}{c/(c + d)}$$

CASE-CONTROL STUDY

Odds ratio =
$$\frac{\dfrac{a/(a + c)}{c/(a + c)}}{\dfrac{b/(b + d)}{d/(b + d)}} = \frac{a/c}{b/d} = \frac{ad}{bc}$$

Figure 6.3 ■ Calculation of relative risk from a cohort study and odds ratio (estimated relative risk) from a case-control study.

$[a/(a + b)]$ and unexposed $[c/(c + d)]$ members of the cohort. It was also possible to calculate the relative risk:

Relative risk

$$= \frac{\text{Incidence of disease in the exposed}}{\text{Incidence of disease in the unexposed}}$$

$$= \frac{a/(a + b)}{c/(c + d)}$$

The case-control study, on the other hand, began with the selection of a group of cases of atypical fracture $(a + c)$ and a group of controls with other fractures $(b + d)$. There is no way of knowing disease rates because these groups are determined not by nature but by the investigators' selection criteria. Therefore, it is not possible to compute the incidence of disease among people exposed and not exposed to bisphosphonates; and it is not possible to calculate a relative risk. What does have meaning, however, is the relative frequency of exposure to bisphosphonates among cases and controls.

One approach to comparing the frequency of exposure among cases and controls provides a measure of risk that is conceptually and mathematically similar to relative risk. The **odds ratio** is defined as the odds that a case is exposed divided by the odds that a control is exposed:

$$\frac{\left(\dfrac{a}{a + c}\right)}{\left(\dfrac{c}{a + c}\right)}$$
$$\overline{\quad\dfrac{\left(\dfrac{b}{b + d}\right)}{\left(\dfrac{d}{b + d}\right)}\quad}$$

Which simplifies to:

$$\frac{\left(\dfrac{a}{c}\right)}{\left(\dfrac{b}{d}\right)},$$

where odds are the ratios of two probabilities, the probability of an event divided by 1 − the probability of that event.

The odds ratio can be further simplified to:

$$\frac{ad}{bc}$$

Referring back to Figure 6.3, the odds ratio can be obtained by multiplying diagonally across the table and dividing these cross-products.

The meaning of the odds ratio is analogous to that of relative risk obtained from cohort studies. If the frequency of exposure is higher among cases, the odds ratio will exceed 1, indicating increased risk. The stronger the association is between the exposure and disease, the higher the odds ratio. Conversely, if the frequency of exposure is lower among cases, the odds ratio will be <1, indicating protection. Because of the similarity of the information conveyed by an odds ratio and the relative risk, and the meaning more readily attached to relative risk, odds ratios are often reported as **estimated relative risks**.

An odds ratio is approximately equal to a relative risk when the incidence of disease is low. To see this mathematically, look at the formula for relative risk in Figure 6.3. If the number of cases in the exposed group (a) is small relative to the number of non-cases in that group (b) then $a/(a + b)$ is approximately equal to a/b. Similarly, if the number of cases in the non-exposed group (c) is small relative to non-cases in that group (d), then $c/(c + d)$ is approximated by c/d. Then, relative risk = a/b divided by c/d, which simplified to ad/bc, the odds ratio.

How low must the rates be for the odds ratio to be an accurate estimate of relative risk? The answer depends on the size of the relative risk (7). In general, bias in the estimate of relative risk becomes large enough to matter as disease rates in unexposed people become greater than about 1/100 or perhaps 5/100. As outcomes become more frequent, the odds ratio tends to overestimate the relative risk when it is >1 and underestimate the relative risk when it is <1. Fortunately, most diseases, particularly those examined by means of case-control studies, have considerably lower rates.

Earlier in this chapter, we described why case-control studies should be about incident (new onset) cases, not prevalent ones. Nevertheless, **prevalence odds ratios** are commonly calculated for prevalence studies and reported in the medical literature. The prevalence odds ratio is a measure of association but not a very informative one, not only because of difficulty distinguishing factors related to incidence versus duration but also because the rare disease assumption is less likely to be met.

CONTROLLING FOR EXTRANEOUS VARIABLES

The greatest threat to the validity of observational (cohort and case-control) studies is that the groups being compared might be systematically different in factors related to both exposure and disease—that is, there is confounding. In Chapter 5, we described various ways of controlling for extraneous variables when looking for independent effects of exposure on disease in observational studies. All of these approaches—exclusion, matching, stratified analyses, and modeling—are also used in case-control studies, often in combination. Of course, this can only be done for characteristics that were already suspected to affect the exposure–disease relationship and were measured in the study.

Because mathematical modeling is almost always used to control for extraneous variables, in practice, calculations of odds ratios are much more complicated than the cross product of a two by two table. An odds ratio calculated directly from a 2×2 table is referred to as a crude odds ratio because it has not taken into account variables other than exposure and disease. After adjustment for the effects of these other variables, it is called an adjusted odds ratio.

The implicit reason for case-control studies is to find causes. However, even when extraneous variables have been controlled for by state-of-the-science methods, the possibility remains that unmeasured variables are confounding the exposure–disease relationship. Therefore, one has to settle for describing how exposure is related to disease independently of other variables included in the study and be appropriately humble about the possibility that unmeasured variables might account for the results. For these reasons, the results of observational studies are best described as associations, not causes.

INVESTIGATION OF A DISEASE OUTBREAK

Up to this point, we have described use of the case-control method to identify risk factors for chronic diseases. The same method is used to identify risk factors for outbreaks (small epidemics) of acute diseases, typically infectious diseases or poisonings. Often, the microbe or toxin is obvious early in the epidemic, after diagnostic evaluation of cases, but the mode of transmission is not. Information on how the disease was spread is needed to stop the epidemic and to understand possible modes of transmission, which might be useful in the control of future epidemics.

Example

A large outbreak of gastroenteritis, with many cases complicated by hemolytic-uremic syndrome (a potentially fatal condition with acute renal failure, hemolytic anemia, and thrombocytopenia) occurred in Germany in May 2011 (8). During the epidemic, there were 3,816 reported cases, 845 with hemolytic-uremic syndrome. Figure 6.4 shows the epidemic curve, the number of cases over time. The immediate cause, infection with a toxin-producing strain of the bacterium *Escherichia coli* was quickly identified, but the source of the infection was not. Investigators did a case-control study comparing 26 cases of hemolytic-uremic syndrome with 81 controls, matched for age and neighborhood (9). They found that 6/24 cases (25%) and 7/80 controls (9%) were exposed to sprouts, for an odds ratio of 5.8, suggesting that the infection was transmitted by eating contaminated sprouts. (Note that the odds ratio is not exactly the cross-products in this case because the calculation of odds ratio took into account the matching.) However, cucumbers and other produce were also implicated, although less strongly. To take this further, investigators did a small cohort study of people dining in groups at a single restaurant during the epidemic period. Cases were empirically defined as diners who developed bloody diarrhea or hemolytic-uremic syndrome or were found by culture to have the offending organism. Twenty percent of the cohort met these criteria, 26% of whom had hemolytic-uremic syndrome. The relative risk for sprout consumption was 14.2, and no other food was strongly associated with the disease. Sprout consumption accounted for 100% of cases. Investigators traced back the source of sprouts from the distributor that supplied the restaurant to a single producer. However, they could not culture the causal *Escherichia coli* from seeds in the implicated lot. Following the investigation, and after attention to the producer, the epidemic subsided (Fig. 6.4) and incidence returned to the low levels seen before the epidemic.

This example also illustrates how case-control and cohort studies, laboratory studies of the responsible organism, and "shoe-leather" epidemiology during trace-back acted in concert to identify the underlying cause of the epidemic.

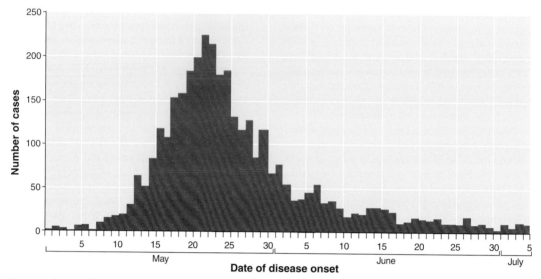

Figure 6.4 ■ Epidemic curve of an outbreak of Shiga-toxin-producing *Escherichia coli* infection in Germany. (Redrawn with permission from Frank C, Werber D, Cramer JP, et al. Epidemic profile of shiga-toxin-producing *Escherichia coli* 0104:H4 outbreak in Germany. N Engl J Med 2011;365:1771–1780.)

Review Questions

Read the following and select the best response.

6.1. In a case-control study of oral contraceptives and myocardial infarction (heart attack), exposure to birth control pills was abstracted from medical records at the time of the myocardial infarction. Results might be biased toward finding an association by all of the following *except:*

A. Physicians might have asked about use of birth control pill use more carefully in cases.

B. Having a myocardial infarction might have led to oral contraceptive use.

C. Physicians might have been more likely to record birth control use in cases.

D. Medical record abstractors might have looked for evidence of oral contraceptive use more carefully if they knew a patient had had a myocardial infarction.

E. Patients might have recalled exposure more readily when they had a heart attack.

6.2. Investigators in Europe did a case-control study, nested in a multicountry cohort of more than 520,000 participants, of vitamin D concentration and the risk of colon cancer. They studied 1,248 cases of incident colon cancer arising in the cohort and an equal number of controls, sampled from the same cohort and matched by age, sex, and study center. Vitamin D was measured in blood samples taken years before diagnosis. Vitamin D levels were lower in patients with colon cancer, independent of a rich array of potentially confounding variables. The study results could be described by any of the following *except:*

A. Vitamin D levels were associated with colorectal cancer.

B. Vitamin D deficiency was a risk factor for colorectal cancer.

C. Nesting the study in a large cohort was a strength of the study.

D. The results might have been confounded with unmeasured variables related to vitamin D levels and colorectal cancer.

E. Vitamin D deficiency was a cause of colorectal cancer.

6.3. Which of the following is the most direct result of a case-control study?

    A. Prevalence
    B. Risk difference
    C. Relative risk
    D. Incidence
    E. Odds ratio

6.4. The epidemic curve for an acute infectious disease describes:

    A. The usual incubation period for the causal agent
    B. A comparison of illness over time in exposed versus non-exposed people
    C. The onset of illness in cases over time
    D. The duration of illness, on average, in affected individuals
    E. The distribution of time from infection to first symptoms

6.5. Which of the following is the best reason for doing a case-control analysis of a cohort study?

    A. Case-control studies are a feasible way of controlling for confounders not found in the cohort dataset.
    B. Case-control studies can provide all the same information more easily.
    C. Case-control studies can determine incidence of disease in exposed and non-exposed members of the cohort.
    D. Case-control studies are in general stronger than cohort studies.

6.6. The best way to identify cases is to obtain them from:

    A. A sample from the general (dynamic) population
    B. Primary care physicians' offices
    C. A community
    D. A cohort representative of the population
    E. A hospital

6.7. What is the best reason to include multiple control groups in a case-control study?

    A. To obtain a stronger estimate of relative risk
    B. There are a limited number of cases and an ample number of potential controls.
    C. To control for confounding
    D. To increase the generalizability of the result
    E. The main control group may be systematically different from cases (other than on the exposure of interest).

6.8. Case-control studies can be used to study all of the following *except:*

    A. The early symptoms of stomach cancer
    B. Risk factors for sudden infant death syndrome
    C. The incidence of suicide in the adult population
    D. The protective effect of aspirin
    E. Modes of transmission of an infectious disease

6.9. In a case-control study of exercise and sudden cardiac death, matching would be useful:

    A. To control for all potential confounding variables in the study
    B. To make cases and controls similar to each other with respect to a few major characteristics
    C. To make it possible to examine the effects of the matched variables on estimated relative risk
    D. To test whether the right controls were chosen for the cases in the study
    E. To increase the generalizability of the study

6.10. In a case-control study of whether prolonged air travel is a risk factor for venous thrombo-embolism, 60 out of 100 cases and 40 out of 100 controls had prolonged air travel. What was the crude odds ratio from this study?

    A. 0.44
    B. 1.5
    C. 2.25
    D. 3.0
    E. Not possible to calculate

6.11. A population-based case-control study would be especially useful for studying:

    A. The population attributable risk of disease
    B. Multiple outcomes (diseases)
    C. The incidence of rare diseases
    D. The prevalence of disease
    E. Risk factors for disease

6.12. The prevalence odds ratio of rheumatoid arthritis provides an estimate of:

    A. The relative risk of arthritis
    B. The attributable risk of arthritis
    C. Risk factors for the duration of arthritis
    D. The association between a patient characteristic and prevalence of arthritis
    E. Risk factors for the incidence of arthritis

6.13. In an outbreak of acute gastroenteritis, a case-control study would be especially useful for identifying:

A. Characteristics of the people affected
B. The number of people affected over time
C. The microbe or toxin causing the outbreak
D. The mode of transmission
E. Where the causative agent originated

6.14. Sampling cases and controls from a defined population or cohort accomplishes which of the following?

A. It is the only way of including incident (new) cases of disease.
B. It avoids the need for inclusion and exclusion criteria.
C. It tends to include cases and controls that are similar to each other except for exposure.
D. It matches cases and controls on important variables.
E. It ensures that the results are generalizable.

6.15. Case-control studies would be useful for answering all of the following questions *except:*

A. Do cholesterol-lowering drugs prevent coronary heart disease?

B. Are complications more common with fiberoptic cholecystectomy than with conventional (open) surgery?
C. Is drinking alcohol a risk factor for breast cancer?
D. How often do complications occur after fiberoptic cholecystectomy?
E. How effective are antibiotics for otitis media?

6.16. In a case-control study of airplane flight and thrombophlebitis, all of the following conditions should be met for the odds ratio to be a reasonable estimate of relative risk *except:*

A. Controls were sampled from the same population as cases.
B. Cases and controls met the same inclusion and exclusion criteria.
C. Other variables that might be related to air travel and thrombosis were controlled for.
D. Cases and controls were equally susceptible to developing thrombophlebitis (e.g., were equally mobile, weight, recent trauma, previous VTE) other than for air travel.
E. The incidence of thrombophlebitis was more than 5/100.

Answers are in Appendix A.

REFERENCES

1. Schilcher J, Michaelsson K, Aspenberg P. Bisphosphonate use and atypical fractures of the femoral head. New Engl J Med 2011;364:1728–1737.
2. Sulheim S, Holme I, Ekeland A, et al. Helmet use and risk of head injuries in alpine skiers and snowboarders. JAMA 2006;295:919–924.
3. Knol MJ, Vandenbroucke JP, Scott P, et al. What do case-control studies estimate? Survey of methods and assumptions in published case-control research. Am J Epidemiol 2008;168:1073–1081.
4. Phillips MR, Yang G, Zhang Y, et al. Risk factors for suicide in China: a national case-control psychological autopsy study. Lancet 2002;360:1728–1736.
5. Psaty BM, Koepsell TD, LoGerfo JP, et al. Beta-blockers and primary prevention of coronary heart disease in patients with high blood pressure. JAMA 1989;261:2087–2094.
6. Hamilton W, Peters TJ, Bankhead C, et al. Risk of ovarian cancer in women with symptoms in primary care: population-based case-control study. BMJ 2009;339:b2998. doi:10.1136/bmj.b2998
7. Feinstein AR. The bias caused by high value of incidence for p1 in the odds ratio assumption that 1-p1 is approximately equal to 1. J Chron Dis 1986;39:485–487.
8. Frank C, Werber D, Cramer JP, et al. Epidemic profile of shiga-toxin-producing *Escherichia coli* 0104:H4 outbreak in Germany. N Engl J Med 2011;365:1771–1780.
9. Buchholz U, Bernard H, Werber D et al. German outbreak of *Escherichia coli* 0104:H4 associated with sprouts. N Engl J Med 2011;365:1763–1770.

Chapter 7

Prognosis

He, who would rightly distinguish those that will survive or die, as well as those that will be subject to disease a longer or shorter time, ought, from his knowledge and attention, to be able to form an estimate of all symptoms, and rationally to weigh their powers by comparison.

—*Hippocrates*
460–375 B.C.

KEY WORDS

Prognosis	Case report
Prognostic factors	Clinical prediction
Clinical course	rules
Natural history	Training set
Zero time	Test set
Inception cohort	Validation
Stage migration	Prognostic
Event	stratification
Survival analysis	Sampling bias
Kaplan-Meier analysis	Migration bias
Time-to-event	Dropouts
analysis	Measurement bias
Censored	Sensitivity analysis
Hazard ratios	Best-case/worst-case
Case series	analysis

When people become sick, they have a great many questions about how their illness will affect them. Is it dangerous? Could I die of it? Will there be pain? How long will I be able to continue my present activities? Will it ever go away altogether? Most patients and their families want to know what to expect, even in situations where little can be done about their illness.

Prognosis is the prediction of the course of disease following its onset. This chapter reviews the ways in which the course of disease can be described. The intention is to give readers a better understanding of a difficult but indispensable task—predicting patients' futures as closely as possible. The objective is to avoid expressing prognoses with vagueness when unnecessary and with certainty when misleading.

Doctors and patients want to know the general course of the illness, but they want to go further and tailor this information to their particular situation as much as possible. For example, even though ovarian cancer is usually fatal in the long run, women with this cancer may live from a few months to many years, and they want to know where on this continuum their particular case is likely to fall.

Studies of prognosis are similar to cohort studies of risk. Patients are assembled who have a particular disease or illness in common, they are followed forward in time, and clinical outcomes are measured. Patient characteristics that are associated with an outcome of the disease, called prognostic factors, are identified. Prognostic factors are analogous to risk factors, except that they represent a different part of the disease spectrum, from disease to outcomes. Case-control studies of people with the disease who do and do not have a bad outcome can also estimate the relative risk associated with various prognostic factors, but they are unable to provide information on outcome rates (see Chapter 6).

DIFFERENCES IN RISK AND PROGNOSTIC FACTORS

Risk and prognostic factors differ from each other in several ways.

The Patients Are Different

Studies of risk factors usually deal with healthy people, whereas studies of prognostic factors are of sick people.

The Outcomes Are Different

For risk, the event being counted is usually the onset of disease. For prognosis, consequences of disease are counted, including death, complications, disability, and suffering.

The Rates Are Different

Risk factors are usually for low-probability events. Yearly rates for the onset of various diseases are on the order of 1/1,000 to 1/100,000 or less. As a result, relationships between exposure and disease are difficult to confirm in the course of day-to-day clinical experiences, even for astute clinicians. Prognosis, on the other hand, describes relatively frequent events. For example, several percent of patients with acute myocardial infarction die before leaving the hospital.

The Factors May be Different

Variables associated with an increased risk are not necessarily the same as those marking a worse prognosis. Often, they are considerably different for a given disease. For example, the number of well-established risk factors for cardiovascular disease (hypertension, smoking, dyslipidemia, diabetes, and family history of coronary heart disease) is inversely related to the risk of dying in the hospital after a first myocardial infarction (Fig. 7.1) (1).

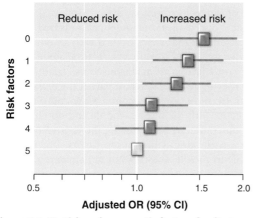

Figure 7.1 ■ Risk and prognostic factors for first myocardial infarction. (Redrawn with permission from Canto JC, Kiefe CI, Rogers WJ, et al. Number if coronary heart disease risk factors and mortality in patients with first myocardial infarction. JAMA 2011;306:2120–2127.)

Clinicians can often form good estimates of short-term prognosis from their own personal experience. However, they may be less able to sort out, without the assistance of research, the various factors that are related to long-term prognosis or the complex ways in which prognostic factors are related to one another.

CLINICAL COURSE AND NATURAL HISTORY OF DISEASE

Prognosis can be described as either the clinical course or natural history of disease. The term clinical course describes the evolution (prognosis) of a disease that has come under medical care and has been treated in a variety of ways that affect the subsequent course of events. Patients usually receive medical care at some time in the course of their illness when they have diseases that cause symptoms such as pain, failure to thrive, disfigurement, or unusual behavior. Examples include type 1 diabetes mellitus, carcinoma of the lung, and rabies. After such a disease is recognized, it is likely to be treated.

The prognosis of disease without medical intervention is termed the natural history of disease. Natural history describes how patients fare if nothing is done about their disease. A great many health conditions do not come under medical care, even in countries with advanced health care systems. They remain unrecognized because they are asymptomatic (e.g., many cancers of the prostate are occult and slow growing) and are, therefore, unrecognized in life. For others, such as osteoarthritis, mild depression, or low-grade anemia, people may consider their symptoms to be one of the ordinary discomforts of daily living, not a disease and, therefore, not seek medical care for them.

Example

Irritable bowel syndrome is a common condition that involves abdominal pain and disturbed bowel habits not caused by other diseases. How often do patients with this condition visit doctors? In a British cohort of 3,875 people without irritable bowel syndrome at baseline, 15% developed the syndrome over the next 10 years (2). Of these, only 17% consulted their primary care physician with related symptoms at least once in 10 years, and 4% had consulted in the past year. In another study, characteristics of the abdominal complaints did not account for whether patients with irritable bowel syndrome sought health care for their symptoms (3).

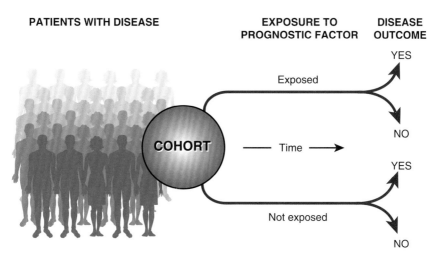

PATIENTS WITH DISEASE   EXPOSURE TO   DISEASE
                                 PROGNOSTIC FACTOR   OUTCOME

Figure 7.2 ■ Design of a cohort study of risk.

ELEMENTS OF PROGNOSTIC STUDIES

Figure 7.2 shows the basic design of a cohort study of prognosis. At best, studies of prognosis are of a defined clinical or geographic population, begin observation at a specified point in time in the course of disease, follow-up all patients for an adequate period of time, and measure clinically important outcomes.

Patient Sample

The purpose of representative sampling from a defined population is to assure that study results have the greatest possible generalizability. It is sometimes possible to study prognosis in a complete sample of patients with new-onset disease in large regions. In some countries, the existence of national medical records makes population-based studies of prognosis possible.

Example

Dutch investigators studied the risk of complications of pregnancy in women with type 1 diabetes mellitus (4). The sample included all of the 323 women in the Netherlands with type 1 diabetes who had become pregnant during a 1-year period and had been under care in one of the nation's 118 hospitals. Most pregnancies were planned, and during pregnancy, most women took folic acid supplements and had good control of their blood sugar. Neverthe-

less, complication rates in newborns were much higher than in the general population. Neonatal morbidity (one or more complications) occurred in 80% of infants and rates of congenital malformations and unusually large newborns (macrosomia) were three-fold to 12-fold higher than in the general population. This study suggests that good control of blood sugar alone was not sufficient to prevent complications of pregnancy in women with type 1 diabetes.

Even without national medical records, population-based studies are possible. In the United States, the Network of Organ Sharing collects data on all patients with transplants, and the Surveillance, Epidemiology, and End Results (SEER) program collects incidence and survival data on all patients with new-onset cancers in several large areas of the country, comprising 28% of the U.S. population. For primary care questions, in the United States and elsewhere, individual practices in communities have banded together into "primary care research networks" to collect research data on their patients' care.

Most studies of prognosis, especially for less common diseases, are of local patients. For these studies, it is especially important to provide the information that users can rely on to decide whether the results generalize to their own situation: patients' characteristics (e.g., age, severity of disease, and comorbidity), the setting where they were found (e.g., primary care practices, community hospitals, or referral centers), and how they were sampled (e.g., complete, random, or convenience sampling). Often, this information is sufficient to establish wide generalizability, for example, in studies of community acquired pneumonia or thrombophlebitis in a local hospital.

Zero Time

Cohorts in prognostic studies should begin from a common point in time in the course of disease, called zero time, such as at the time of the onset of symptoms, diagnosis, or the beginning of treatment. If observation begins at different points in the course of disease for the various patients in a cohort, the description of their prognosis will lack precision, and the timing of recovery, recurrence, death, and other outcome events will be difficult to interpret or will be misleading. The term inception cohort is used to describe a group of patients that is assembled at the onset (inception) of their disease.

Prognosis of cancer is often described separately according to patients' clinical stage (extent of spread) at the beginning of follow-up. If it is, a systematic change in how stage at zero time is established can result in a different prognosis for each stage even if the course of disease is unchanged for each patient in the cohort. This has been shown to happen during staging of cancer—assessing the extent of disease, with higher stages corresponding to more advanced cancer, which is done for the purposes of prognosis and choice of treatment. Stage migration occurs when a newer technology is able to detect the spread of cancer better than an older staging method. Patients who used to be classified in a lower stage are, with the newer technology, classified as being in a higher (more advanced) stage. Removal of patients with more advanced disease from lower stages results in an apparent improvement in prognosis for each stage, regardless of whether treatment is more effective or prognosis for these patients as a whole is better. Stage migration has been called the "Will Rogers phenomenon" after the humorist who said of the geographic migration in the United States during the economic depression of the 1930s, "When the Okies left Oklahoma and moved to California, they raised the average intelligence in both states" (5).

Example

Positron emission tomography (PET) scans, a sensitive test for metastases, are now used to stage non–small cell lung cancers. Investigators compared cancer stages before and after PET scans were in general use and found a 5.4% decline in the number of patients with stage III disease (cancer spread within the chest) and a 8.4% increase in patients with stage IV disease (distant metastases) (6). PET staging was associated with better survival in stage III and stage IV disease, but not earlier stages. The authors concluded that stage migration was responsible for at least some of the apparent improvement in survival in patients with stage III and stage IV lung cancer that occurred after PET scan staging was introduced.

Follow-Up

Patients must be followed for a long enough period of time for most of the clinically important outcome events to have occurred. Otherwise, the observed rate will understate the true one. The appropriate length of follow-up depends on the disease. For studies of surgical site infections, the follow-up period should last for a few weeks, and for studies of the onset of AIDS and its complications in patients with HIV infection, the follow-up period should last several years.

Outcomes of Disease

Descriptions of prognosis should include the full range of manifestations of disease that would be considered important to patients. This means not only death and disease but also pain, anguish, and the inability to care for one's self or pursue usual activities. The 5 Ds—death, disease, discomfort, disability, and dissatisfaction—are a simple way to summarize important clinical outcomes (see Table 1.2).

In their efforts to be "scientific," physicians tend to value precise or technologically measured outcomes, sometimes at the expense of clinical relevance. As discussed in Chapter 1, clinical effects that cannot be directly perceived by patients, such as radiologic reduction in tumor size, normalization of blood chemistries, improvement in ejection fraction, or change in serology, are not clinically useful ends in themselves. It is appropriate to substitute these biologic phenomena for clinical outcomes only when the two are known to be related to each other. Thus, in patients with pneumonia, short-term persistence of abnormalities on chest radiographs may not be alarming if the patient's fever has subsided, energy has returned, and cough has diminished.

Ways to measure patient-centered outcomes are now used in clinical research. Table 7.1 shows a simple measure of quality of life used in studies of cancer

Table 7.1

A Simple Measure of Quality of Life. The Eastern Collaborative Oncology Group's Performance Scale

Performance Status	Definition
0	Asymptomatic
1	Symptomatic, fully ambulatory
2	Symptomatic, in bed <50% of the day
3	Symptomatic, in bed >50% of the day
4	Bedridden
5	Dead

Adapted with permission from Oken MM, Creech RH, Tomey DC, et al. Toxicity and response criteria of the Eastern Oncology Group. Am J Clin Oncol 1982;5:649–655.

treatment. There are also research measures for performance status, health-related quality of life, pain, and other aspects of patient well-being.

DESCRIBING PROGNOSIS

It is convenient to summarize the course of disease as a single rate—the proportion of people experiencing an event during a fixed time period. Some rates used for this purpose are shown in Table 7.2. These

Table 7.2

Rates Commonly Used to Describe Prognosis

Rate	Definition[a]
5-year survival	Percent of patients surviving 5 years from some point in the course of their disease
Case fatality	Percent of patients with a disease who die of it
Disease-specific mortality	Number of people per 10,000 (or 100,000) population dying of a specific disease
Response	Percent of patients showing some evidence of improvement following an intervention
Remission	Percent of patients entering a phase in which disease is no longer detectable
Recurrence	Percent of patients who have return of disease after a disease-free interval

[a]Time under observation is either stated or assumed to be sufficiently long so that all events that will occur have been observed.

rates have in common the same basic components of incidence: events arising in a cohort of patients over time.

A Trade-Off: Simplicity versus More Information

Summarizing prognosis by a single rate has the virtue of simplicity. Rates can be committed to memory and communicated succinctly. Their drawback is that relatively little information is conveyed. Large differences in prognosis can be hidden within similar summary rates.

Figure 7.3 shows 5-year survival rates for patients with four conditions. For each condition, about 10% of the patients are alive at 5 years. However, the clinical courses are otherwise quite different in ways that are very important to patients. Early survival in patients with dissecting aneurysms is very poor, but if they survive the first few months, their risk of dying is much less affected by having had the aneurysm (Fig. 7.3A). Patients with locally invasive, non–small cell lung cancer experience a relatively constant mortality rate throughout the 5 years following diagnosis (Fig. 7.3B). The life of patients with amyotrophic lateral sclerosis (ALS, Lou Gehrig disease, a slowly progressive paralysis) and respiratory difficulties is not immediately threatened, but as neurologic function continues to decline over the years, the inability to breathe without assistance leads to death (Fig. 7.3C). Figure 7.3D is a benchmark. Only at age 100 years do people in the general population have a 5-year survival rate comparable to that of patients with the three diseases.

Survival Analysis

When interpreting prognosis, it is preferable to know the likelihood, on average, that patients with a given condition will experience an outcome at any point in time. Prognosis expressed as a summary rate does not contain this information. However, figures can show information about average time to event for any point in the course of disease. By **event**, we mean a dichotomous clinical outcome that can occur only once. In the following discussion, we take the common approach of describing outcomes in terms of "survival," but the same methods apply to the reverse (time to death) and to any other outcome event such as cancer recurrence, cure of infection, freedom from symptoms, or arthritis becoming inactive.

Survival of a Cohort

The most straightforward way to learn about survival is to assemble a cohort of patients who have the

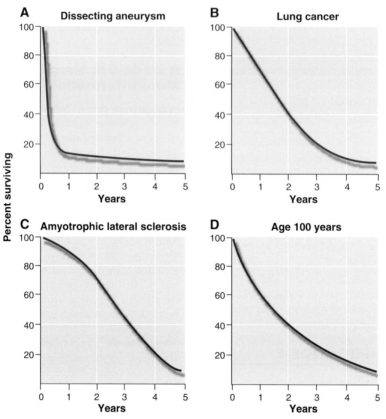

Figure 7.3 ■ A limitation of 5-year survival rates: Four conditions with the same 5-year survival rate of 10%.

condition of interest and are at the same point in the course of their illness (e.g., onset of symptoms, diagnosis, or beginning of treatment), and then keep them all under observation until all experience the outcome or not. For a small cohort, one might then represent these patients' clinical course, as shown in Figure 7.4A. The plot of survival against time displays steps corresponding to the death of each of the 10 patients in the cohort. If the number of patients were increased, the size of the steps would diminish. If a very large number of patients were studied, the figure would approximate a smooth curve (Fig. 7.4B). This information could then be used to predict the year-by-year, or even week-by-week, prognosis of similar patients.

Unfortunately, obtaining the information in this way is impractical for several reasons. Some of the patients might drop out of the study before the end of the follow-up period, perhaps because of another illness, a move from the study area, or dissatisfaction with the study. These patients would have to be excluded from the cohort even though considerable effort had been exerted to gather data on them until

the point at which they dropped out. Also, it would be necessary to wait until all of the cohort's members had reached each point in follow-up before the probability of surviving to that point could be calculated. Because patients ordinarily become available for a study over a period of time, at any point in calendar time, there would be a relatively long follow-up for patients who had entered the study first, but only brief experience with those who had entered more recently. The last patient who entered the study would have to reach each year of follow-up before any information on survival to that year would be available.

Survival Curves

To make efficient use of all available data from each patient in the cohort, survival analysis has been developed to *estimate* the survival of a cohort over time. The usual method is called Kaplan-Meier analysis, after its originators. Survival analysis can be applied to any outcomes that are dichotomous and occur only once during follow-up (e.g., time to

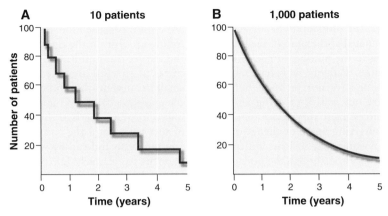

Figure 7.4 ■ Survival of two cohorts, small and large, when all members are observed for the full period of follow-up.

coronary event or to recurrence of cancer). A more general term, useful when an event other than survival is described, is time-to-event analysis.

Figure 7.5 shows a simplified survival curve. On the vertical axis is the estimated probability of surviving, and on the horizontal axis is the period of time from the beginning of observation (zero time).

The probability of surviving to any point in time is estimated from the cumulative probability of surviving each of the time intervals that preceded it. Time intervals can be made as small as necessary; in Kaplan-Meir analyses, the intervals are between each new event, such as death, and the preceding one, however short or long that is. Most of the time,

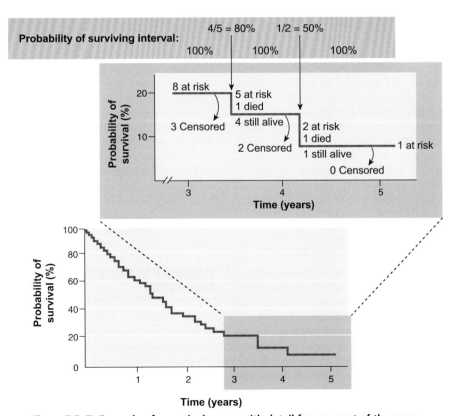

Figure 7.5 ■ Example of a survival curve, with detail for one part of the curve.

no one dies and the probability of surviving is 1. When a patient dies, the probability of surviving at that moment is calculated as the ratio of the number of patients surviving to the number at risk of dying at that point in time. Patients who have already died, dropped out, or have not yet been followed up to that point are not at risk of dying and are, therefore, not used to estimate survival for that time. The probability of surviving does not change during intervals in which no one dies, so it is recalculated only when there is a death. Although the probability at any given interval is not very accurate, because either nothing has happened or there has been only one event in a large cohort, the overall probability of surviving up to each point in time (the product of all preceding probabilities) is remarkably accurate. When patients are lost from the study at any point in time, they are referred to as **censored** and are no longer counted in the denominator from that point forward.

A part of the survival curve in Figure 7.5 (from 3 to 5 years after zero time) is presented in detail to illustrate the data used to estimate survival: patients at risk, patients no longer at risk (censored), and patients experiencing outcome events at each point in time.

Variations on basic survival curves increase the amount of information they convey. Including the numbers of patients at risk at various points in time gives some idea of the contribution of chance to the observed rates, especially toward the end of follow-up. The vertical axis can show the proportion with, rather than without, the outcome event; the resulting curve will sweep upward and to the right. The precision of survival estimates, which declines with time because fewer and fewer patients are still under observation, can be shown by confidence intervals at various points in time (see Chapter 11). Tics are sometimes added to the survival curves to indicate each time a patient is censored.

Interpreting Survival Curves

Several points must be kept in mind when interpreting survival curves. First, the vertical axis represents the *estimated* probability of surviving for members of the cohort, not the cumulative incidence of surviving if all members of the cohort were followed up.

Second, points on a survival curve are the best estimate, for a given set of data, of the probability of survival for members of a cohort. However, the precision of these estimates depends on the number of patients on whom the estimate is based, as do all observations of samples. One can be more confident that the estimates on the left-hand side of the curve are sound, because more patients are at risk early in follow-up. But on the right-hand side, at the tail of the curve, the number of patients on whom estimates of survival are based may become relatively small because deaths, dropouts, and late entrants to the study, so that fewer and fewer patients are followed for that length of time. As a result, estimates of survival toward the end of the follow-up period are imprecise and can be strongly affected by what happens to relatively few patients. For example, in Figure 7.5, only one patient was under observation at year 5. If that one remaining patient happened to die, the probability of surviving would fall from 8% to zero. Clearly, this would be a too literal reading of the data. Therefore, estimates of survival at the tails of survival curves must be interpreted with caution.

Finally, the shape of many survival curves gives the impression that outcome events occurs more frequently early in follow-up than later on, when the slope approaches a plateau. But this impression is deceptive. As time passes, rates of survival are being applied to a diminishing number of patients, causing the slope of the curve to flatten even if the rate of outcome events did not change.

As with any estimate, Kaplan-Meier estimates of time to event depend on assumptions. It is assumed that being censored is not related to prognosis. To the extent that this is not true, a survival analysis may yield biased estimates of survival in cohorts. The Kaplan-Meier method may not be accurate enough if there are competing risks—more than one kind of outcome event—and the outcomes are not independent of each other such that one event changes the probability of experiencing the other. For example, patients with cancer who develop an infection related to aggressive chemotherapy and drop out for that reason may have had a different chance of dying of the cancer. There are other methods for estimating cumulative incidence in the presence of competing risks.

IDENTIFYING PROGNOSTIC FACTORS

Often, studies go beyond a simple description of prognosis in a homogeneous group of patients to compare prognosis in patients with different characteristics, that is, they identify prognostic factors. Multiple survival curves, one for patients with each of the characteristics, are represented on the same figure where they can be visually (and statistically) compared.

Patients with renal cell carcinoma, like many other cancers, have widely different chances of surviving over the several years after diagnosis. Prognosis varies according to characteristics of the cancer and patient, such as stage (how far the cancer has spread, from being limited to the kidney at one extreme to metastases to distant organs at the other), grade (how abnormal the cancer cells appear), and performance status (how well patients are able to care for themselves). A study combined these three characteristics into five prognostic groups (Fig. 7.6) (7). In the most favorable group, more than 90% of patients were alive at 8 years, whereas in the least favorable group, all were dead at 3 years. This information might be especially useful in helping patients and doctors understand what lies ahead, and it is much more informative than simply saying that "overall, 70% of patients with renal cell carcinoma survive 5 years."

The effects of one prognostic factor relative to the effects of another can be summarized from data in a time-to-even analysis by a hazard ratio, which is analogous to a risk ratio (relative risk). Also, survival curves can be compared after taking into account other factors related to prognosis so that the independent effect of just one variable is examined.

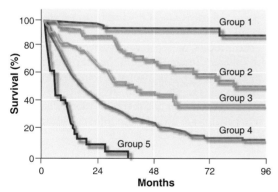

Figure 7.6 ■ Example of prognostic stratification. Survival from surgery in a patient with renal cell cancer according to prognostic strata. (Redrawn with permission from Zisman A, Pantuck AJ, Dorey F, et al. Improved prognostification for renal cell carcinoma using an integrated staging system. J Clin Oncol 2001;19:1649–1657.)

CASE SERIES

A case series is a description of the course of disease in a small number of cases, a few dozen at most. An even smaller report, with fewer than 10 patients, is called a case report. Cases are typically found at a clinic or referral center and then followed forward in time to describe the course of disease and backward in time to describe what came earlier.

Such reports can make an important contribution to understanding of disease, primarily by describing experiences with newly defined syndromes or uncommon conditions. The reason for introducing case series into a chapter about prognosis is that they may masquerade as true cohort studies even though they do not have comparable strengths.

Physicians in emergency departments see patients with bites from North American rattlesnakes. These bites are relatively uncommon at any one place, making it difficult to carry out large cohort studies of their clinical course, so physicians must rely mainly on case series. An example is a description of the clinical course of all 24 children managed at a children's hospital in California during a 10-year period (8). Nineteen of the children were actually injected with venom, and they were managed with the aggressive use of antivenin. Three had surgical treatment to remove soft-tissue debris or relieve tissue pressure. There were no serious reactions to antivenin, and all patients left the hospital without functional impairment.

Physicians caring for children with rattlesnake bites would be grateful for this and other case series if there were no better information to guide their care, but that is not to say that the case series provided a complete and fully reliable picture of snake-bite care. Of all children bitten in that region, some may have been doing so well after a bite that they were not sent to the referral center. Others might have been doing so badly that they were rushed to the nearest hospital or even died before reaching a hospital at all. In other words, the case series does not describe the clinical course of all children from the time of snakebite (the inception) but rather a selected sample of children who happened to come under care at that particular hospital. In effect, case series describe the clinical course of prevalent, not necessarily a representative sample of incident cases, so they are "false" cohorts.

CLINICAL PREDICTION RULES

A combination of variables can provide a more precise prognosis than any of these variables taken one at a time. As discussed in Chapter 4, clinical prediction rules estimate the probability of outcomes (either prognosis or diagnosis) according to a set of patient characteristics defined by history, physical examination, and simple laboratory tests. They are "rules" because they are often tied to recommendations about further diagnostic evaluation or treatment. To make prediction rules workable in clinical settings, they depend on data that are available in the usual care of patients and scoring, the basis for the prediction, that has been simplified.

Example

Atrial fibrillation causes an increased risk of stroke. Clots form in the atria in the absence of regular, organized contractions and, if dislodged, can travel to the brain causing an embolic stroke. This complication can be prevented by anticoagulation but at the risk of bleeding. Clinicians and patients must weigh the risk of stroke in the absence of treatment against the risk of bleeding complications with treatment. To assist in this decision, a clinical prediction rule called CHADS2 has been developed and validated (9). A set of five readily available clinical observations are used to separate patients with atrial fibrillation into six risk strata with a 14-fold difference in risk of stroke (Table 7.3). The aggressiveness of anticoagulation is in turn tied to the CHADS2 score (10). For example, typical recommendations based on risk of stroke and effectiveness of anticoagulation are that patients with a CHADS2 score of 0 have no anticoagulation, those with a score of 1 are treated with aspirin or oral anticoagulation, and those with a score of at least 2 are treated with oral anticoagulation, the most aggressive treatment.

Table 7.3

The CHADS2 Score and Risk of Stroke According to CHADS2 Score

☐ Diagnosis of heart failure, past or current (1 point)
☐ Hypertension treated or untreated (1 point)
☐ Age ≥75 years (1 point)
☐ Diabetes mellitus (1 point)
☐ Secondary prevention in patients with prior ischemic stroke, transient ischemic attack, or thromboembolism (2 points)

CHADS2 score = total point count

CHADS2 Points	Stroke Risk per 100 Person-Years
0	0.49
1	1.52
2	2.50
3	5.27
4	6.02
5–6	6.88

Reproduced as published in UpToDate, Calculation: Atrial Fibrillation CHADS(2) Score for Stroke Risk, with permission from MedCalc 3000 by Foundation Internet, Pittsburgh, PA.

A clinical prediction rule should be developed in one setting and tested in others—with different patients, physicians, and usual care practices—to assure that predictions are good for a broad range of settings and not just for where it was developed, because it might have been the result of the particular characteristics of that setting. The data used to develop the prediction rule is called the training set, and the data used to assess its validity is called the test set, which is used for validation of the prediction rule.

The process of separating patients into groups with different prognosis, as in the previous example, is called prognostic stratification. In this case, atrial fibrillation is the disease and stroke is the outcome. The concept is similar to risk stratification (Chapter 4), where patients are divided into different strata of risk for developing disease.

BIAS IN COHORT STUDIES

In cohort studies of risk or prognosis, bias can alter the description of the course of disease. Bias can also create apparent differences between groups when differences do not actually exist in nature or obscure differences when they really do exist. These biases have their counterparts in case-control studies as well.

They are a separate consideration from confounding and effect modification (Chapter 5).

There are an almost infinite variety of systematic errors, many of which are given specific names, but some are more basic. They can be recognized more easily when one knows where they are most likely to occur in the course of a study. With that in mind, we describe some possibilities for bias in cohort studies and discuss them in relation to the following study of prognosis.

Example

Bell's palsy is the sudden, one-sided, unexplained onset of weakness of the face in the area innervated by the facial nerve. Often, the cause is unknown, although some cases are associated with herpes simplex or herpes zoster infections, diabetes, pregnancy, and a variety of other conditions. What is the clinical course? Investigators in Denmark followed up 1,701 patients with Bell palsy once a month until function returned or 1 year (11). Recovery reached its maximum within 3 weeks in 85% of patients and in 3 to 5 months in the remaining 15%. By that time, 71% of patients had recovered fully; for the rest, the remaining loss of function was slight in 12%, mild in 13%, and severe in 4%. Recovery was related to younger age, less initial palsy, and earlier onset of recovery.

When thinking about the validity of this study, one should consider at least the following.

Sampling Bias

Sampling bias has occurred when the patients in a study are not like other patients with the condition. Were patients in this study like others with Bell palsy? The answer depends on the user's perspective. Patients were "from the Copenhagen area" and apparently under the care of an ear, nose, and throat specialist, so the results generalize to other referred patients (as long as we accept that Bell palsy in Denmark is similar to this condition in other parts of the world). However, mild cases might not have been included because they were managed by local clinicians and quickly recovered or not brought to medical attention at all, which limits the applicability in primary care settings.

Sampling bias can also be misleading when prognosis is compared across groups and sampling has produced groups that are systematically different with respect to prognosis, even before the factor of interest is considered. In the Bell palsy example, older patients might have had a worse prognosis because they are the ones who had an underlying herpes virus infection, not because of their age.

Is this not confounding? Strictly speaking, it is not because the study is for the purpose of prediction, not to identify independent "causes" of recovery. Also, it is not plausible to consider such phenomena as severity of palsy or onset of recovery as causes because they are probably part of the chain of events leading from disease to recovery. But to the extent that one wants to show that prognostic factors are independent predictors of outcome, the same approaches as are used for confounding (Chapter 5) can be used to establish independence.

Migration Bias

Migration bias is present when some patients drop out of the study during follow-up and they are systematically different from those who remain. It is often the case that some members of the original cohort leave a study over time. (Patients are assured that this is their right as part of the ethical conduct of research on humans.) If dropout occurs randomly, such that the characteristics of lost patients are on average similar to patients who remain, then there would be no bias. This is so regardless of whether the number of dropouts is large or similar in the cohorts being compared, but ordinarily the characteristics of lost patients are not the same as those who remain in a study. Dropping out tends to be related to prognosis. For example, patients who are doing especially well or badly with their Bell palsy may be more likely to leave the study, as would those who need care for other illnesses, for whom the extra visits related to the study would be burdensome. This would distort the main (descriptive) results of the study—rate and completeness of recovery. If the study also aims to identify prognostic factors (e.g., recovery in old versus young patients), that also could be biased by patients dropping out, for the same reasons.

Migration bias might be seen as an example of selection bias because patients who were still in the study when outcomes were measured were selected from all those who began in the study. Migration bias might be considered an example of measurement bias because patients who migrate out of the study are no longer available when outcomes are measured.

Measurement Bias

Measurement bias is present when members of the cohort are not all assessed similarly for outcome. In the Bell palsy study, all members of the cohort were examined by a common protocol every month until they were no longer improving, ruling out this possibility. If it had been left to individual patients and physicians whether, when, and how they were examined, this would have diminished confidence in the description of time to and completeness of recovery. Measurement bias also comes into play if prognostic groups are compared and patients in one group have a systematically better chance of having outcomes detected than those in another. Some outcomes, such as death, cardiovascular catastrophes, and major cancers, are so obvious that they are unlikely to be missed. But for less clear-cut outcomes, including specific cause of death, subclinical disease, side effects, or disability, measurement bias can occur because of differences in the methods with which the outcome is sought or classified.

Measurement bias can be minimized in three general ways: (i) examine all members of the cohort equally for outcome events; (ii) if comparisons of prognostic groups are made, ensure that researchers are unaware of the group to which each patient belongs; and (iii) set up careful rules for deciding if an outcome event has occurred (and follow the rules). To help readers understand the extent of these kinds of biases in a given study, it is usual practice to include, with reports of the study, a flow diagram describing how the number of participants changed as the study progressed and why. It is also helpful to compare the characteristics of patients in and out of the study after sampling and follow-up.

Bias from "Non-differential" Misclassification

Until now, we have been discussing how the results of a study can be biased when there are systematic differences in how exposure or disease groups are classified. But bias can also result if misclassification is "non-differential," that is, it occurs similarly in the groups being compared. In this case, the bias is toward finding no effect.

Example

When cigarette smoking is assessed by simply asking people whether they smoke, there is substantial misclassification relative to a gold standard such as the presence or absence of cigarette products in saliva. Yet in a cohort study of cigarette smoking and coronary heart disease (CHD), misclassification of smoking could not be different in people who did or did not develop CHD because the outcome was not known at the time exposure was assessed. Even so, to the extent that smoking is incorrectly classified, it reduces whatever differences in CHD rates in smokers and non-smokers that might have existed if all patients had been correctly classified, making a "null" effect more likely. At the extreme, if classifying smoking status were totally at random, there could be no association between smoking and CHD.

BIAS, PERHAPS, BUT DOES IT MATTER?

Clinical epidemiology is not an error-finding game. Rather, it is meant to characterize the credibility of a study so that clinicians can decide how much to rely on its results when making high-stakes decisions about patients. It would be irresponsible to ignore results of studies that meet high standards, just as clinical decisions need not be bound by the results of weak studies.

With this in mind, it is not enough to recognize that bias might be present in a study. One must go on to determine if bias is actually present in the particular study. Beyond that, one must decide whether the consequences of bias are sufficiently large that they change the conclusions in a clinically important way. If damage to the study's conclusions is not very great, then the presence of bias is of little practical consequence and the study is still useful.

SENSITIVITY ANALYSIS

One way to decide how much bias might change the conclusions of a study is to do a sensitivity analysis, that is, to show how much larger or smaller the observed results might have been under various assumptions about the missing data or potentially biased measurements. A best-case/worst-case analysis tests the effects of the most extreme possible assumptions but is an unreasonably severe test for the effects of bias in most situations. More often, sensitivity analyses test the effects of somewhat unlikely values, as in the following example.

Example

Poliomyelitis has been eradicated in many parts of the world but late effects of infection continue. Some patients develop post-polio syndrome (muscle weakness, pain, and fatigue) many years after the original infection. To describe the rate of post-polio syndrome, investigators identified a cohort of 939 patients who had had poliomyelitis in the 1950 s (12). Up to 40 years later, they were able to get information about symptoms for 551 members of the cohort, and in them the rate of post-polio syndrome was 137 of 551 (25%). Understandably, after so many years, 388 patients could not be followed-up.

If the missing members of the cohort had different rates of post-polio syndrome from those who were followed-up, how much could they have biased the observed rate of post-polio syndrome? If patients who were not followed up were twice as likely to get post-polio

syndrome as those who were, the true rate would have been (137 + 194)/939 = 35%. (That is, all 137 patients known to have the syndrome plus 50% of those who were not followed up divided by all members of the original cohort.) If the missing patients were half as likely to get the syndrome, the true rate would have been (137 + 48)/939 = 20%. Thus, even with an improbably large difference in post-polio syndrome rates in missing patients, the true rate would still have been in the 20% to 35% range, a useful approximation for clinical use.

More or less extreme differences could have been assumed for the missing patients to explore how "sensitive" the study result were to missing members of the cohort. Sensitivity analysis is a useful way of estimating how much various kinds of bias could have affected the results of studies of all kinds—cohort and case-control studies of risk or prognosis, the accuracy of diagnostic tests, or clinical trials of the effectiveness of treatment or prevention.

Review Questions

Read the following and select the best response.

7.1. For a study of the risk of esophageal cancer in patients with Barrett esophagus (a precancerous lesion), which of the following times in the course of disease is the best example of zero time?

A. Diagnosis of Barrett esophagus for each patient
B. Death of each patient
C. Diagnosis of esophageal cancer for each patient
D. Calendar time when the first patient is enrolled in the study
E. Calendar time when no patient remains in the study

7.2. A cohort study describes the recurrence of seizure within 1 year in children hospitalized with a first febrile seizure. It compared recurrence in children who had infection versus immunization as an underlying cause for fever at the time of the first seizure. Some

of the children were no longer in the study when outcome (a second seizure) was assessed at 1 year. Which of the following would have the greatest effect on study results?

A. Why the children dropped out
B. When in the course of follow-up the children left the study
C. Whether dropping out was related to prognosis
D. Whether the number of children dropping out is similar in the groups

7.3. A cohort study of prostate cancer care compares rates of incontinence in patients who were treated with surgery versus medical care alone. Incontinence is assessed from review of medical records. Which of the following is *not* an example of measurement bias?

A. Men were more likely to tell their surgeon about incontinence.
B. Surgeons were less likely to record complications of their surgery in the record.

C. Men who got surgery were more likely to have follow-up visits.
D. Chart abstractors used their judgment is deciding whether incontinence was present or not.
E. Rates of incontinence were higher in the men who got surgery.

7.4. A clinical prediction rule has been developed to classify the prognosis of community-acquired pneumonia. Which of the following is most characteristic of such a clinical prediction rule?

A. Calculating a score is simple.
B. The clinical data are readily available.
C. Multiple prognostic factors are included.
D. The results are used to guide further management of the patient.
E. All of the above.

7.5. A study describes the clinical course of patients who have an uncommon neurologic disease. Patients are identified at a referral center that specializes in this disease. Their medical records are reviewed for patients' characteristics, treatments, and their current disease status. Which of the following best describes this kind of study?

A. Cohort study
B. Case-control study
C. Case series
D. Cross-sectional study
E. A randomized controlled trial

7.6. A study used time-to-event analysis to describe the survival from diagnosis of 100 patients with congestive heart failure. By the third year, 60 patients have been censored. Which of the following would *not* be a reason for one of these patients being censored?

A. The patient died of another cause before year 3.
B. The patient decided not to continue in the study.
C. The patient developed another disease that could be fatal.
D. The patient had been enrolled in the study for less than 3 years.

7.7. Which of the following kinds of studies *cannot* be used to identify prognostic factors?

A. Prevalence study
B. Time-to-event analysis
C. Case-control study
D. Cohort study

7.8. Which of the following best describes the information in a survival curve?

A. An unbiased estimate of survival even if some patients leave the study
B. The estimated probability of survival from zero time
C. The proportion of a cohort still alive at the end of follow-up
D. The rate at which original members of the cohort leave the study
E. The cumulative survival of a cohort over time

7.9. Which of the following is the most appropriate sample for a study of prognosis?

A. Members of the general population
B. Patients in primary care in the community
C. Patients admitted to a community hospital
D. Patients referred to a specialist
E. It depends on who will use the results of the study.

7.10. Investigators wish to describe the clinical course of multiple sclerosis. They take advantage of a clinical trial, already completed, in which control patients received usual care. Patients in the trial had been identified at referral centers, had been enrolled at the time of diagnosis, and had met rigorous entry criteria. After 10 years, all patients had been examined yearly and remained under observation, and 40% were still able to walk. Which of the following most limits the credibility of this study?

A. Inconsistent zero time
B. Generalizability
C. Measurement bias
D. Migration bias
E. Failure to use time-to-event methods

7.11. Many different clinical prediction rules have been developed to assess the severity of community-acquired pneumonia. Which of the following is the most important reason for choosing one to use?

A. The prediction rule classifies patients into groups with very different prognosis.
B. The prediction rule has been validated in different settings.
C. Many variables are included in the rule.
D. Prognostic factors include state-of-the-science diagnostic tests.
E. The score is calculated using computers.

7.12. In a study of patients who smoke and developed peripheral arterial disease, the hazard ratio for amputation in patients who continued to smoke, relative to those who quit smoking, is 5. Which of the following best characterizes the hazard ratio?

A. In this study, it is the rate of continued smoking divided by the rate of quitting.
B. It can be estimated from a case-control study of smoking and amputation.
C. It cannot be adjusted for the presence or absence of other factors related to prognosis.
D. It conveys information similar to relative risk.
E. It is calculated from the cumulative incidence of amputation in smokers and quitters.

7.13. In a time-to-event analyses, the event:

A. Can occur only once
B. Is dichotomous
C. Both A and B
D. Neither A nor B

Answers are in Appendix A.

REFERENCES

1. Canto JG, Kiefe CI, Rogers WJ, et al. Number if coronary heart disease risk factors and mortality in patients with first myocardial infarction. JAMA 2011;306:2120–2127.
2. Talley NJ, Zinsmeister AR, Van Dyke C, et al. Epidemiology of colonic symptoms and the irritable bowel syndrome. Gastroenterology 1991;101:927–934.
3. Ford AC, Forman D, Bailey AG, et al. Irritable bowel syndrome: A 10-year natural history of symptoms and factors that influence consultation behavior. Am J Gastroenterol 2007; 103:1229–1239.
4. Evers IM, de Valk HW, Visser GHA. Risk of complications of pregnancy in women with type 1 diabetes: Nationwide prospective study in the Netherlands. BMJ 2004;328:915–918.
5. Feinstein AR, Sosin DM, Wells CK. The Will Rogers phenomenon: stage migration and new diagnostic techniques as a source of misleading statistics for survival in cancer. N Engl J Med 1985;312:1604–1608.
6. Chee KG, Nguyen DV, Brown M, et al. Positron emission tomography and improved survival in patients with lung cancer. The Will Rogers phenomenon revisited. Arch Intern Med 2008;168:1541–1549.
7. Zisman A, Pantuck AJ, Dorey F, et al. Improved prognostification for renal cell carcinoma using an integrated staging system. J Clin Oncol 2001;19:1649–1657.
8. Shaw BA, Hosalkar HS. Rattlesnake bites in children: antivenin treatment and surgical indications. J Bone Joint Surg Am 2002;84-A(9):1624.
9. Gage BF, Waterman AD, Shannon W, et al. Validation of clinical classification schemes for predicting stroke. Results from the National Registry of Atrial Fibrillation. JAMA 2001; 285:2864–2870.
10. Go AS, Hylek EM, Chang Y, et al. Anticoagulation therapy for stroke prevention in atrial fibrillation. How well do randomized trials translate into clinical practice? JAMA 2003;290:2685–2692.
11. Peitersen E. Bell's palsy: the spontaneous course of 2,500 peripheral facial nerve palsies of different etiologies. Acta Otolaryngol 2002;(549):4–30.
12. Ramlow J, Alexander M, LaPorte R, et al. Epidemiology of post-polio syndrome. Am J Epidemiol 1992;136:769–785.

Chapter 8

Diagnosis

Appearances to the mind are of four kinds. Things either are what they appear to be; or they neither are, nor appear to be; or they are, and do not appear to be; or they are not, yet appear to be. Rightly to aim in all these cases is the wise man's task.

—Epictetus[†]
2nd century A.D.

KEY WORDS

Diagnostic test
True positive
True negative
False positive
False negative
Gold standard
Reference standard
Criterion standard
Sensitivity
Specificity
Cutoff point
Receiver operator
    characteristic
    (ROC) curve
Spectrum
Bias
Predictive value
Positive predictive
    value

Negative predictive
    value
Posterior (posttest)
    probability
Accuracy
Prevalence
Prior (pretest)
    probability
Likelihood ratio
Probability
Odds
Pretest odds
Posttest odds
Parallel testing
Serial testing
Clinical prediction
    rules
Diagnostic decision-
    making rules

Clinicians spend a great deal of time diagnosing complaints or abnormalities in their patients, generally arriving at a diagnosis after applying various diagnostic tests. Clinicians should be familiar with basic principles when interpreting diagnostic tests. This chapter deals with those principles.

A diagnostic test is ordinarily understood to mean a test performed in a laboratory, but the principles discussed in this chapter apply equally well to clinical information obtained from history, physical examination, and imaging procedures. They also apply when a constellation of findings serves as a diagnostic test. Thus, one might speak of the value of prodromal neurologic symptoms, headache, nausea, and vomiting in diagnosing classic migraine, or of hemoptysis and weight loss in a cigarette smoker as an indication of lung cancer.

SIMPLIFYING DATA

In Chapter 3, we pointed out that clinical measurements, including data from diagnostic tests, are expressed on nominal, ordinal, or interval scales. Regardless of the kind of data produced by diagnostic tests, clinicians generally reduce the data to a simpler form to make them useful in practice. Most ordinal scales are examples of this simplification process. Heart murmurs can vary from very loud to barely audible, but trying to express subtle gradations in the intensity of murmurs is unnecessary for clinical decision making. A simple ordinal scale—grades I to VI—serves just as well. More often, complex data are reduced to a simple dichotomy (e.g., present/absent, abnormal/normal, or diseased/well). This is done particularly when test results are used to help determine treatment decisions, such as the degree of anemia that requires transfusion. For any given test result, therapeutic decisions are either/or decisions; either treatment is begun or it is withheld. When there are gradations of therapy according to the test result, the data are being treated in an ordinal fashion.

[†]A 19th Century physician and proponent of the "numerical method" (relying on counts, not impressions) to understand the natural history of diseases such as typhoid fever.

The use of blood pressure data to decide about therapy is an example of how information can be simplified for practical clinical purposes. Blood pressure is ordinarily measured to the nearest 1 mm Hg (i.e., on an interval scale). However, most hypertension treatment guidelines, such as those of the Joint National Committee on the Detection, Evaluation, and Treatment of Hypertension (1), choose a particular level (e.g., 140 mm Hg systolic pressure or 90 mm Hg diastolic pressure) at which to initiate drug treatment. In doing so, they transformed interval data into dichotomous data. To take the example further, turning the data into an ordinal scale, the Joint National Committee also recommends that physicians choose a treatment plan according to whether the patient's blood pressure is "prehypertension" (systolic 120 to 139 mm Hg or diastolic 80 to 89 mm Hg), "stage 1 hypertension" (systolic 140 to 159 mm Hg or diastolic 90 to 99 mm Hg), or "stage 2 hypertension" (systolic ≥160 mm Hg or diastolic ≥100 mm Hg).

THE ACCURACY OF A TEST RESULT

Diagnosis is an imperfect process, resulting in a probability rather than a certainty of being right. The doctor's certainty or uncertainty about a diagnosis has been expressed by using terms such as "rule out" or "possible" before a clinical diagnosis. Increasingly, clinicians express the likelihood that a patient has a disease as a probability. That being the case, it behooves the clinician to become familiar with the mathematical relationships between the properties of diagnostic tests and the information they yield in various clinical situations. In many instances, understanding these issues will help the clinician reduce diagnostic uncertainty. In other situations, it may only increase understanding of the degree of uncertainty. Occasionally, it may even convince the clinician to increase his or her level of uncertainty.

A simple way of looking at the relationships between a test's results and the true diagnosis is shown in Figure 8.1. The test is considered to be either positive (abnormal) or negative (normal), and the disease is either present or absent. There are then four possible types of test results, two that are correct (true)

Figure 8.1 ■ The relationship between a diagnostic test result and the occurrence of disease. There are two possibilities for the test result to be correct (true positive and true negative) and two possibilities for the result to be incorrect (false positive and false negative).

and two that are wrong (false). The test has given the correct result when it is positive in the presence of disease (true positive) or negative in the absence of the disease (true negative). On the other hand, the test has been misleading if it is positive when the disease is absent (false positive) or negative when the disease is present (false negative).

The Gold Standard

A test's accuracy is considered in relation to some way of knowing whether the disease is truly present or not—a sounder indication of the truth often referred to as the gold standard (or reference standard or criterion standard). Sometimes the standard of accuracy is itself a relatively simple and inexpensive test, such as a rapid streptococcal antigen test (RSAT) for group A streptococcus to validate the clinical impression of strep throat or an antibody test for human immunodeficiency virus infection. More often, one must turn to relatively elaborate, expensive, or risky tests to be certain whether the disease is present or absent. Among these are biopsy, surgical exploration, imaging procedures, and of course, autopsy.

For diseases that are not self-limited and ordinarily become overt over several months or even years after a test is done, the results of follow-up can serve as a gold standard. Screening for most cancers and chronic, degenerative diseases fall into this category. For them, validation is possible even if on-the-spot confirmation of a test's performance is not feasible because the immediately available gold standard is too risky, involved, or expensive. If follow-up is used, the length of the follow-up period must be long enough for the disease to declare itself, but not so long that new cases can arise after the original testing (see Chapter 10).

Because it is almost always more costly, more dangerous, or both to use more accurate ways of establishing the truth, clinicians and patients prefer simpler tests to the rigorous gold standard, at least initially. Chest x-rays and sputum smears are used to determine the cause of pneumonia, rather than bronchoscopy and lung biopsy for examination of the diseased lung tissue. Electrocardiograms and blood tests are used first to investigate the possibility of acute myocardial infarction, rather than catheterization or imaging procedures. The simpler tests are used as proxies for more elaborate but more accurate or precise ways of establishing the presence of disease, with the understanding that some risk of misclassification results. This risk is justified by the safety and convenience of the simpler tests. But simpler tests are only useful when the risks of misclassification are known and are acceptably low. This requires a sound comparison of their accuracy to an appropriate standard.

Lack of Information on Negative Tests

The goal of all clinical studies aimed at describing the value of diagnostic tests should be to obtain data for all four of the cells shown in Figure 8.1. Without all these data, it is not possible to fully evaluate the accuracy of the test. Most information about the value of a diagnostic test is obtained from clinical, not research, settings. Under these circumstances, physicians are using the test in the care of patients. Because of ethical concerns, they usually do not feel justified in proceeding with more exhaustive evaluation when preliminary diagnostic tests are negative. They are naturally reluctant to initiate an aggressive workup, with its associated risk and expense, unless preliminary tests are positive. As a result, data on the number of true negatives and false negatives generated by a test (cells c and d in Fig. 8.1) tend to be much less complete in the medical literature than data collected about positive test results.

This problem can arise in studies of screening tests because individuals with negative tests usually are not subjected to further testing, especially if the testing involves invasive procedures such as biopsies. One method that can get around this problem is to make use of stored blood or tissue banks. An investigation of prostate-specific antigen (PSA) testing for prostate cancer examined stored blood from men who subsequently developed prostate cancer and men who did not develop prostate cancer (2). The results showed that for a PSA level of 4.0 ng/mL, sensitivity over the subsequent 4 years was 73% and specificity was 91%. The investigators were able to fill in all four cells

without requiring further testing on people with negative test results. (See the following text for definitions of sensitivity and specificity.)

Lack of Information on Test Results in the Nondiseased

Some types of tests are commonly abnormal in people without disease or complaints. When this is so, the test's performance can be grossly misleading when the test is applied to patients with the condition or complaint.

Example

Magnetic resonance imaging (MRI) of the lumbar spine is used in the evaluation of patients with low back pain. Many patients with back pain show herniated intervertebral discs on MRI, and the pain is often attributed to the finding. But, how often are vertebral disc abnormalities found in people who do not have back pain? Several studies done on subjects without a history of back pain or sciatica have found herniated discs in 22% to 58% and bulging discs in 24% to 79% of asymptomatic subjects with mean ages of 35 to more than 60 years old (3). In other words, vertebral disc abnormalities are common and may be a coincidental finding in a patient with back pain.

Lack of Objective Standards for Disease

For some conditions, there are simply no hard-and-fast criteria for diagnosis. Angina pectoris is one of these. The clinical manifestations were described nearly a century ago, yet there is still no better way to substantiate the presence of angina pectoris than a carefully taken history. Certainly, a great many objectively measurable phenomena are related to this clinical syndrome, for example, the presence of coronary artery stenosis on angiography, delayed perfusion on a thallium stress test, and characteristic abnormalities on electrocardiograms both at rest and with exercise. All are more commonly found in patients believed to have angina pectoris, but none is so closely tied to the clinical syndrome that it can serve as the standard by which the condition is considered present or absent.

Other examples of medical conditions difficult to diagnose because of the lack of simple gold standard tests include hot flashes, Raynaud's disease, irritable bowel syndrome, and autism. In an effort to standardize practice, expert groups often develop lists of symptoms and other test results that can be used in combination to diagnose the clinical condition. Because there is no gold standard, however, it is possible that these lists are not entirely correct. Circular reasoning can occur—the validity of a laboratory test is established by comparing its results to a clinical diagnosis based on a careful history of symptoms and a physical examination, but once established, the test is then used to validate the clinical diagnosis gained from history and physical examination!

Consequences of Imperfect Gold Standards

Because of such difficulties, it is sometimes not possible for physicians in practice to find information on how well the tests they use compare with a thoroughly trustworthy standard. They must choose as their standard of validity another test that admittedly is imperfect, but is considered the best available. This may force them into comparing one imperfect test against another, with one being taken as a standard of validity because it has had longer use or is considered superior by a consensus of experts. In doing so, a paradox may arise. If a new test is compared with an old (but imperfect) standard test, the new test may seem worse even though it is actually better. For example, if the new test were more sensitive than the standard test, the additional patients identified by the new test would be considered false positives in relation to the old test. Similarly, if the new test is more often negative in patients who really do not have the disease, results for those patients would be considered false negatives compared with the old test. Thus, a new test can perform no better than an established gold standard test, and it will seem inferior when it approximates the truth more closely unless special strategies are used.

Example

Computed tomographic ("virtual") colonoscopy was compared to traditional (optical) colonoscopy in screening for colon cancer and adenomatous polyps that can be precursors of cancer (4). Both tests were performed on every patient without the clinician

interpreting each test knowing the results of the other test. Traditional colonoscopy is usually considered the gold standard for identifying colon cancer or polyps in asymptomatic adults. However, virtual colonoscopy identified more colon cancers and adenomatous polyps (especially those behind folds in the colon) than the traditional colonoscopy. In order not to penalize the new test in comparison to the old, the investigators ingeniously created a new gold standard—a repeat optical colonoscopy after reviewing the results of both testing procedures—whenever there was disagreement between the tests.

SENSITIVITY AND SPECIFICITY

Figure 8.2 summarizes some relationships between a diagnostic test and the actual presence of disease. It is an expansion of Figure 8.1, with the addition of some useful definitions. Most of the remainder of this chapter deals with these relationships in detail.

Example

Figure 8.3 illustrates these relationships with an actual study (5). Deep venous thrombosis (DVT) in the lower extremities is a serious condition that can lead to pulmonary embolism; patients with DVT should receive anticoagulation. However, because anticoagulation has risks, it is important to differentiate between patients with and without DVT. Compression ultrasonography is highly sensitive and specific for proximal thrombosis and has been used to confirm or rule out DVT. Compression ultrasonography is expensive and dependent on highly trained personnel, so a search for a simpler diagnostic test was undertaken. Blood tests to identify markers of endogenous fibrinolysis, D-dimer assays, were developed and evaluated for the diagnosis of DVT. Figure 8.3 shows the performance of a D-dimer assay in the diagnosis of DVT. The gold standard in the study was the result of compression ultrasonography and/or a 3-month follow-up.

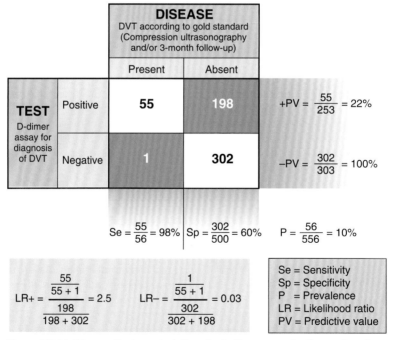

Figure 8.2 ■ Diagnostic test characteristics and definitions. Se = sensitivity; Sp = specificity; P = prevalence; PV = predictive value; LR = likelihood ratio. Note that LR+ calculations are the same as Se/(1 − Sp) and calculations for LR− are the same as (1 − Se)/Sp.

Figure 8.3 ■ Diagnostic characteristics of a D-dimer assay in diagnosing deep venous thrombosis (DVT). (Data from Bates SM, Kearon C, Crowther M, et al. A diagnostic strategy involving a quantitative latex D-dimer assay reliably excludes deep venous thrombosis. Ann Intern Med 2003;138:787–794.)

Definitions

As can be seen in Figure 8.2, sensitivity is defined as the proportion of people with the disease who have a positive test for the disease. A sensitive test will rarely miss people with the disease. Specificity is the proportion of people without the disease who have a negative test. A specific test will rarely misclassify people as having the disease when they do not.

Applying these definitions to the DVT example (Fig. 8.3), we see that 55 of the 56 patients with DVT had positive D-dimer results—for a sensitivity of 98%. However, of the 500 patients who did not have DVT, D-dimer results were correctly negative for only 302, for a specificity of 60%.

Use of Sensitive Tests

Clinicians should take the sensitivity and specificity of a diagnostic test into account when selecting a test. A sensitive test (i.e., one that is usually positive in the presence of disease) should be chosen when there is an important penalty for missing a disease. This would be so, for example, when there is reason to suspect a dangerous but treatable condition, such as tuberculosis, syphilis, or Hodgkin lymphoma, or in a patient suspected of having DVT. Sensitive tests are also helpful during the early stages of a diagnostic workup, when several diagnoses are being considered, to reduce the number of possibilities. Diagnostic tests are used in these situations to rule out diseases with a negative result of a highly sensitive test (as in the DVT example). As another example, one might choose the highly sensitive HIV antibody test early in the evaluation of lung infiltrates and weight loss to rule out an AIDS-related infection. In summary, a highly sensitive test is most helpful to the clinician when the test result is negative.

Use of Specific Tests

Specific tests are useful to confirm (or "rule in") a diagnosis that has been suggested by other data. This is because a highly specific test is rarely positive in the absence of disease; it gives few false-positive results. (Note that in the DVT example, the D-dimer test was not specific enough [60%] to initiate treatment after a positive test. All patients with positive results underwent compression ultrasonography, a much more specific test.) Highly specific tests are particularly needed when false-positive results can harm the patient physically, emotionally, or financially. Thus, before patients are subjected to cancer chemotherapy, with all its attendant risks, emotional trauma, and financial costs, tissue diagnosis (a highly spe-

cific test) is generally required. In summary, a highly specific test is most helpful when the test result is positive.

Trade-Offs between Sensitivity and Specificity

It is obviously desirable to have a test that is both highly sensitive and highly specific. Unfortunately, this is often not possible. Instead, whenever clinical data take on a range of values, there is a trade-off between the sensitivity and specificity for a given diagnostic test. In those situations, the location of a cutoff point, the point on the continuum between normal and abnormal, is an arbitrary decision. As a consequence, for any given test result expressed on a continuous scale, one characteristic, such as sensitivity, can be increased only at the expense of the other (e.g., specificity). Table 8.1 demonstrates this interrelationship for the use of B-type natriuretic peptide (BNP) levels in the diagnosis of congestive heart failure among patients presenting to emergency departments with acute dyspnea (6). If the cutoff level of the test were set too low (≥50 pg/mL), sensitivity is high (97%), but the trade-off is low specificity (62%), which would require many patients without congestive heart failure to undergo further testing for it. On the other hand, if the cutoff level were set too high (≥150 pg/mL), more patients with congestive heart failure would be missed. The authors suggested that an acceptable compromise would be a cutoff level of 100 pg/mL, which has a sensitivity of 90% and a specificity of 76%. There is no way, using a BNP test alone, that one can improve both the sensitivity and specificity of the test at the same time.

Table 8.1

Trade-Off between Sensitivity and Specificity When Using BNP Levels to Diagnose Congestive Heart Failure		
BNP Level (ph/mL)	**Sensitivity (%)**	**Specificity (%)**
50	97	62
80	93	74
100	90	76
125	87	79
150	85	83

Adapted with permission from Maisel AS, Krishnaswamy P, Nowak RM, et al. Rapid measurement of B-type natriuretic peptide in the emergency diagnosis of heart failure. N Engl J Med 2002;347: 161–167.

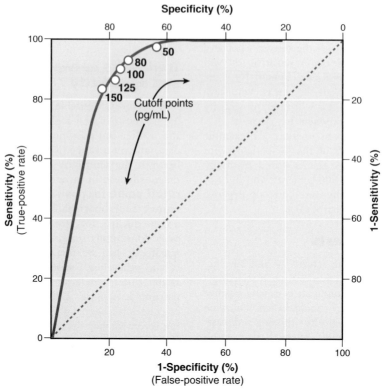

Figure 8.4 ■ A receiver operator characteristic (ROC) curve. The accuracy of B-type natriuretic peptide (BNP) in the emergency diagnosis of heart failure with various cutoff levels of BNP between dyspnea due to congestive heart failure and other causes. (Adapted with permission from Maisel AS, Krishnaswamy P, Nowak RM, et al. Rapid measurement of B-type natriuretic peptide in the emergency diagnosis of heart failure. N Engl J Med 2002;347:161–167.)

The Receiver Operator Characteristic (ROC) Curve

Another way to express the relationship between sensitivity and specificity for a given test is to construct a curve, called a receiver operator characteristic (ROC) curve. An ROC curve for the BNP levels in Table 8.1 is illustrated in Figure 8.4. It is constructed by plotting the true-positive rate (sensitivity) against the false-positive rate (1 – specificity) over a range of cutoff values. The values on the axes run from a probability of 0 to 1 (0% to 100%). Figure 8.4 illustrates visually the trade-off between sensitivity and specificity.

Tests that discriminate well crowd toward the upper left corner of the ROC curve; as the sensitivity is progressively increased (the cutoff point is lowered), there is little or no loss in specificity until very high levels of sensitivity are achieved. Tests that perform less well have curves that fall closer to the diagonal running from lower left to upper right. The

diagonal shows the relationship between true-positive and false-positive rates for a useless test—one that gives no additional information to what was known before the test was performed, equivalent to making a diagnosis by flipping a coin.

The ROC curve shows how severe the trade-off between sensitivity and specificity is for a test and can be used to help decide where the best cutoff point should be. Generally, the best cutoff point is at or near the "shoulder" of the ROC curve, unless there are clinical reasons for minimizing either false negatives or false positives.

ROC curves are particularly valuable ways of comparing different tests for the same diagnosis. The overall accuracy of a test can be described as the area under the ROC curve; the larger the area, the better the test. Figure 8.5 compares the ROC curve for BNP to that of an older test, ventricular ejection fraction determined by electrocardiography (7). BNP is both more sensitive and more specific, with a larger area

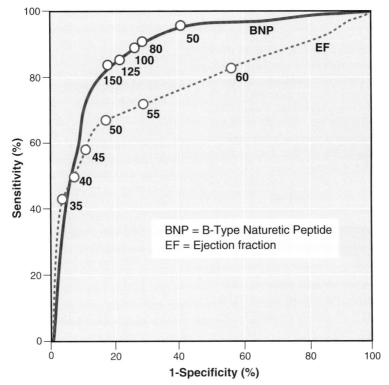

Figure 8.5 ■ **ROC curves for the BNP and left ventricular ejection fractions by echocardiograms in the emergency diagnosis of congestive heart failure in patients presenting with acute dyspnea.** Overall, BNP is more sensitive and more specific than ejection fractions, resulting in more area under the curve. (Redrawn with permission from Steg PG, Joubin L, McCord J, et al. B-type natriuretic peptide and echocardiographic determination of ejection fraction in the diagnosis of congestive heart failure in patients with acute dyspnea. Chest 2005;128:21–29.)

under the curve (0.89) than that for ejection fraction (0.78). It is also easier and faster to obtain in an emergency setting—test characteristics important in clinical situations when quick results are needed.

Obviously, tests that are both sensitive and specific are highly sought after and can be of enormous value. However, practitioners must frequently work with tests that are not both highly sensitive and specific. In these instances, they must use other means of circumventing the trade-off between sensitivity and specificity. The most common way is to use the results of several tests together, as discussed later in this chapter.

ESTABLISHING SENSITIVITY AND SPECIFICITY

Often, a new diagnostic test is described in glowing terms when first introduced, only to be found

wanting later when more experience with it has accumulated. Initial enthusiasm followed by disappointment arises not from any dishonesty on the part of early investigators or unfair skepticism by the medical community later. Rather, it is related to limitations in the methods by which the properties of the test were established in the first place. Sensitivity and specificity may be inaccurately described because an improper gold standard has been chosen, as discussed earlier in this chapter. In addition, two other issues related to the selection of diseased and nondiseased patients can profoundly affect the determination of sensitivity and specificity as well. They are the **spectrum** of patients to which the test is applied and **bias** in judging the test's performance. Statistical uncertainty, related to studying a relatively small number of patients, also can lead to inaccurate estimates of sensitivity and specificity.

Spectrum of Patients

Difficulties may arise when the patients used to describe the test's properties are different from those to whom the test will be applied in clinical practice. Early reports often assess the test's characteristics among people who are clearly diseased compared with people who are clearly not diseased, such as medical student volunteers. The test may be able to distinguish between these extremes very well but perform less well when differences are subtler. Also, patients with disease often differ in severity, stage, or duration of the disease, and a test's sensitivity will tend to be higher in more severely affected patients.

Example

Ovarian cancer, the fourth most common non-skin cancer in women, has spread beyond the ovary by the time it is clinically detected in most patients, and 5-year survival rates for such patients are about 30%. Because there is no effective screening test for ovarian cancer, guidelines were developed for early referral of patients with pelvic masses to Ob-Gyn specialists, with the hope of catching the disease at a curable stage. A study was done of the guidelines' accuracy in patients evaluated for a pelvic mass (8). In postmenopausal patients, the overall guideline sensitivity was 93% and specificity was 60%. However, when examined by cancer stage, sensitivity for early stage was lower than for late stage disease, 80% versus 98%. Ten of the 14 primary ovarian cancers missed by using the guidelines were the earliest stage I. Thus, the sensitivity for the guidelines to detect ovarian cancer depended on the particular mix of stages of patients with disease used to describe the test characteristics. Ironically, in the case of ovarian cancer, sensitivity of the guidelines was lowest for the stage that would be clinically most useful.

Some people in whom disease is suspected may have other conditions that cause a positive test, thereby increasing the false-positive rate and decreasing specificity. In the example of guidelines for ovarian cancer evaluation, specificity was low for all cancer stages (60%). One reason for this is that levels of the cancer marker, CA-125, recommended by guidelines, are elevated by many diseases and conditions other than ovarian cancer. These extraneous conditions decreased the specificity and increased the false-positive rate of the guidelines. Low specificity of diagnostic and screening tests is a major problem for ovarian cancer and can lead to surgery on many women without cancer.

Disease spectrum and prevalence of disease are especially important when a test is used for screening instead of diagnosis (see Chapter 10 for a more detailed discussion of screening). In theory, the sensitivity and specificity of a test are independent of the prevalence of diseased individuals in the sample in which the test is being evaluated. (Work with Fig. 8.2 to confirm this for yourself.) In practice, however, several characteristics of patients, such as stage and severity of disease, may be related to both the sensitivity and the specificity of a test and to the prevalence because different kinds of patients are found in high- and low-prevalence situations. Screening for disease illustrates this point; screening involves the use of the test in an asymptomatic population in which the prevalence of the disease is generally low and the spectrum of disease favors earlier and less severe cases. In such situations, sensitivity tends to be lower and specificity higher than when the same test is applied to patients suspected of having the disease, more of whom have advanced disease.

Example

A study was made of the sensitivity and specificity of the clinical breast examination for breast cancer in about 750,000 women (9). When the clinical breast examination was used as a *diagnostic* test on women with breast complaints, the sensitivity and specificity for breast cancer were 85% and 73%, respectively. However, when the same examination was used as a *screening* test on women who had no breast symptoms, sensitivity fell to 36% and specificity rose to 96%.

Bias

The sensitivity and specificity of a test should be established independently of the means by which the true diagnosis is established. Otherwise, there could be a biased assessment of the test's properties. As already pointed out, if the test is evaluated using data obtained during the course of a clinical evaluation of patients suspected of having the disease in question, a positive test may prompt the clinician to continue pursuing the diagnosis, increasing the likelihood that the disease will be found. On the other hand, a negative test may cause the clinician to abandon further testing, making it more likely that the disease, if present, will be missed.

Therefore, when the sensitivity and specificity of a test are being assessed, the test result should not be part of the information used to establish the diagnosis. In studying DVT diagnosis by D-dimer assay (discussed earlier), the investigators made sure that the physicians performing the gold standard tests (ultrasonography and follow-up assessment) were unaware of the results of the D-dimer assays so that the results of the D-dimer assays could not influence (bias) the interpretation of ultrasonography (10).

In the course of routine clinical care, this kind of bias can be used to advantage, especially if the test result is subjectively interpreted. Many radiologic imaging interpretations are subjective, and it is easy to be influenced by the clinical information provided. All clinicians have experienced having imaging studies overread because of a clinical impression or, conversely, of going back over old studies in which a finding was missed because a clinical fact was not communicated at the time and, therefore, attention was not directed to a particular area. Both to minimize and to take advantage of these biases, some radiologists prefer to read imaging studies twice, first without, then with the clinical information.

All the biases discussed tend to increase the agreement between the test and the gold standard. That is, they tend to make the test seem more accurate than it actually is.

Chance

Values for sensitivity and specificity are usually estimated from observations on relatively small samples of people with and without the disease of interest. Because of chance (random variation) in any one sample, particularly if it is small, the true sensitivity and specificity of the test can be misrepresented, even if there is no bias in the study. The particular values observed are compatible with a range of true values, typically characterized by the "95% confidence intervals" (see Chapter 12).[†] The width of this range of values defines the precision of the estimates

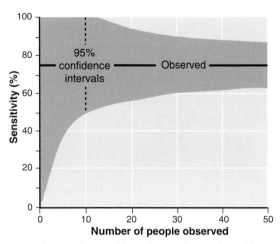

Figure 8.6 ■ The precision of an estimate of sensitivity. The 95% confidence interval for an observed sensitivity of 75%, according to the number of people observed.

of sensitivity and specificity. Therefore, reported values for sensitivity and specificity should not be taken too literally if a small number of patients is studied.

Figure 8.6 shows how the precision of estimates of sensitivity increases as the number of people on which the estimate is based increases. In this particular example, the observed sensitivity of the diagnostic test is 75%. Figure 8.6 shows that if this estimate is based on only 10 patients, by chance alone, the true sensitivity could be as low as 45% and as high as nearly 100%. When more patients are studied, the 95% confidence interval narrows and the precision of the estimate increases.

PREDICTIVE VALUE

Sensitivity and specificity are properties of a test that should be taken into account when deciding whether to use the test. However, once the results of a diagnostic test are available, whether positive or negative, the sensitivity and specificity of the test are no longer relevant because these values are obtained in persons known to have or not to have the disease. But if one knew the disease status of the patient, it would not be necessary to order the test! For the clinician, the dilemma is to determine if the patient has the disease, given the results of a test. (In fact, clinicians are usually more concerned with this question than the sensitivity and specificity of the test.)

Definitions

The probability of disease, given the results of a test, is called the predictive value of the test (see Fig. 8.2).

[†]The 95% confidence interval of a proportion is easily estimated by the following formula, based on the binomial theorem:

$$p \pm 2\sqrt{\frac{p(1-p)}{N}}$$

where p is the observed proportion and N is the number of people observed. To be more exact, multiply by 1.96 instead of 2.

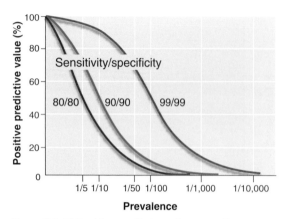

Figure 8.7 ■ **Positive predictive value according to sensitivity, specificity, and prevalence of disease.**

Positive predictive value is the probability of disease in a patient with a positive (abnormal) test result. **Negative predictive value** is the probability of *not* having the disease when the test result is negative (normal). Predictive value answers the question, "If my patient's test result is positive (negative), what are the chances that my patient does (does not) have the disease?" Predictive value is sometimes called **posterior (or posttest) probability**, the probability of disease *after* the test result is known. Figure 8.3 illustrates these concepts. Of the 253 patients with positive D-dimer assays, only 55 (22%) had DVT (positive predictive value). The negative predictive value of the test was much better, almost 100%.

The term **accuracy** is sometimes used to summarize the overall value of a test. Accuracy is the proportion of all test results, both positive and negative, that is correct. For the DVT example in Figure 8.3, the accuracy of D-dimer assays was 64%. (Calculate this for yourself.) The area under the ROC curve is another useful summary measure of the information provided by a test result. However, these summary measures usually are too crude to be useful clinically because specific information about the component parts—sensitivity, specificity, and predictive value at specific cutoff points—is lost when they are aggregated into a single number.

Determinants of Predictive Value

The predictive value of a test is not a property of the test alone. It is determined by the sensitivity and specificity of the test and the prevalence of disease in the population being tested, when **prevalence** has its customary meaning, the proportion of persons in a defined population at a given point in time having

the condition in question. Prevalence is also called **prior (or pretest) probability**, the probability of disease before the test result is known. (For a full discussion of prevalence, see Chapter 2.)

The more sensitive a test is the better will be its negative predictive value (the more confident the clinician can be that a negative test result rules out the disease being sought). Conversely, the more specific the test is, the better will be its positive predictive value (the more confident the clinician can be that a positive test confirms or rules in the diagnosis being sought). Because predictive value is also influenced by prevalence, it is not independent of the setting in which the test is used. Positive results, even for a very specific test, when applied to patients with a low likelihood of having the disease, will be largely false positives. Similarly, negative results, even for a very sensitive test, when applied to patients with a high chance of having the disease, are likely to be false negatives. In summary, the interpretation of a positive or negative diagnostic test result varies from setting to setting, according to the prevalence of disease in the particular setting.

It is not intuitively obvious why prevalence should affect interpretation of a test result. For those who are skeptical, it might help to consider how a test would perform at the extremes of prevalence. Remember that no matter how sensitive and specific a test might be (short of perfection), there will still be a small proportion of patients who are misclassified by it. Imagine a population in which no one has the disease. In such a group, all positive results, even for a very specific test, will be false positives. Therefore, as the prevalence of disease in a population approaches zero, the positive predictive value of a test also approaches zero. Conversely, if everyone in a population tested has the disease, all negative results will be false negatives, even for a very sensitive test. As prevalence approaches 100%, negative predictive value approaches zero. Another way for skeptics to convince themselves of these relationships is to work with Figure 8.3, holding sensitivity and specificity constant, changing prevalence, and calculating the resulting predictive values.

Figure 8.7 illustrates the effect of prevalence on positive predictive value for a test at different but generally high levels of sensitivity and specificity. When the prevalence of disease in the population tested is relatively high—more than several percent—the test performs well. But at lower prevalences, the positive predictive value drops to nearly zero (negative predictive value improves), and the test is virtually useless. (The figure illustrates why positive predictive value of a test is so much better in diagnostic studies, which often can evaluate tests with a few hundred patients, than in screening studies, which usually must use tens of thousands of patients, because of the difference of underlying prevalence of disease in the two situations.) As sensitivity and specificity fall, the influence of prevalence on predictive value becomes more pronounced.

It is sometimes possible in clinical situations to manipulate prevalence of a disease so that a diagnostic test becomes more useful.

Example

As indicated earlier in this chapter, DVT, a potentially dangerous cause of leg pain, is difficult to diagnose without specialized testing. Many patients with leg pain do not have DVT, and it is important to differentiate patients who do and do not have DVT because treatment for it (anticoagulation) is risky. It would be helpful to have a quick and easy diagnostic test that can rule out DVT, but, as is clear from Figure 8.3, D-dimer assays are sensitive but not specific. However, even a test with relatively poor specificity might work reasonably well in a group of patients with a low prevalence of disease. An effort was made to rule out DVT and improve negative predictive value by assigning patients to groups with differing probabilities (prevalences) of DVT before applying the diagnostic test. In a synthesis of 14 studies evaluating the use of D-dimer assays in more than 8,000 patients, investigators found that the overall prevalence of DVT was 19% (11). Using a simple validated clinical rule involving several clinical findings and history items, patients were stratified into groups of low (5%), medium (17%), and high (53%) probabilities (prevalence) of DVT and then tested with high-sensitivity D-dimer assays. Sensitivity was high (95% to 98%) in all the groups, but specificity varied according to DVT prevalence: 58% among patients with low probability, 41% among those with medium probability, and 36% among those with high probability. Although specificity of 58% is not very high, when the D-dimer assay results were negative among patients with a low clinical probability of DVT, the negative predictive value was >99%—fewer than 1% of patients in this group were diagnosed with DVT after at least 3 months of follow-up. Thus, the test was especially useful for excluding DVT in patients with a low probability of DVT (about 40% of all patients) without further testing. This is an example of how a negative result of a non-specific test becomes clinically useful when used in a group of patients with a very low prevalence of disease.

As is clear from the example and Figure 8.6, prevalence is usually more important than sensitivity and specificity in determining predictive value. One reason why this is so is that prevalence can vary over a much wider range than sensitivity and specificity can. Prevalence of disease can vary from 1 in 1 million to <1 in 10, depending on the age, gender, risk factors, and clinical findings of the patient. Consider the difference in prevalence of liver disease in healthy, young adults who do not use drugs, are not sexually promiscuous, and consume only occasional alcohol as compared to jaundiced intravenous drug users who have multiple sex partners. In contrast, sensitivity and specificity of diagnostic tests usually vary over a much narrower range, from about 50% to 99%.

Estimating Prevalence (Pretest Probability)

Because prevalence of disease is such a powerful determinant of how useful a diagnostic test will be, clinicians should consider the probability of disease before ordering a test. But how can a doctor estimate the prevalence or probability of a particular disease in patients? Until recently, they tended to rely on clinical observations and their experience to estimate (usually implicitly) the pretest probability of most diseases. Studies have shown that these estimates are often inaccurate (perhaps because doctors tend to remember recent or remarkable patients and, consequently, give them too much weight when making estimates).

For several infectious diseases, such as influenza and methicillin-resistant *Staphylococcus aureus* infection, periodic studies and tracking systems by the Centers for Disease Control and Prevention alert clinicians about changing prevalence. Large clinical computer databanks also provide quantitative estimates of the probability of disease, given various combinations of clinical findings. Although the resulting estimates of prevalence are not likely to be very precise, using estimates from the medical literature is bound to be more accurate than implicit judgment alone.

Increasing the Pretest Probability of Disease

Within the clinical setting, there are several ways in which the probability of a disease can be increased before using a diagnostic test. Considering the relationship between the predictive value of a test and prevalence, it is obviously to the physician's advantage to apply diagnostic tests to patients with an increased likelihood of having the disease being sought. In fact, diagnostic tests are most helpful when the presence of disease is neither very likely nor very unlikely.

Specifics of the Clinical Situation

The specifics of the clinical situation are clearly a strong influence on the decision to order tests. Symptoms, signs, and disease risk factors all raise or lower the probability of finding a disease. For some diseases, clinical-decision rules made up of simple history and physical examinations produce groups of patients with known prevalence or incidence of disease, as shown in the DVT example. A young woman with chest pain is more likely to have coronary disease if she has typical angina and hypertension and she smokes. As a result, an abnormal ECG stress test is more likely to represent coronary disease in such a woman than in a similar woman with nonspecific chest pain and no coronary risk factors.

The value of applying diagnostic tests to persons more likely to have a particular illness is intuitively obvious to most doctors. Nevertheless, with the increasing availability of diagnostic tests, it is easy to adopt a less selective approach when ordering tests. However, the less selective the approach, the lower the prevalence of the disease is likely to be and the lower will be the positive predictive value of the test.

Example

The probability of coronary artery disease (CAD) based on the results of an ECG exercise (stress) test varies according to the pretest probability of CAD, which differs according to age, gender, symptoms, and risk factors. Figure 8.8 demonstrates posttest probabilities after stress tests among men with different ages, symptoms, and risk factors (i.e., different pretest probabilities of CAD). The elliptical curves show the results for probabilities of CAD after positive and negative test results. An asymptomatic 45-year-old man has a very low pretest probability of CAD, which rises little (to <10%) after a positive test and decreases to practically zero after a negative test. At the other extreme, for a 55-year-old man with typical angina who has a 93% pretest probability of CAD, a positive test raises the probability of CAD to nearly 100%, whereas a negative test reduces the posttest probability to about 75%—hardly reassuring to either the patient or the doctor; further testing will likely occur regardless of the test result in this patient, making the test useless. Stress testing is most useful in a 45-year-old man with atypical chest pain who has a pretest 51% probability of CAD. A positive test raises the posttest probability of CAD to about 75%, which argues for more invasive and definitive testing, whereas a negative test lowers the probability of CAD to about 10%.

Because of the prevalence effect, physicians must interpret similar stress test results differently in different clinical situations. A positive test usually will be misleading if it is used to search for unsuspected disease in low-prevalence situations, as sometimes has been done among young joggers and on "executive physicals" of young healthy persons. The opposite applies to an older man with typical angina. In this case, a negative stress test result is too often false negative to exclude disease. As is clear in Figure 8.8, a diagnostic test is most useful in intermediate situations, in which prevalence (pretest probability) is neither very high nor very low.

Selected Demographic Groups

In a given setting, physicians can increase the yield of diagnostic tests by applying them to demographic groups known to be at higher risk for a disease. The pretest probability of CAD in a 55-year-old man complaining of atypical angina chest pain is 65%; in a 35-year-old woman with the same kind of pain, it is 12% (12). Similarly, a sickle cell test would obviously have a higher positive predictive value among African Americans than among whites of Norwegian descent.

Referral Process

Referral to teaching hospital wards, clinics, and emergency departments increases the chance that significant disease will underlie patients' complaints. Therefore, relatively more aggressive use of diagnostic tests might be justified in these settings. (The need for

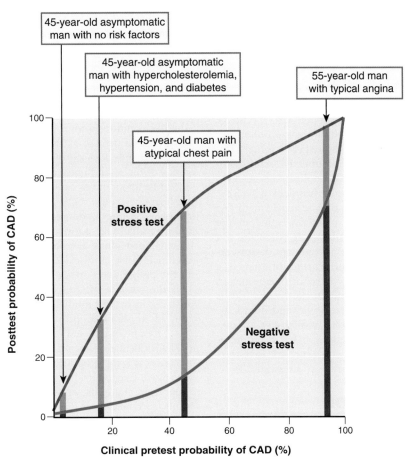

Figure 8.8 ■ Posttest probabilities of coronary artery disease among men with different pretest probabilities who underwent ECG exercise (stress) tests. The top of the light pink bars indicate posttest probabilities of CAD after positive tests and the top of the red bars indicate posttest probabilities of CAD after negative tests. (Redrawn with permission from Patterson RE, Horowitz SF. Importance of epidemiology and biostatistics in deciding clinical strategies for using diagnostic tests: a simplified approach using examples from coronary artery disease. J Am Coll Cardiol 1989;13:1653–1665.)

speedy diagnosis also promotes quicker use of diagnostic tests.) In primary care practice, on the other hand, and particularly among patients without complaints, the chance of finding disease is considerably smaller, and tests should be used more sparingly.

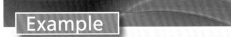

Example

While practicing in a military clinic, one author saw hundreds of people with headache, rarely ordered diagnostic tests, and never encountered a patient with a severe underlying cause

of headache. (It is unlikely that important conditions were missed because the clinic was virtually the only source of medical care for these patients, and the soldiers remained in the military community for many months.) However, during the first week back in a medical residency at a teaching hospital, a patient with a headache similar to the ones managed in the military was found to have a cerebellar abscess!

Because clinicians may work at different points along the prevalence spectrum at various times in their clinical practices, they should bear in mind that the intensity of their diagnostic evaluations may need to be adjusted to suit the specific setting.

Implications for Interpreting the Medical Literature

Published descriptions of diagnostic tests often include, in addition to sensitivity and specificity, some conclusions about the interpretation of a positive or negative test (the test's predictive value). This is done to provide information directly useful to clinicians, but the data for these publications are often gathered in university teaching hospitals where the prevalence of serious disease is relatively high. As a result, statements about predictive value in the medical literature may be misleading when the test is applied in less highly selected settings. Occasionally, authors compare the performance of a test in a number of patients known to have the disease and an equal number of patients without the disease. This is an efficient way to describe sensitivity and specificity. However, any reported positive predictive value from such studies means little because it has been determined for a group of patients in which the investigators artificially set the prevalence of disease at 50%.

LIKELIHOOD RATIOS

Likelihood ratios are an alternative way of describing the performance of a diagnostic test. They summarize the same kind of information as sensitivity and specificity and can be used to calculate the probability of disease after a positive or negative test (positive or negative predictive value). The main advantage of likelihood ratios is that they can be used at multiple levels of test results.

Odds

Because the use of likelihood ratios depends on odds, to understand them, it is first necessary to distinguish odds from probability. Odds and probability contain the same information, but they express it differently. Probability, which is used to express sensitivity, specificity, and predictive value, is the proportion of people in whom a particular characteristic, such as a positive test, is present. Odds, on the other hand, is the ratio of two probabilities, the probability of an event to that of 1 – the probability of the event. The two can be interconverted using simple formulas:

$$Odds = Probability\ of\ event$$
$$\div\ (1 - Probability\ of\ event)$$
$$Probability = Odds \div (1 + Odds)$$

These terms should be familiar to most readers because they are used in everyday conversation. For example, we may say that the odds are 4:1 that the New England Patriots football team will win tonight or that they have an 80% probability of winning.

Definitions

The likelihood ratio for a particular value of a diagnostic test is defined as the probability of that test result in people with the disease divided by the probability of the result in people without disease (see Fig. 8.2). Likelihood ratios express how many times more (or less) likely a test result is to be found in diseased, compared with nondiseased, people. For dichotomous results (both positive and negative), two types of likelihood ratios describe the test's ability to discriminate between diseased and nondiseased people. In the case of a test's positive likelihood ratio (LR+), it is the ratio of the proportion of diseased people with a positive test result (sensitivity) to the proportion of nondiseased people with a positive result (1 – specificity). A test's negative likelihood ratio (LR–) is calculated when the test result is negative. In that case, it is the proportion of diseased people with a negative test result (1 – sensitivity) divided by the proportion of nondiseased people with a negative test result (specificity) (see Fig. 8.2).

In the DVT example (Fig. 8.3), the data can be used to calculate likelihood ratios for DVT in the presence of a positive or negative D-dimer assay. A positive test is about 2.5 times more likely to be found in the presence of DVT than in the absence of it. If the D-dimer assay was negative, the likelihood ratio for this negative test is 0.03.

Use of Likelihood Ratios

Likelihood ratios must be used with odds, not probability. Therefore, the first step is to convert pretest probability (prevalence) to pretest odds, as outlined earlier:

$$Odds = Probability\ of\ event$$
$$\div\ (1 - Probability\ of\ event)$$

Likelihood ratios can then be used to convert pretest odds to posttest odds, by means of the following formula:

$$Pretest\ odds \times Likelihood\ ratio = Posttest\ odds$$

Posttest odds can, in turn, be converted back to a probability, using the formula:

$$Probability = Odds \div (1 + Odds)$$

In these relationships, pretest odds contain the same information as prior or pretest probability (prevalence), likelihood ratios the same as sensitivity/specificity, and posttest odds the same as positive predictive value (posttest probability).

Why Use Likelihood Ratios?

Why master the concept of likelihood ratios when they are much more difficult to understand than prevalence, sensitivity, specificity, and predictive value? The main advantage of likelihood ratios is that they make it possible to go beyond the simple and clumsy classification of a test result as either abnormal or normal, as is done when describing the accuracy of a diagnostic test only in terms of sensitivity and specificity at a single cutoff point. Obviously, disease is more likely in the presence of an extremely abnormal test result than it is for a marginally abnormal one. With likelihood ratios, it is possible to summarize the information contained in test results at different levels. One can define likelihood ratios for each of an entire range of possible values. In this way, information represented by the degree of abnormality is not discarded in favor of just the crude presence or absence of it.

In computing likelihood ratios across a range of test results, a limitation of sensitivity and specificity is overcome. Instead of referring to the ability of the test to identify all individuals with a given result or worse, it refers to the ability of a *particular* test result to identify people with the disease. The same is true for the calculation of specificity. Thus, for tests with a range of results, LRs can report information at each level. In general, tests with LRs further away from 1.0 are associated with few false positives and few false negatives (>10 for LR+ and <0.1 for LR−), whereas those with LRs close to 1.0 give much less accurate results (2.1 to 5.0 for LR+ and 0.5 to 0.2 for LR−).

In summary, likelihood ratios can accommodate the common and reasonable clinical practice of putting more weight on extremely high (or low) test results than on borderline ones when estimating the probability (or odds) that a particular disease is present.

Example

Pleural effusions are routinely evaluated when the cause is not clear, to determine if the effusion is a transudate (body fluids passing through a membrane and with few cells or debris) or an exudate (with cellular material and debris), which may indicate inflammatory or malignant disease and often requires further diagnostic evaluation. Traditionally, one way to differentiate the two was to measure the protein in pleural fluid and serum; if the ratio of pleural fluid protein to serum protein was >0.50, the pleural fluid was identified as an exudate. However, the single cut-point may obscure important diagnostic information. This possibility was examined in a study of 1,448 patients with pleural fluids known to be either exudates or transudates (13). Table 8.2 shows the distribution of pleural fluid findings according to the ratio of pleural fluid protein to serum protein, along with calculated likelihood ratios. Not surprisingly, at high values of pleural fluid protein to serum protein ratios, almost all specimens were exudates and the likelihood ratios were high, whereas at the other extreme, the opposite was true. Overall, ratios close to the traditional cut-point indicated that the distinction between exudates and transudates was uncertain. Also, using the traditional cut-point of 0.50, there was more misclassification below than above the cut-point.

Table 8.2

Distribution of Ratios for Pleural Fluid Protein to Serum Protein in Patients with Exudates and Transudates, with Calculation of Likelihood Ratios

Ratio of Pleural Fluid Protein to Serum Protein	Number of Patients with Test Result		Likelihood Ratio
	Exudates	Transudates	
>0.70	475	1	168.65
0.66–0.70	150	1	53.26
0.61–0.65	117	6	6.92
0.56–0.60	102	12	3.02
0.50–0.55	70	14	1.78
0.46–0.50	47	34	0.49
0.41–0.45	27	34	0.28
0.36–0.40	13	37	0.12
0.31–0.35	8	44	0.06
≤0.30	19	182	0.04

Reproduced with permission from Heffner JE, Sahn SA, Brown LK. Multilevel likelihood ratios for identifying exudative pleural effusions. Chest 2002;121:1916–1920.

The likelihood ratio has several other advantages over sensitivity and specificity as a description of test performance. As is clear from Table 8.2, the information contributed by the test is summarized in one number corresponding to each level of test result. Also, likelihood ratios are particularly well suited for describing the overall odds of disease when a series of diagnostic tests is used (see the following text).

Calculating Likelihood Ratios

Figure 8.9A demonstrates two ways of arriving at posttest probability: by calculation and with a nomogram. Figure 8.9B makes the calculations using the DVT example in Figure 8.3 and shows that the calculated posttest probability (22%) is the same as the positive predictive value calculated arrived at by the nomogram in the figure. Although the process is conceptually simple and each individual calculation is easy, the overall effort is a bit daunting. To make it easy, several computerized programs for diagnostic test calculators that also construct the associated nomogram are available free on the Web. The nomogram shows the difference between pre- and posttest odds, but it requires having the nomogram easily available.

These calculations demonstrate a disadvantage of likelihood ratios. One must use odds, not probabilities, and most of us find thinking in terms of odds more difficult than probabilities. Also, the conversion from probability to odds and back requires math, Internet access, or the use of a nomogram, which can complicate calculating posttest odds and predictive value during the routine course of patient care.

Table 8.3 displays a simplified approach. Likelihood ratios of 2, 5, and 10 increase the probability of disease approximately 15%, 30%, and 45%, respectively, and the inverse of these (likelihood ratios of 0.5, 0.2, and 0.1) decrease the probability of disease similarly 15%, 30%, and 45% (14). Bedside use of likelihood ratios is easier when the three specific likelihood ratios and their effect (multiples of 15) on posttest probability are remembered, especially when the clinician can estimate the probability of disease in the patient before the test is done. Using this algorithm in the DVT example (Fig. 8.3), the probability of disease with a LR+ of 2.5 would be approximately 25% (the underlying 10% prevalence plus about 15%). This is a little higher estimate than that obtained with the mathematical calculation, but it is close enough to conclude that a patient with a positive D-dimer assay needs some other test to confirm the presence of DVT.

A) Mathematical approach
1) Convert pretest probability (prevalence) to pretest odds
    Pretest odds = prevalence/(1 − prevalence)
2) Multiply pretest odds by likelihood ratio to obtain posttest odds
    Pretest odds × likelihood ratio = posttest odds
3) Convert posttest odds to posttest probability (predictive value)
    Posttest probability = posttest odds/(1 + posttest odds)

B) Using a likelihood ratio nomogram
Place a straight edge at the correct prevalence and likelihood ratio values and read off the posttest probability where the straight edge crosses the line.

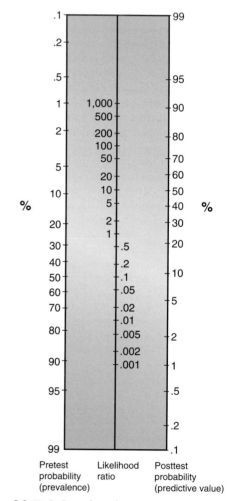

Figure 8.9 ■ **A.** Formula and nomogram using test likelihood ratios to determine posttest probability of disease.

A) Mathematical approach

1) Convert pretest probability (prevalence) to pretest odds
    .10/(1−.10) = .111

2) Multiply pretest odds by likelihood ratio of positive test
    .11 x 2.5 = 0.278

3) Convert posttest odds to posttest probability
    (positive predictive value)
        0.278/(1 + 0.278) = .22 = 22%

B) Using a likelihood ratio nomogram
The pretest probability is 10% and the LR+ is 2.5. Place a ruler to intersect these 2 values and it crosses the posttest probability line at about 22%.

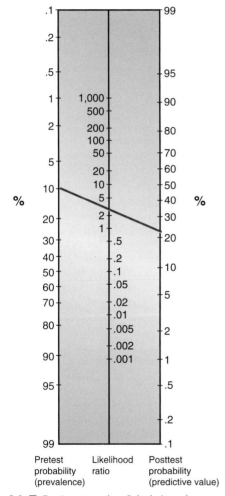

Figure 8.9 ■ B. An example: Calculating the posttest probability of a positive D-dimer assay test for DVT (see Fig. 8.3). (Adapted with permission from Fagan TJ. Nomogram for Bayes's theorem. N Eng J Med 1975;293:257.)

Table 8.3

Simple "Rule of Thumb" for Determining Effect of Likelihood Ratios on Disease Probability	
Likelihood Ratio	**Approximate Change in Disease Probability (%)**
10	+45
9	+40
8	—
7	—
6	+35
5	+30
4	+25
3	+20
2	+15
1	No Change
0.5	−15
0.4	−20
0.3	−25
0.2	−30
0.1	−45

Adapted with permission from McGee S. Simplifying likelihood ratios. J Gen Intern Med 2002;17:646–649.

MULTIPLE TESTS

Because clinicians commonly use imperfect diagnostic tests with <100% sensitivity and specificity and intermediate likelihood ratios, a single test frequently results in a probability of disease that is neither high nor low enough for managing the patient (e.g., somewhere between 10% and 90%). Usually, it is not acceptable to stop the diagnostic process at such a point. Would a physician or patient be satisfied with the conclusion that the patient has even a 20% chance of having carcinoma of the colon? Or that an asymptomatic, 45-year-old man with multiple risk factors has about a 30% chance of coronary heart disease after a positive ECG stress test? Even for less deadly diseases, tests resulting in intermediate posttest probabilities require more investigation. The physician is ordinarily bound to raise or lower the probability of disease substantially in such situations—unless, of course, the diagnostic possibilities are all trivial, nothing could be done about the result, or the risk of proceeding further is prohibitive. When these exceptions do not apply, the clinician will want to find a way to rule in or rule out the disease more decisively.

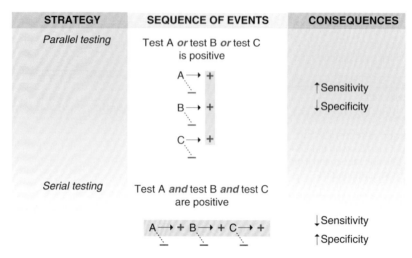

| STRATEGY | SEQUENCE OF EVENTS | CONSEQUENCES |

Figure 8.10 ■ Parallel and serial testing. In parallel testing, all tests are done at the same time. In serial testing, each subsequent test is done only when the previous test result is positive.

When multiple different tests are performed and all are positive or all are negative, the interpretation is straightforward. All too often, however, some are positive and others are negative. Interpretation is then more complicated. This section discusses the principles by which multiple tests are applied and interpreted.

Multiple diagnostic tests can be applied in two basic ways (Fig. 8.10). They can be used in **parallel testing** (i.e., all at once), and a positive result of any test is considered evidence for disease. Or they can be done in **serial testing** (i.e., consecutively), with the decision to order the next test in the series based on the results of the previous test. For serial testing, all tests must give a positive result in order for the diagnosis to be made because the diagnostic process is stopped with a negative result.

Parallel Testing

Physicians usually order tests in parallel when rapid assessment is necessary, as in hospitalized or emergency patients, or for ambulatory patients who cannot return easily because they are not mobile or have come from a long distance for evaluation.

Multiple tests in parallel generally increase the sensitivity and, therefore, the negative predictive value for a given disease prevalence, above those of each individual test. On the other hand, specificity and positive predictive value are lower than for each individual test. That is, disease is less likely to be missed. (Parallel testing is probably one reason why referral centers seem to diagnose disease that local physicians miss.) However, false-positive diagnoses are also more likely to be made (thus, the propensity for overdiagnosing in such centers as well). In summary, parallel testing is particularly useful when the clinician is faced with the need for a very sensitive testing strategy but has available only two or more relatively insensitive tests that measure different clinical phenomena. By using the tests in parallel, the net effect is a more sensitive diagnostic strategy. The price, however, is further evaluation or treatment of some patients without the disease.

Example

Neither of two tests used for diagnosing ovarian cancer, CA-125 and transvaginal ultrasound, is a sensitive test when used alone. A study was done in which 28,506 women underwent both tests in a trial of ovarian cancer screening (15). If either test result was abnormal (a parallel testing strategy), women were referred for further evaluation. Positive predictive values were determined for each test individually as well as when both tests were abnormal (a serial testing strategy). The authors did not calculate sensitivities and specificities of the tests; to do so, they would have needed to include any cases of ovarian cancer that occurred in the

Table 8.4

Test Characteristics of CA-125 and Transvaginal Ultrasound (TVU)			
Test	**Sensitivity[a] (%)**	**Specificity[a] (%)**	**Positive Predictive Value (%)**
Abnormal CA-125 (≥35 U/mL)	55.2	98.7	4.0
Abnormal TVU	75.8	95.4	1.6
Abnormal CA-125 or TVU	100.0	94.1	1.7
Abnormal CA-125 and TVU	31.0	99.9	26.5

[a]Sensitivity and specificity estimated without interval cancers (see text).
Data from Buys SS, Partridge E, Greene M, et al. Ovarian cancer screening in the Prostate, Lung, Colorectal and Ovarian (PLCO) cancer screening trial: findings from the initial screen of a randomized trial. Am J Obstet Gynecol 2005;193:1630–1639.

women in the interval between the first and next screening round. However, it is possible to roughly estimate the values for sensitivity and specificity from the information in the paper. Table 8.4 shows the positive predictive values as well as estimated sensitivities and specificities of the tests. Using the two tests in parallel raised the estimated sensitivity to about 100%, but the positive predictive value was lower (1.7%) than when using the tests individually. Because follow-up evaluation of abnormal screening tests for ovarian cancer often involves abdominal surgery, tests with high positive predictive values are important. The low positive predictive value resulting from a parallel testing strategy meant that almost all women who required follow-up evaluation—many of whom underwent surgery—did not have ovarian cancer. The authors examined what would have happened if a serial testing strategy had been used (requiring both tests to be positive before further evaluation); positive predictive value rose to 26.5%, but at the cost of lowering the estimated sensitivity to 31%, so low that 20 of 29 cancers would have been missed using this strategy.

Clinical Prediction Rules

A modification of parallel testing occurs when clinicians use the combination of multiple tests, some with positive and some with negative results, to arrive at a diagnosis. Usually, they start by taking a history and doing a physical examination. They may also order laboratory tests. The results of the combined testing from history, physical examination, and laboratory tests are then used to make a diagnosis. This process, long an implicit part of clinical medicine, has been examined systematically for an increasing number of diagnoses. For some medical conditions, certain history items, physical findings, and laboratory results are particularly important in their predictive power for making a diagnosis. The resulting test combinations are called clinical prediction rules or diagnostic decision-making rules, which divides patients into groups with different prevalences.

Example

Pharyngitis is among the most common complaints in office practice, but it is not straight forward which patients should be treated with antibiotics for group A streptococcus. The gold standard for group A streptococcus diagnosis is a throat culture, but because results are not available immediately (and because only about 10% of adult patients with sore throats have strep throat), methods to decrease the need for culture have been sought. A clinical prediction rule was studied (16), with different risks of streptococcal infection according to the score (Table 8.5). The authors then applied six different management strategies according to the score results and showed the trade-offs in terms of sensitivity, specificity, unnecessary use of antibiotics, clinic staff effort, and cost. The clinical prediction rule identified patients with a low enough likelihood of group A streptococcus that they were not subjected to further diagnostic or treatment efforts, an approach now incorporated into guidelines of several organizations.

Table 8.5

An Example of a Diagnostic Decision-Making Rule: Predictors of Group A Streptococcus (GAS) Pharyngitis. Modified Centor Score

Criteria	Points
Temperature >38°C (100.4°F)	1
Absence of cough	1
Swollen, tender anterior cervical nodes	1
Tonsillar swelling or exudate	1
Age	1
3–14 years	1
15–44 years	0
≥45 years	−1

Score	Probability of a Positive Culture for GAS (%)
≤0	1–2.5
1	5–10
2	11–17
3	28–35
≥4	51–53

Adapted with permission from McIsaac WJ, Kellner JD, Aufricht P, et al. Empirical validation of guidelines for the management of pharyngitis in children and adults. JAMA 2004;291:1587–1595.

Serial Testing

Serial testing maximizes specificity and positive predictive value but lowers sensitivity and the negative predictive value, as demonstrated in Table 8.4. One ends up surer that positive test results represent disease but runs an increased risk that disease will be missed. Serial testing is particularly useful when none of the individual tests available to a clinician is highly specific.

Physicians most often use serial testing strategies in clinical situations where rapid assessment of patients is not required, such as in office practices and hospital clinics in which ambulatory patients are followed over time. (In acute care settings, time is the enemy of a serial testing approach.) Serial testing is also used when some of the tests are expensive or risky, with these tests being employed only after simpler and safer tests suggest the presence of disease. For example, maternal age, blood tests, and ultrasound are used to identify pregnancies at higher risk of delivering a baby with Down syndrome. Mothers found to be at high risk by those tests are then offered chorionic villus sampling or amniocentesis, both of which entail risk of fetal loss. Serial testing leads to less laboratory use than parallel testing because additional evaluation is contingent on prior test results. However, serial testing takes more time because additional tests are ordered only after the results of previous ones become available. Usually, the test that is less risky, less invasive, easier to do, and cheaper should be done first. If these factors are not in play, performing the test with the highest specificity is usually more efficient, requiring fewer patients to undergo both tests.

Serial Likelihood Ratios

When a series of tests is used, an overall probability can be calculated using the likelihood ratio for each test result, as shown in Figure 8.11. The prevalence of disease before testing is first converted to pretest odds. As each test is done, the posttest odds of one become the pretest odds for the next. In the end, a new probability of disease is found that takes into

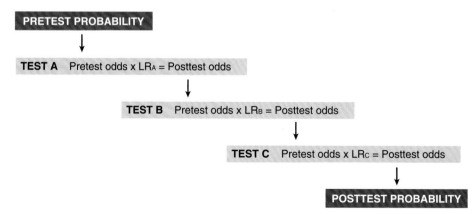

Figure 8.11 ■ Use of likelihood ratios in serial testing. As each test is completed, its posttest odds become the pretest odds for the subsequent test.

account the information contributed by all the tests in the series.

Assumption of Independence

When multiple tests are used, the accuracy of the final result depends on whether the additional information contributed by each test is somewhat independent of that already available from the preceding ones so that the next test does not simply duplicate known information. For example, in the diagnosis of endocarditis, it is likely that fever (an indication of inflammation), a new heart murmur (an indication of valve destruction), and Osler nodes (an indication of emboli) each add independent, useful information. In the example of pharyngitis, the investigators used statistical techniques to ensure that each diagnostic

test included in the decision rule contributed independently to the diagnosis. To the degree that the two tests are not contributing independent information, multiple testing is less useful. For example, if two tests are used in parallel with 60% and 80% sensitivities, and the better test identifies all the cases found by the less sensitive test, the combined sensitivity cannot be higher than 80%. If they are completely independent of each other, then the sensitivity of parallel testing would be 92% (80% + [60% × 20%]).

The premise of independence underlies the entire approach to the use of multiple tests. However, it seems unlikely that tests for most diseases are fully independent of each other. If the assumption that the tests are completely independent is wrong, calculation of the probability of disease from several tests would tend to overestimate the tests' value.

Review Questions

Questions 8.1–8.10 are based on the following example. For each question, select the best answer.

A study was made of symptoms and physical findings in 247 patients evaluated for sinusitis. The final diagnosis was made according to x-ray findings (gold standard) (17). Ninety-five patients had sinusitis, and 49 of them also had facial pain. One hundred fifty-two did not have sinusitis, and 79 of these patients had facial pain.

8.1. What is the sensitivity of facial pain for sinusitis in this study?

A. 38%
B. 48%
C. 52%
D. 61%

8.2. What is the specificity?

A. 38%
B. 48%
C. 52%
D. 61%

8.3. If the doctor thought the patient had sinusitis because the patient had facial pain, for what percent of patients would she be correct?

A. 38%
B. 48%
C. 52%
D. 61%

8.4. If the doctor thought the patient did not have sinusitis because the patient did not have facial pain, for what percent of patients would she be correct?

A. 38%
B. 48%
C. 52%
D. 61%

8.5. How common was sinusitis in this study?

A. 38%
B. 48%
C. 52%
D. 61%

8.6. What is the posttest probability of sinusitis in patients with facial pain in this study?

A. 38%
B. 48%
C. 52%
D. 61%

Both the positive and negative likelihood ratios for facial pain were 1.0. When clinicians asked several other questions about patient symptoms and took physical examination results into account, the likelihood ratios for their overall clinical impressions as to whether patients had sinusitis were as follows: "high probability," LR 4.7; "intermediate probability," LR 1.4, and "low probability," LR 0.4.

8.7. What is the probability of sinusitis in patients assigned a "high probability" by clinicians?

A. ~10%
B. ~20%
C. ~45%
D. ~75%
E. ~90%

8.8. What is the probability of sinusitis in patients assigned an "intermediate probability" by clinicians?

A. ~10%
B. ~20%
C. ~45%
D. ~75%
E. ~90%

8.9. What is the probability of sinusitis in patients assigned a "low probability" by clinicians?

A. ~10%
B. ~20%
C. ~45%
D. ~75%
E. ~90%

8.10. Given the answers for questions 8.7–8.9, which of the following statements is *incorrect*?

A. A clinical impression of "high probability" of sinusitis is more useful in the management of patients than one of "low probability."
B. A clinical impression of "intermediate probability" is approximately equivalent to a coin toss.

C. Predictive value of facial pain will be higher in a clinical setting in which the prevalence of sinusitis is 10%.

For questions 8.11 and 8.12, select the best answer.

8.11. Which of the following statements is most correct?

A. Using diagnostic tests in parallel increases specificity and lowers positive predictive value.
B. Using diagnostic tests in series increases sensitivity and lowers positive predictive value.
C. Using diagnostic tests in parallel increases sensitivity and positive predictive value.
D. Using diagnostic tests in series increases specificity and positive predictive value.

8.12. Which of the following statements is most correct?

A. When using diagnostic tests in parallel or series, each test should contribute information independently.
B. When using diagnostic tests in series, the test with the lowest sensitivity should be used first.
C. When using diagnostic tests in parallel, the test with the highest specificity should be used first.

Answers are in Appendix A.

REFERENCES

1. Chobanian AV, Bakris GL, Black HR, et al. The Seventh Report of the Joint National Committee on Prevention, Detection, Evaluation, and Treatment of High Blood Pressure: The JNC 7 Report. JAMA 2003:289:2560–2571.
2. Gann PH, Hennekens CH, Stampfer MJ. A prospective evaluation of plasma prostate-specific antigen for detection of prostatic cancer. JAMA 1995;273:289–294.
3. Wheeler SG, Wipf JE, Staiger TO, et al. Approach to the diagnosis and evaluation of low back pain in adults. In: Basow DS, ed. UpToDate. Waltham, MA; UpToDate; 2011.
4. Pickhardt PJ, Choi JR, Hwang I, et al. Computed tomographic virtual colonoscopy to screen for colorectal neoplasia in asymptomatic adults. N Engl J Med 2003;349:2191–2200.
5. Bates SM, Kearon C, Crowther M, et al. A diagnostic strategy involving a quantitative latex D-dimer assay reliably excludes deep venous thrombosis. Ann Intern Med 2003;138: 787–794.
6. Maisel AS, Krishnaswamy P, Nowak RM, et al. Rapid measurement of B-type natriuretic peptide in the emergency diagnosis of heart failure. N Engl J Med 2002;347:161–167.
7. Steg PG, Joubin L, McCord J, et al. B-type natriuretic peptide and echocardiographic determination of ejection fraction in the diagnosis of congestive heart failure in patients with acute dyspnea. Chest 2005;128:21–29.
8. Dearking AC, Aletti GD, McGree ME, et al. How relevant are ACOG and SGO guidelines for referral of adnexal mass? Obstet Gynecol 2007;110:841–848.
9. Bobo JK, Lee NC, Thames SF. Findings from 752,081 clinical breast examinations reported to a national screening program from 1995 through 1998. J Natl Cancer Inst 2000;92: 971–976.
10. Bates SM, Grand'Maison A, Johnston M, et al. A latex D-dimer reliably excludes venous thromboembolism. Arch Intern Med 2001;161:447–453.

11. Wells PS, Owen C, Doucette S, et al. Does this patient have deep vein thrombosis? The rational clinical examination. JAMA 2006;295:199–207.

12. Garber AM, Hlatky MA. Stress testing for the diagnosis of coronary heart disease. In Basow DS, ed. UpToDate. Waltham, MA; UpToDate; 2012.

13. Heffner JE, Sahn SA, Brown LK. Multilevel likelihood ratios for identifying exudative pleural effusions. Chest 2002;121:1916–1920.

14. McGee S. Simplifying likelihood ratios. J Gen Intern Med 2002;17:646–649.

15. Buys SS, Partridge E, Greene M, et al. Ovarian cancer screening in the Prostate, Lung, Colorectal and Ovarian (PLCO) cancer screening trial: findings from the initial screen of a randomized trial. Am J Obstet Gynecol 2005;193:1630–1639.

16. McIsaac WJ, Kellner JD, Aufricht P, et al. Empirical validation of guidelines for the management of pharyngitis in children and adults. JAMA 2004;291:1587–1595.

17. Williams JW, Simel DL, Roberts L, et al. Clinical evaluation for sinusitis. Making the diagnosis by history and physical examination. Ann Intern Med 1992;117:705–710.

Treatment

Treatments should be given "not because they ought to work, but because they do work."
—L.H. Opie
1980

KEY WORDS

Hypotheses
Treatment
Intervention
Comparative
  effectiveness
Experimental studies
Clinical trials
Randomized
  controlled trials
Equipoise
Inclusion criteria
Exclusion criteria
Comorbidity
Large simple trials
Practical clinical trials
Pragmatic clinical
  trials
Hawthorne effect
Placebo
Placebo effect
Random allocation
Randomization
Baseline
  characteristics
Stratified
  randomization
Compliance
Adherence
Run-in period
Cross-over
Blinding

Masking
Allocation
  concealment
Single-blind
Double-blind
Open label
Composite outcomes
Health-related quality
  of life
Health status
Efficacy trials
Effectiveness trials
Intention-to-treat
  analysis
Explanatory analyses
Per-protocol
Superiority trials
Non-inferiority trials
Inferiority margin
Cluster randomized
  trials
Cross-over trials
Trials of $N = 1$
Confounding by
  indication
Phase I trials
Phase II trials
Phase III trials
Postmarketing
  surveillance

After the nature of a patient's illness has been established and its expected course predicted, the next question is, what can be done about it? Is there a treatment that improves the outcome of disease? This chapter describes the evidence used to decide whether a well-intentioned treatment is actually effective.

IDEAS AND EVIDENCE

The discovery of effective new treatments requires both rich sources of promising possibilities and rigorous ways of establishing that the treatments are, in fact, effective (Fig. 9.1).

Ideas

Ideas about what might be a useful treatment arise from virtually any activity within medicine. These ideas are called hypotheses to the extent that they are assertions about the natural world that are made for the purposes of empiric testing.

Some therapeutic hypotheses are suggested by the mechanisms of disease at the molecular level. Drugs for antibiotic-resistant bacteria are developed through knowledge of the mechanism of resistance and hormone analogues are variations on the structure of native hormones. Other hypotheses about treatments have come from astute observations by clinicians, shared with their colleagues in case reports. Others are discovered by accident: The drug minoxidil, which was developed for hypertension, was found to improve male pattern baldness; and tamoxifen, developed for contraception, was found to prevent breast cancer in high-risk women. Traditional medicines, some of which are supported by centuries of experience,

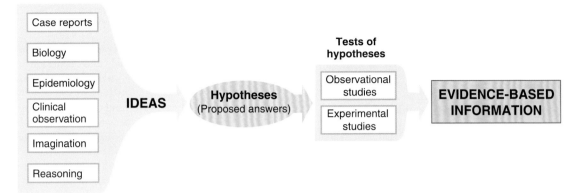

Figure 9.1 ■ Ideas and evidence.

may be effective. Aspirin, atropine, and digitalis are examples of naturally occurring substances that have become established as orthodox medicines after rigorous testing. Still other ideas come from trial and error. Some anticancer drugs have been found by methodically screening huge numbers of substances for activity in laboratory models. Ideas about treatment, but more often prevention, have also come from epidemiologic studies of populations. The Framingham Study, a cohort study of risk factors for cardiovascular diseases, was the basis for clinical trials of lowering blood pressure and serum cholesterol.

Testing Ideas

Some treatment effects are so prompt and powerful that their value is self-evident even without formal testing. Clinicians do not have reservations about the effectiveness of antibiotics for bacterial meningitis, or diuretics for edema. Clinical experience is sufficient.

In contrast, many diseases, including most chronic diseases, involve treatments that are considerably less dramatic. The effects are smaller, especially when an effective treatment is tested against another effective treatment. Also outcomes take longer to develop. It is then necessary to put ideas about treatments to a formal test, through clinical research, because a variety of circumstances, such as coincidence, biased comparisons, spontaneous changes in the course of disease, or wishful thinking, can obscure the true relationship between treatment and outcomes.

When knowledge of the pathogenesis of disease, based on laboratory models or physiologic studies in humans, has become extensive, it is tempting to predict effects in humans on this basis alone. However, relying solely on current understanding of mechanisms without testing ideas using strong clinical research on intact humans can lead to unpleasant surprises.

Example

Control of elevated blood sugar has been a keystone in the care of patients with diabetes mellitus, in part to prevent cardiovascular complications. Hyperglycemia is the most obvious metabolic abnormality in patients with diabetes. Cardiovascular disease is common in patients with diabetes, and observational studies have shown an association between elevated blood sugar and cardiovascular events. To study the effects of tight control of blood sugar on cardiovascular events, the ACCORD Trial randomized 10,251 patients with type 2 diabetes mellitus and other risk factors for cardiovascular disease to either intensive therapy or usual care (1). Glucose control was substantially better in the intensive therapy group but surprisingly, after 3.7 years in the trial, patients assigned to intensive therapy had 21% more deaths. They also had more hypoglycemic episodes and more weight gain. Results were similar after 5 years of follow-up. Increased mortality with "tight" control, which was contrary to conventional thinking about diabetes (but consistent with other trial results), has prompted less aggressive goals for blood glucose control and more aggressive treatment of other risk factors for cardiovascular disease, such as blood pressure, smoking, and dyslipidemia.

This study illustrates how treatments that make good sense, based on what is known about the disease at the time, may be found to be ineffective when put to a rigorous test in humans. Knowledge of pathogenesis, worked out in laboratory models, may be disappointing in human studies because the laboratory studies are in highly simplified settings. They usually exclude or control for many real-world influences on disease such as variation in genetic endowment, the physical and social environment, and individual behaviors and preferences.

Clinical experience and tradition also need to be put to a test. For example, bed rest has been advocated for a large number of medical conditions. Usually, there is a rationale for it. For example, it has been thought that the headache following lumbar puncture might result from a leak of cerebrospinal fluid through the needle track causing stretching of the meninges. However, a review of 39 trials of bed rest for 15 different conditions found that outcome did not improve for any condition. Outcomes were worse with bed rest in 17 trials, including not only lumbar puncture, but also acute low back pain, labor, hypertension during pregnancy, acute myocardial infarction, and acute infectious hepatitis (2).

Of course, it is not always the case that ideas are debunked. The main point is that promising treatments have to be tested by clinical research rather than accepted into the care of patients on the basis of reasoning alone.

STUDIES OF TREATMENT EFFECTS

Treatment is any intervention that is intended to improve the course of disease after it is established. Treatment is a special case of interventions in general that might be applied at any point in the natural history of disease, from disease prevention to palliative care at the end of life. Although usually thought of as medications, surgery, or radiotherapy, health care interventions can take any form, including relaxation therapy, laser surgery, or changes in the organization and financing of health care. Regardless of the nature of a well-intentioned intervention, the principles by which it is judged superior to other alternatives are the same.

Comparative effectiveness is a popular name for a not-so-new concept, the head-to-head comparison of two or more interventions (e.g., drugs, devices, tests, surgery, or monitoring), all of which are believed to be effective and are current options for care. Comparison is not just for effectiveness, but also for all clinically important end results of the interventions—both beneficial and harmful. Results can help clinicians and patients understand all of the consequences of choosing one or another course of action when both have been considered reasonable alternatives.

Observational and Experimental Studies of Treatment Effects

Two general methods are used to establish the effects of interventions: observational and experimental studies. The two differ in their scientific strength and feasibility.

In observational studies of interventions, investigators simply observe what happens to patients who for various reasons do or do not get exposed to an intervention (see Chapters 5–7). Observational studies of treatment are a special case of studies of prognosis in general, in which the prognostic factor of interest is a therapeutic intervention. What has been said about cohort studies applies to observational studies of treatment as well. The main advantage of these studies is feasibility. The main drawback is the possibility that there are systematic differences in treatment groups, other than the treatment itself, that can lead to misleading conclusions about the effects of treatment.

Experimental studies are a special kind of cohort study in which the conditions of study—selection of treatment groups, nature of interventions, management during follow-up, and measurement of outcomes—are specified by the investigator for the purpose of making unbiased comparisons. These studies are generally referred to as clinical trials. Clinical trials are more highly controlled and managed than cohort studies. The investigators are conducting an experiment, analogous to those done in the laboratory. They have taken it upon themselves (with their patients' permission) to isolate for study the unique contribution of one factor by holding constant, as much as possible, all other determinants of the outcome.

Randomized controlled trials, in which treatment is randomly allocated, are the standard of excellence for scientific studies of the effects of treatment. They are described in detail below, followed by descriptions of alternative ways of studying the effectiveness of interventions.

RANDOMIZED CONTROLLED TRIALS

The structure of a randomized controlled trial is shown in Figure 9.2. All elements are the same as for a cohort study except that treatment is assigned by randomization rather than by physician and patient choice. The "exposures" are treatments, and the "outcomes" are any possible end result of treatment (such as the 5 Ds described in Table 1.2).

The patients to be studied are first selected from a larger number of patients with the condition of

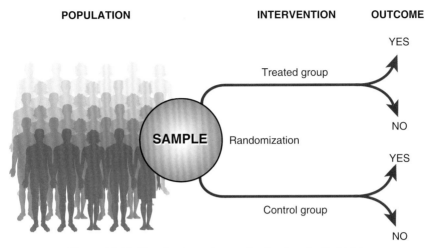

POPULATION   **INTERVENTION**   **OUTCOME**

Figure 9.2 ■ **The structure of a randomized controlled trial.**

interest. Using randomization, the patients are then divided into two (or more) groups of comparable prognosis. One group, called the experimental group, is exposed to an intervention that is believed to be better than current alternatives. The other group, called a control (or comparison) group, is treated the same in all ways except that its members are not exposed to the experimental intervention. Patients in the control group may receive a placebo, usual care, or the current best available treatment. The course of disease is then recorded in both groups, and differences in outcome are attributed to the intervention.

The main reason for structuring clinical trials in this way is to avoid confounding when comparing the respective effects of two or more kinds of treatments. The validity of clinical trials depends on how well they have created equal distribution of all determinants of prognosis, other than the one being tested, in treated and control patients.

Individual elements of clinical trials are described in detail in the following text.

Ethics

Under what circumstances is it ethical to assign treatment at random, rather than as decided by the patient and physician? The general principle, called equipoise, is that randomization is ethical when there is no compelling reason to believe that either of the randomly allocated treatments is better than the other. Usually it is believed that the experimental intervention *might* be better than the control but that has not been conclusively established by strong research. The primary outcome must be benefit; treatments cannot be randomly allocated to discover whether one is more harmful than the other. Of course, as with any human research, patients must fully understand the consequences of participating in the study, know that they can withdraw at any time without compromising their health care, and freely give their consent to participate. In addition, the trial must be stopped whenever there is convincing evidence of effectiveness, harm, or futility in continuing.

Sampling

Clinical trials typically require patients to meet rigorous inclusion and exclusion criteria. These are intended to increase the homogeneity of patients in the study, to strengthen internal validity, and to make it easier to distinguish the "signal" (treatment effect) from the "noise" (bias and chance).

Among the usual inclusion criteria is that patients really do have the condition being studied. To be on the safe side, study patients must meet strict diagnostic criteria. Patients with unusual, mild, or equivocal manifestations of disease may be left out in the process, restricting generalizability.

Of the many possible exclusion criteria, several account for most of the losses:

1. Patients with comorbidity (diseases other than the one being studied) are typically excluded because the care and outcome of these other diseases can muddy the contrast between experimental and comparison treatments and their outcomes.
2. Patients are excluded if they are not expected to live long enough to experience the outcome events of interest.
3. Patients with contraindications to one of the treatments cannot be randomized.

4. Patients who refuse to participate in a trial are excluded, for ethical reasons described earlier in the chapter.
5. Patients who do not cooperate during the early stages of the trial are also excluded. This avoids wasted effort and the reduction in internal validity that occurs when patients do not take their assigned intervention, move in and out of treatment groups, or leave the trial altogether.

For these reasons, patients in clinical trials are usually a highly selected, biased sample of all patients with the condition of interest. As heterogeneity is restricted, the internal validity of the study is improved; in other words, there is less opportunity for differences in outcome that are not related to treatment itself. However, exclusions come at the price of diminished generalizability: Patients in the trial are not like most other patients seen in day-to-day care.

Example

Figure 9.3 summarizes how patients were selected for a randomized controlled trial of asthma management (3). Investigators invited 1,410 patients with asthma in 81 general practices in Scotland to participate. Only 458 of those invited, about one-third, agreed to participate and could be contacted. An additional 199 were excluded, mainly because they did not meet eligibility criteria, leaving 259 patients (18% of those invited) to be randomized. Although the study invited patients from community practices, those who actually participated in the trial were highly selected and perhaps unlike most patients in the community.

Because of the high degree of selection in trials, it may require considerable faith to generalize the results of clinical trials to ordinary practice settings.

If there are not enough patients with the disease of interest, at one time and place, to carry out a scientifically sound trial, then sampling can be from multiple sites with common inclusion and exclusion criteria. This is done mainly to achieve adequate sample size, but it also increases generalizability, to the extent that the sites are somewhat different from each other.

Large simple trials are a way of overcoming the generalizability problem. Trial entry criteria are simplified so that most patients developing the study condition are eligible. Participating patients have to have accepted random allocation of treatment, but their care is otherwise the same as usual, without a great deal of extra testing that is part of some trials. Follow-up is for a simple, clinically important outcome, such as discharge from the hospital alive. This approach not only improves generalizability, it also makes it easier to recruit large numbers of participants at a reasonable cost so that moderate effect sizes (large effects are unlikely for most clinical questions) can be detected.

Practical clinical trials (also called pragmatic clinical trials) are designed to answer real-world questions in the actual care of patients by including the kinds of patients and interventions found in ordinary patient care settings.

Example

Severe ankle sprains are a common problem among patients visiting emergency departments. Various treatments are in common use. The Collaborative Ankle Support Trial Group enrolled 584 patients with severe ankle sprain in eight emergency departments in the United Kingdom in a randomized trial of four commonly used treatments: tubular compression bandage and three types of mechanical support (4). Quality of ankle function at 3 months was best after a below-the-knee cast was used for 10 days and worst when a tubular compression bandage was used; the tubular compression bandage was being used in 75% of centers in the United Kingdom at the time. Two less effective forms of mechanical support were several times more expensive than the cast. All treatment groups improved over time and there was no difference in outcome among them at 9 months.

Practical trials are different from typical efficacy trials where, in an effort to increase internal validity, severe restrictions are applied to enrollment, intervention, and adherence, limiting the relevance of their results for usual patient care decisions. Large simple trials may be of practical questions too, but practical trials need not be so large.

Intervention

The intervention can be described in relation to three general characteristics: generalizability, complexity, and strength.

First, is the intervention one that is likely to be implemented in usual clinical practice? In an effort

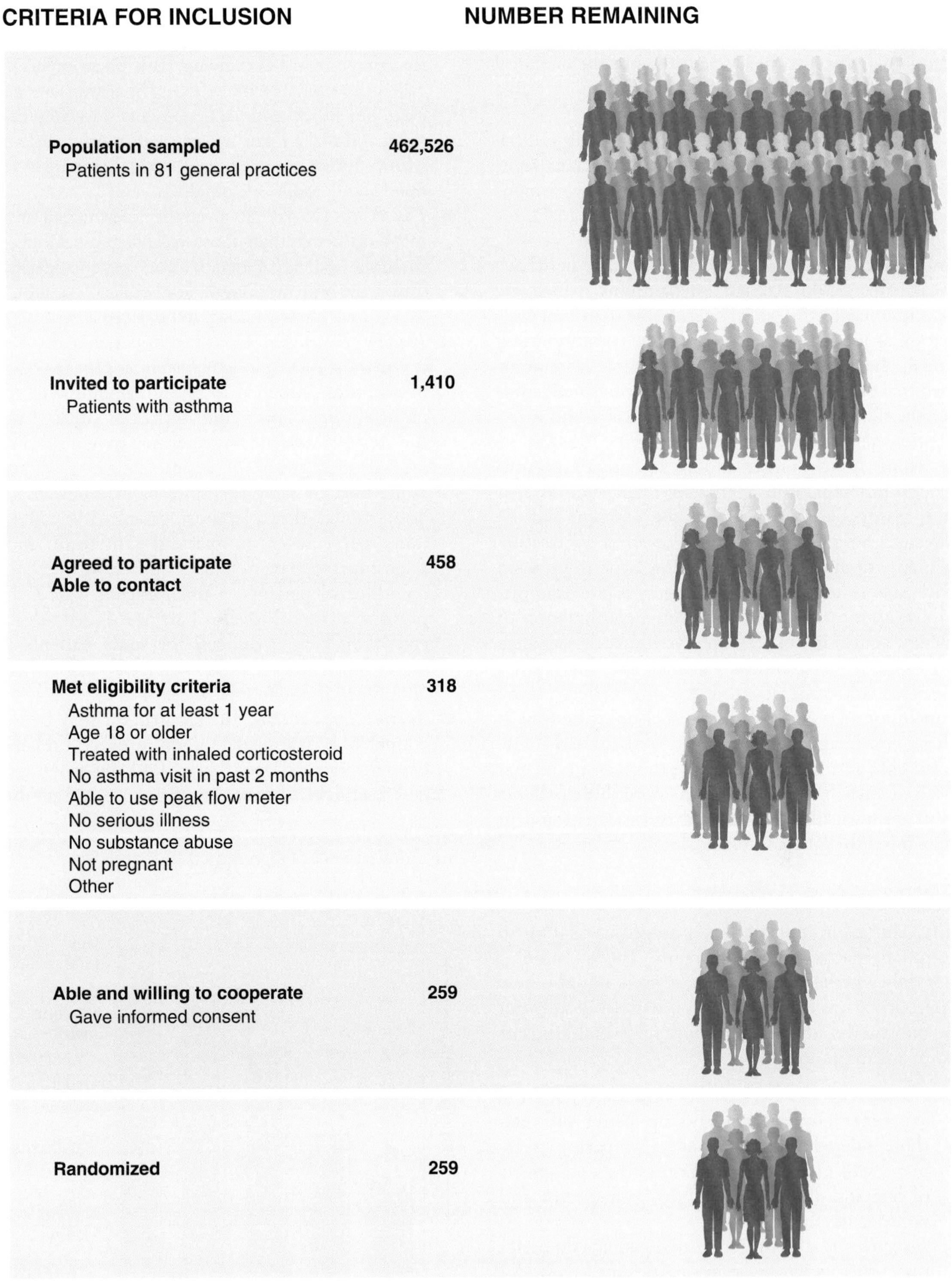

CRITERIA FOR INCLUSION   NUMBER REMAINING

Population sampled   462,526
  Patients in 81 general practices

Invited to participate   1,410
  Patients with asthma

Agreed to participate   458
Able to contact

Met eligibility criteria   318
  Asthma for at least 1 year
  Age 18 or older
  Treated with inhaled corticosteroid
  No asthma visit in past 2 months
  Able to use peak flow meter
  No serious illness
  No substance abuse
  Not pregnant
  Other

Able and willing to cooperate   259
  Gave informed consent

Randomized   259

Figure 9.3 ■ **Sampling of patients for a randomized controlled trial of asthma management.** (Data from Hawkins G, McMahon AD, Twaddle S, et al. Stepping down inhaled corticosteroids in asthma: randomized controlled trial. BMJ 2003;326: 1115–1121.)

to standardize the intervention so that it can be easily described and reproduced in other settings, investigators may cater to their scientific, not their clinical colleagues by studying treatments that are not feasible in usual practice.

Second, does the intervention reflect the normal complexity of real-world treatment? Clinicians regularly construct treatment plans with many components. Single, highly specific interventions make for tidy science because they can be described precisely and applied in a reproducible way, but they may have weak effects. Multifaceted interventions, which are often more effective, are also amenable to careful evaluation as long as their essence can be communicated and applied in other settings. For example, a randomized trial of fall prevention in acute care hospitals studied the effects of a fall risk assessment scale, with interventions tailored to each patient's specific risks (5).

Third, is the intervention in question sufficiently different from alternative managements that it is reasonable to expect that the outcome will be affected? Some diseases can be reversed by treating a single, dominant cause. Treating hyperthyroidism with radioisotope ablation or surgery is one example. However, most diseases arise from a combination of factors acting in concert. Interventions that change only one of them, and only a small amount, cannot be expected to result in strong treatment effects. If the conclusion of a trial evaluating such interventions is that a new treatment is not effective when used alone, it should come as no surprise. For this reason, the first trials of a new treatment tend to enroll those patients who are most likely to respond to treatment and to maximize dose and compliance.

Comparison Groups

The value of an intervention is judged in relation to some alternative course of action. The question is not only whether a comparison is used, but also how appropriate it is for the research question. Results can be measured against one or more of several kinds of comparison groups.

- *No Intervention.* Do patients who are offered the experimental treatment end up better off than those offered nothing at all? Comparing treatment with no treatment measures the total effects of care and of being in a study, both specific and nonspecific.
- *Being Part of a Study.* Do treated patients do better than other patients who just participate in a study? A great deal of special attention is directed toward patients in clinical trials. People have a tendency to change their behavior when they are the target of

special interest and attention because of the study, regardless of the specific nature of the intervention they might be receiving. This phenomenon is called the Hawthorne effect. The reasons are not clear, but some seem likely: Patients want to please them and make them feel successful. Also, patients who volunteer for trials want to do their part to see that "good" results are obtained.

- *Usual Care.* Do patients given the experimental treatment do better than those receiving usual care—whatever individual doctors and patients decide? This is the only meaningful (and ethical) question if usual care is already known to be effective.
- *Placebo Treatment.* Do treated patients do better than similar patients given a placebo—an intervention intended to be indistinguishable (in physical appearance, color, taste, or smell) from the active treatment but does not have a specific, known mechanism of action? Sugar pills and saline injections are examples of placebos. It has been shown that placebos, given with conviction, relieve severe, unpleasant symptoms, such as postoperative pain, nausea, or itching, in about one-third of patients, a phenomenon called the placebo effect. Placebos have the added advantage of making it difficult for study patients to know which intervention they have received (see "Blinding" in the following text).
- *Another Intervention.* The comparator may be the current best treatment. The point of a "comparative effectiveness" study is to find out whether a new treatment is better than the one in current use.

Changes in outcome related to these comparators are cumulative, as diagrammed in Figure 9.4.

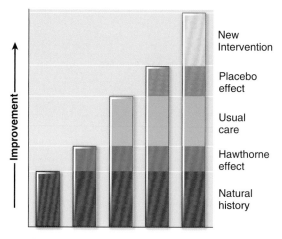

Figure 9.4 ■ Total effects of treatment are the sum of spontaneous improvement (natural history) as well as nonspecific and specific responses.

Allocating Treatment

To study the effects of a clinical intervention free of confounding, the best way to allocate patients to treatment groups is by means of random allocation (also referred to as randomization). Patients are assigned to either the experimental or the control treatment by one of a variety of disciplined procedures—analogous to flipping a coin—whereby each patient has an equal (or at least known) chance of being assigned to any one of the treatment groups.

Random allocation of patients is preferable to other methods of allocation because only randomization has the ability to create truly comparable groups. All factors related to prognosis, regardless of whether they are known before the study takes place or have been measured, tend to be equally distributed in the comparison groups.

In the long run, with a large number of patients in a trial, randomization usually works as just described. However, random allocation does not guarantee that the groups will be similar; dissimilarities can arise by chance alone, particularly when the number of patients randomized is small. To assess whether "bad luck" has occurred, authors of randomized controlled trials often present a table comparing the frequency in the treated and control groups of a variety of characteristics, especially those known to be related to outcome. These are called baseline characteristics because they are present before randomization and, therefore, should be equally distributed in the treatment groups.

Example

Table 9.1 shows some of the baseline characteristics for a study of liberal versus restrictive blood transfusion in high-risk patients after hip surgery. The 2,016 enrolled patients were at increased risk because of risk factors for cardiovascular disease or anemia after surgery. The primary outcome was death or the inability to walk across a room without human assistance (6). Table 9.1 lists several characteristics already known, from other studies or clinical experience, to be related to one or both of these outcomes. Each of these characteristics was similarly distributed in the two treatment groups. These comparisons, at least for the several characteristics that were measured, strengthen the belief that randomization was carried out properly and actually produced groups with similar risk for death or inability to walk unassisted.

Table 9.1

Example of a Table Comparing Baseline Characteristics: A Randomized Trial of Liberal versus Restrictive Transfusion in High-Risk Patients after Hip Surgery

Characteristics	Percent with Characteristic for Each Group	
	% Liberal (1,007 Patients)	% Restricted (1,009 Patients)
Age (mean)	81.8	81.5
Male	24.8	23.7
Any cardiovascular disease	63.3	62.5
Tobacco use <600 mg/d	11.6	11.3
Anesthesiology risk score	3.0	2.9
General anesthesia	54.0	56.2
Lived in nursing home	10.3	10.9

Data from Carson JL, Terrin ML, Noveck H, et al. Liberal or restrictive transfusion in high-risk patients after hip surgery. N Engl J Med 2011; 365:2453–2462.

It is reassuring to see that important prognostic variables are nearly equally distributed in the groups being compared. If the groups are substantially different in a large trial, it suggests that something has gone wrong with the randomization process. Smaller differences, which are expected because of chance, can be controlled for during data analyses (see Chapter 5).

In some situations, especially small trials, to reduce the risk of bad luck, it is best to make sure that at least some of the characteristics known to be strongly associated with outcome occur equally in treated and control patients. Patients are gathered into groups (strata) that have similar levels of a prognostic factor (e.g., age for most chronic diseases) and are randomized separately within each of the strata, a process called stratified randomization (Fig. 9.5). The final groups are sure to be comparable, at least for the characteristics that were used to create the strata. Some investigators do not favor stratified randomization, arguing that whatever differences arise from bad luck are unlikely to be large and can be adjusted for mathematically after the data have been collected.

Differences Arising after Randomization

Not all patients in clinical trials participate as originally planned. Some are found to not have the disease

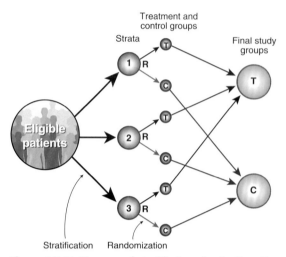

Figure 9.5 ■ **Diagram of stratified randomization. T = treated group, C = control group, and R = randomization.**

they were thought to have when they entered the trial. Others drop out, do not take their medications, are taken out of the study because of side effects or other illnesses, or somehow obtain the other study treatment or treatments that are not part of the study at all. In this way, treatment groups that might have been comparable just after randomization become less so as time passes.

Patients May Not Have the Disease Being Studied

It is sometimes necessary (both in clinical trials and in practice) to begin treatment before it is certain whether the patient actually has the disease for which the treatment is designed.

Example

Hydrocortisone may improve survival from septic shock, especially in patients with abnormal adrenal response to shock, as measured by an inappropriately small rise in plasma cortisol after administration of corticotropin. Treatment must begin before the results of the test are available. Investigators in Israel and Europe studied whether hydrocortisone improved survival to 28 days in patients with septic shock (7). Patients were randomized to hydrocortisone or placebo, and treatment was begun before results of the corticotrophin

test were available. Of 499 patients with septic shock enrolled in the trial, 233 (47%) had adrenal insufficiency. The main analysis was of this subgroup, those who it was believed might respond to hydrocortisone, not of all patients randomized. Among patients with poor response to corticotrophin, there was no difference in survival in patients treated with hydrocortisone, compared with placebo.

Because response to corticotrophin was a characteristic that existed before randomization, it had been randomly allocated, so the advantages of a randomized controlled trial were preserved. However, the inefficiency of enrolling and gathering data on patients who would not contribute to the study's results could not be avoided. Also, the number of patients in the study was reduced, making it more difficult to detect differences in survival if they existed. Nevertheless, this kind of trial has the important advantage of providing information on both the consequences of a decision that a clinician must make before all the relevant information is available as well as effectiveness of treatment in the subset of patients most likely to respond (see the Intention-to-Treat and Explanatory Trials section in this chapter).

Compliance

Compliance is the extent to which patients follow medical advice. The term adherence is preferred by some people because it connotes a less subservient relationship between patient and doctor. Compliance is another characteristic that comes into play after randomization.

Although noncompliance suggests a kind of willful neglect of good advice, other factors also contribute. Patients may misunderstand which drugs and doses are intended, run out of prescription medications, confuse various preparations of the same drug, or have no money or insurance to pay for drugs. Taken together, non-compliance may limit the usefulness of treatments that have been shown to work under favorable conditions.

In general, compliance marks a better prognosis, apart from treatment. Patients in randomized trials who were compliant with placebo had better outcomes than those who were not (8).

Compliance is particularly important in medical care outside the hospital. In hospitals, many factors act to constrain patients' personal behavior and render them compliant. Hospitalized patients are generally sicker and more frightened. They are in strange surroundings, dependent upon the skill and attention of the staff for everything, including their life. What is more, doctors, nurses, and pharmacists have developed a well-organized system for ensuring that patients receive what is ordered for them. As a result, clinical experience and medical literature developed on the wards may underestimate the importance of compliance outside the hospital, where most patients and doctors are and where following doctors' orders is less common.

In clinical trials, patients are typically selected to be compliant. During a run-in period, in which placebo is given and compliance monitored, noncompliant patients can be detected and excluded before randomization.

Cross-over

Patients may move from one randomly allocated treatment to another during follow-up, a phenomenon called cross-over. If exchanges between treatment groups take place on a large scale, it can diminish the observed differences in treatment effect compared to what might have been observed if the original groups had remained intact.

Cointerventions

After randomization, patients may receive a variety of interventions other than the ones being studied. For example, in a study of asthma treatment, they may receive not only the experimental drug but also different doses of their usual drugs and make greater efforts to control allergens in the home. If these occur unequally in the two groups and affect outcomes, they can introduce systematic differences between the groups that were not present when the groups were formed.

Blinding

Participants in a trial may change their behavior or reporting of outcomes in a systematic way (i.e., be biased) if they are aware of which patients are receiving which treatment. One way to minimize this effect is by blinding, an attempt to make the various participants in a study unaware of the treatment group patients have been randomized to so that this knowledge cannot cause them to act differently, and thereby diminish the internal validity of the study. Masking is a more appropriate metaphor, but blinding is the time-honored term.

Blinding can take place in a clinical trial at four levels (Fig. 9.6). First, those responsible for allocating patients to treatment groups should not know which treatment will be assigned next making it impossible for them to break the randomization plan. Allocation concealment is a term for this form of blinding. Without it, some investigators might be tempted to enter patients in the trial out of order to ensure that individuals get the treatment that seems best for them. Second, patients should be unaware of

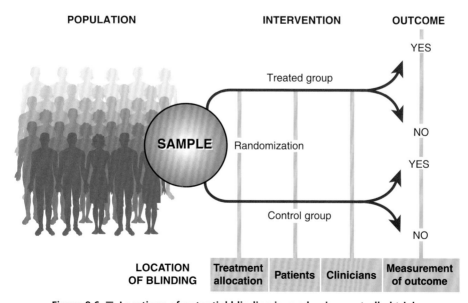

Figure 9.6 ■ **Locations of potential blinding in randomize controlled trials.**

which treatment they are taking so that they cannot change their compliance or reporting of symptoms because of this information. Third, to ensure physicians caring for patients in a study cannot, even subconsciously, manage patients differently, physicians should not know which treatment each patient is on. Finally, when the researchers who assess outcomes are unaware of which treatment individual patients have been offered, that knowledge cannot affect their measurements.

The terms single-blind (patients) and double-blind are sometimes used, but their meanings are ambiguous. It is better simply to describe what was done. A trial in which there is no attempt at blinding is called an *open trial* or, in the case of drug trials, an open label trial.

In drug studies, blinding is often made possible by using a placebo. However, for many important clinical questions, such as the effects of surgery, radiotherapy, diet, or the organization of medical care, blinding of patients and their physicians is difficult if not impossible.

Even when blinding appears to be possible, it is more often claimed than successful. Physiologic effects, such as lowered pulse rate with beta-blocking drugs and gastrointestinal upset or drowsiness with other drugs, may signal to patients whether they are taking the active drug or placebo.

Assessment of Outcomes

Randomized controlled trials are a special case of cohort studies, and what we have already said about measures of effect and biases in cohort studies (Chapter 5) apply to them as well, as do the dangers of substituting intermediate outcomes for clinically important ones (Chapter 1).

Example

A low level of high-density lipoprotein (HDL) cholesterol is a risk factor for cardiovascular disease. The drug niacin raises HDL levels and lowers low-density lipoprotein (LDL) cholesterol and triglycerides (both also risk factors); therefore, taking niacin might contribute to the prevention of cardiovascular disease when taken in addition to a lipid-lowering "statin" drug such as simvastatin, which lowers LDL but not HDL cholesterol or triglycerides. In a randomized controlled trial of adding niacin to simvastatin, patients on niacin had higher HDL and lower LDL cholesterol and triglycerides than patients on simvastatin alone (9). However, rates of the primary outcome, a composite of cardiovascular events (see the following text), was the same in the two treatment groups: 16.4% in the niacin group and 16.2 in the placebo group. The authors concluded that "there was no incremental clinical benefit from the addition of niacin to statin therapy . . . despite significant improvements in HDL cholesterol and triglyceride levels."

Clinical trials may have as their primary outcome a composite outcome, a set of outcomes that are related to each other but are treated as a single outcome variable. For example, in a study of percutaneous repair versus open surgery for mitral regurgitation, the composite outcome was the absence of death, mitral valve surgery, or severe mitral regurgitation 12 months after treatment (10). There are several advantages to this approach. The individual outcomes in the composite may be so highly related to each other, biologically and clinically, that it is artificial to consider them separately. The presence of one (such as death) may prevent the other (such as severe mitral regurgitation) from occurring. With more ways to experience an outcome event, a study is better able to detect treatment effects (see Chapter 11). The disadvantage of composite outcomes is that they can obscure differences in effects for different individual outcomes. In addition, one component may account for most of the result, giving the impression that the intervention affects the others too. All of these disadvantages can be overcome by simply examining effect on each component outcome separately as well as together.

In addition to "hard" outcomes such as survival, remission of disease, and return of function, a trial sometimes measure health-related quality of life by broad, composite measures of health status. A simple quality-of-life measure used by a collaborative group of cancer researchers is shown in Table 9.2. This "performance scale" combines symptoms and function, such as the ability to walk. Others are much more extensive; the Sickness Impact Profile contains more than 100 items and a dozen categories. Still others are specifically developed for individual diseases. The main issue is that the value of a clinical trial is strengthened to the extent that such measures are reported along with hard measures such as death and recurrence of disease.

Table 9.2

A Simple Measure of Quality of Life. The Eastern Collaborative Oncology Group's Performance Scale	
Performance Status	**Definition**
0	Asymptomatic
1	Symptomatic, fully ambulatory
2	Symptomatic, in bed <50% of the day
3	Symptomatic, in bed >50% of the day
4	Bedridden
5	Dead

Table 9.3

Summarizing Treatment Effects	
Summary Measure[a]	**Definition**
Relative risk reduction	$\dfrac{\text{Control event rate} - \text{Treated event rate}}{\text{Control event rate}}$
Absolute risk reduction	Control even rate – Treated event rate
Number needed to treat OR number needed to harm	$\dfrac{1}{\text{Control event rate} - \text{Treatment event rate}}$

[a]For continuous data in which there are measurements at baseline and after treatment, analogous measures are based on the mean values for treated and control groups either after treatment or for the difference between baseline and posttreatment values.

Options for describing effect size in clinical trials are summarized in Table 9.3. The options are similar to summaries of risk and prognosis but related to change in outcome resulting from the intervention.

EFFICACY AND EFFECTIVENESS

Clinical trials may describe the results of an intervention in ideal or in real-world situations (Fig. 9.7).

First, can treatment help under *ideal* circumstances? Trials that answer this question are called efficacy trials. Elements of ideal circumstances include patients who accept the interventions offered to them, follow instructions faithfully, get the best possible care, and do not have care for other

diseases. Most randomized trials are designed in this way.

Second, does treatment help under *ordinary* circumstances? Trials designed to answer this kind of question are called effectiveness trials. All the usual elements of patient care are part of effectiveness trials. Patients may not take their assigned treatment. Some may drop out of the study, and others find ways to take the treatment they were not assigned. The doctors and facilities may not be the best. In short, effectiveness trials describe results as most patients would experience them. The difference between efficacy and effectiveness has been described as the "implementation gap," the gap between ideal care and ordinary care, and is a target for improvement in its own right.

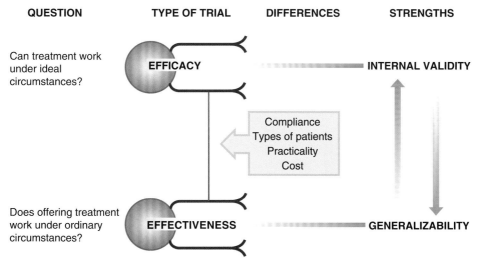

Figure 9.7 ■ Efficacy and effectiveness.

Efficacy trials usually precede effectiveness trial. The rationale is that if treatment under the best circumstances is not effective, then effectiveness under ordinary circumstances is impossible. Also, if an effectiveness trial were done first and it showed no effect, the result could have been because the treatment at its best is just not effective or that the treatment really is effective but was not received.

Intention-to-Treat and Explanatory Trials

A related issue is whether the results of a randomized controlled trial should be analyzed and presented according to the treatment to which the patients were randomized or according to the one they actually received (Fig. 9.8).

One question is: Which treatment choice is best at the time the decision must be made? To answer this question, analysis is according to which group the patients were assigned (randomized), regardless

of whether these patients actually received the treatment they were supposed to receive. This way of analyzing trial results is called an intention-to-treat analysis. An advantage of this approach is that the question corresponds to the one actually faced by clinicians; they either offer a treatment or not. Also, the groups compared are as originally randomized, so this comparison has the full strength of a randomized trial. The disadvantage is that to the extent that many patients do not receive the treatment to which they were randomized, differences in effectiveness will tend to be obscured, increasing the chances of observing a misleadingly small effect or no statistical effect at all. If the study shows no difference, it will be uncertain whether the problem is the treatment itself or that it was not received.

Another question is whether the experimental treatment itself is better. For this question, the proper analysis is according to the treatment each patient actually received, regardless of the treatment

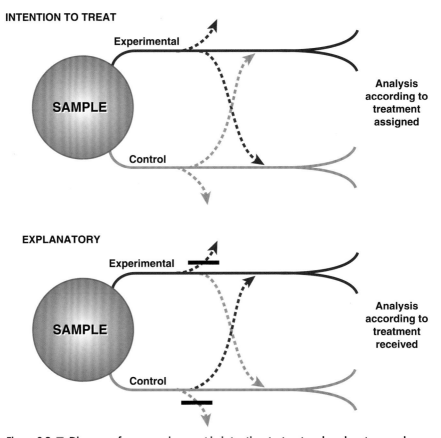

Figure 9.8 ■ Diagram of group assignment in intention-to-treat and explanatory analyses.

to which they were randomized. Trials analyzed in this way are called explanatory analyses (also called per-protocol) because they assess whether actually taking the treatments, rather than just being offered them, makes a difference. The problem with this approach is that unless most patients receive the treatment to which they are assigned, the study no longer represents a randomized trial; it is simply a cohort study. One must be concerned about dissimilarities among groups, other than the experimental treatment, and must use methods such as restriction, matching, stratification, or adjustment to achieve comparability, just as one would for any non-experimental study.

In general, intention-to-treat analyses are more relevant to effectiveness questions, whereas explanatory analyses are consistent with the purposes of efficacy trials, although aspects of the trial other than how they are analyzed matter too. The primary analysis is usually intention-to-treat, but both are reported. Both approaches are legitimate, with the right one depending on the question being asked. To the extent that patients in a trial follow the treatment to which they were randomized, these two analyses will give similar results.

SUPERIORITY, EQUIVALENCE, AND NON-INFERIORITY

Until now, we have been discussing superiority trials, ones that seek to establish that one treatment is *better* than another, but sometimes the most important question is whether a treatment is no less effective than another. A typical example is when a new drug is safer, cheaper, or easier to administer than the established one and would, therefore, be preferable if it were as effective. In non-inferiority trials, the purpose is to show that a new treatment is unlikely to be less effective, at least to a clinically important extent, than the currently accepted treatment, which has been shown in other studies to be more effective than placebo. The question is one-directional—whether a new treatment is not worse—without regard to whether it might be better.

It is statistically impossible to establish that a treatment is not at all inferior to another. However, a study can rule out an effect that is less than a predetermined "minimum clinically important difference," also called an inferiority margin, the smallest difference in effect that is still considered clinically important. The inferiority margin actually takes into account both this clinical difference plus the statistical imprecision of the study. The following is an example of a non-inferiority trial.

Example

Yaws is an infectious disease affecting more that 500,000 children in poor, rural areas of Africa, Asia, and South America. It is a chronic, deforming disease affecting mainly skin, bones, and cartilage. Long-acting penicillin given by injection has been the drug of choice and is cheap and well tolerated. However, there are disadvantages to injection drugs in resource-poor settings, mainly difficulties arranging for the equipment and personnel to give injections and the risk that unsafe injection practices would cause transmission of blood-borne pathogens such as HIV or hepatitis. To identify an effective but more practical alternative, investigators in Papua New Guinea did a randomized controlled non-inferiority trial of a single dose of the oral antibiotic azithromycin versus penicillin injection (11). Non-inferiority was defined as the lower limit of the 95% confidence interval for the difference in rates (see Chapter 11) that was no more than 10% lower for azithromycin than for penicillin. The cure rate was 96% in the azithromycin group and 93% for the penicillin group, and the confidence interval of the difference met the criteria for azithromycin being non-inferior. With evidence that a simpler treatment is as effective as penicillin injection, elimination of this disease, a goal in the 1960s, might again be realistic.

Non-inferiority trials usually require a larger sample size than comparable superiority trials, especially if the inferiority margin is small or one wants to rule out small differences. Also, any aspect of the trial that tends to minimize differences between comparison groups, such as intention-to-treat analyses in trials where many patients have dropped out or crossed over or when measurements of outcomes are imprecise, artificially increase the likelihood of finding non-inferiority regardless of whether it is truly present—that is, they result in a weak test for non-inferiority.

VARIATIONS ON BASIC RANDOMIZED TRIALS

In cluster randomized trials, naturally occurring groups ("clusters") of patients (defined by the doctors, hospitals, clinics, or communities that patients are affiliated with) are randomized, and outcome events are counted in patients according to the treatment their cluster was assigned. Randomization of groups, not the individuals in them, may be preferable for several reasons. It may just be more practical to randomized clusters than individuals. Patients within clusters may be more similar to each other than to patients in other clusters, and this source of variation, apart from the study treatments themselves, should be taken into account in the study. If patients were randomized within clusters, they or their physicians might learn from each other about both treatments and this might affect their behaviors. For example, how successfully could a physician be at randomly treating some patients with urinary tract infection one way and other patients another way? Similarly, could a hospital establish a new plan to prevent intravenous catheter infections in some of its intensive care units and not others when physicians see patients in both settings over time? For these reasons, randomizing clusters rather than patients can be the best approach in some circumstances.

There are other variations on the usual ("parallel group") randomized controlled trials. Cross-over trials expose patients first to one of two randomly allocated treatments and later to the other. If it can be assumed that effects of the first exposure are no longer present by the time of the second exposure, perhaps because treatment is short-lived or there has been a "wash-out" period between exposures, then each patient will have been exposed to each treatment in random order. This controls for differences in responsiveness among patients not related treatment effects.

TAILORING THE RESULTS OF TRIALS TO INDIVIDUAL PATIENTS

Clinical trials describe what happens on average. They involve pooling the experience of many patients who may be dissimilar, both to one another and to the patients to whom the trial results will be generalized. How can estimates of treatment effect be obtained that more closely match individual patients?

Subgroups

Patients in clinical trials can be sorted into subgroups, each with a specific characteristic (or combination of characteristics) such as age, severity of disease, and comorbidity that might cause a different treatment effect. That is, the data are examined for effect modification. The number of such subgroups is limited only by the number of patients in the subgroups, which has to be large enough to provide reasonably stable estimates. As long as the characteristics used to define

the subgroups existed before randomization, patients in each subgroup have been randomly allocated to treatment groups. As a consequence, results in each subgroup represent, in effect, a small trial within a trial. The characteristics of a given patient (e.g., the patient might be elderly and have severe disease but no comorbidity) can be matched more specifically to those of one of the subgroups than it can to the trial as a whole. Treatment effectiveness in the matched subgroup will more closely approximate that of the individual patient and will be limited mainly by statistical risks of false-positive and false-negative conclusions, which are described in Chapter 11.

Effectiveness in Individual Patients

A treatment that is effective on average may not work on an individual patient. Therefore, results of valid clinical research provide a good reason to begin treating a patient, but experience with that patient is a better reason to continue or not continue. When managing an individual patient, it is prudent to ask the following series of questions:

- Is the treatment known (by randomized controlled trials) to be efficacious for any patients?
- Is the treatment known to be effective, on average, in patients like mine?
- Is the treatment working in my patient?
- Are the benefits worth the discomforts and risks (according to the patient's values and preferences)?

By asking these questions and not simply following the results of trials alone, one can guard against ill-founded choice of treatment or stubborn persistence in the face of poor results.

Trials of *N* = 1

Rigorous clinical trials, with proper attention to bias and chance, can be carried out on individual patients, one at a time. The method, called trials of *N* = 1, is an improvement over the time-honored process of trial and error. A patient is given one treatment or another, such as an active treatment or placebo, in random order, each for a brief period of time. The patient and physician are blinded to which treatment is given. Outcomes, such as a simple preference for a treatment or a symptom score, are assessed after each period. After many repetitions patterns of responses are analyzed statistically, much as one would for a more usual randomized controlled trial. This method is useful for deciding on the care of individual patients when activity of disease is unpredictable, response to treatment is prompt, and there is no carryover effect from period to period. Examples of diseases for which the method can be used include migraine headaches, asthma, and fibromyalgia. For all their intellectual appeal, however, trials of $N = 1$ are rarely done and even more rarely published.

ALTERNATIVES TO RANDOMIZED CONTROLLED TRIALS

Randomized controlled trials are the gold standard for studies of the effectiveness of interventions. Only large randomized trials can definitively eliminate confounding as an alternative explanation for observed results.

Limitations of Randomized Trials

However, the availability of several well-conducted randomized controlled trials does not necessarily settle a question. For example, after 21 randomized controlled trials over three decades (one is described in an example earlier in this chapter) the effectiveness of corticosteroids for septic shock remains controversial. The heterogeneity of trial results seems partly related to differences in dose and duration of the drug, the proportion of patients with relative adrenal insufficiency, and whether the outcome is reversal of shock or survival. That is, the trials were of the same general questions but very different specific questions.

Clinical trials also suffer from practical limitations. They are expensive; in 2011, the average cost per patient in drug trials was estimated to be nearly $50,000, and some large trials have cost hundreds of millions of dollars. Logistics can be daunting, especially in maintaining similar methods across sites in multicenter trials and in maintaining the integrity of allocation concealment. Randomization itself remains a hindrance, if not to the conduct of trials at all then to full, unbiased participation. It is particularly difficult to convince patients to be randomized when a practice has become well established in the absence of conclusive evidence of its benefit.

For these reasons, clinical trials are not available to guide clinicians in many important treatment decisions, but clinical decisions must be made nonetheless. What are the alternatives to randomized controlled trials, and how credible are they?

Observational Studies of Interventions

In the absence of a consensus favoring one mode of treatment over others, various treatments are given according to the preferences of each individual patient and doctor. As a result, in the course of ordinary patient care, large numbers of patients are treated in various ways and go on to manifest the effects. When experience with these patients is captured and properly analyzed, it can complement the information available from randomized trials, suggest where new trials are needed, and provide answers where trials are not yet available.

Example

Non–small cell lung cancer is common in the elderly. Palliative chemotherapy for advanced disease prolongs life, yet the elderly receive chemotherapy less often than younger patients, perhaps because of concern that they would be more likely to develop adverse events such as fever and infections, nerve damage, or deep venous thrombosis. To see if elderly patients in the community really are more likely to experience adverse events, everything else being equal, investigators analyzed data from a cohort study of the care and outcomes of lung cancer (12). There was consistent evidence that the older patients who received chemotherapy were selected to be less likely to have adverse events: Fewer got chemotherapy, they had fewer adverse events before treatment, and they received less aggressive therapy. Even so, adverse event rates after chemotherapy were 34% to 70% more frequent in older patients than in younger ones. This effect could not be attributed to other diseases more common with age—they persisted after adjustment for comorbidity—and is more likely to be the result of age-related decrease in organ function. Whether the benefits of treatment outweigh the increased rate of adverse events is a separate question.

Unfortunately, it is difficult to be sure that observational studies of treatment are not confounded. Treatment choice is determined by a great many factors including severity of illness, concurrent diseases, local preferences, and patient cooperation. Patients receiving the various treatments are likely to differ not only in their treatment but in other ways as well.

Especially troubling is confounding by indication (sometimes called "reverse causation"), which occurs when whatever prompted the doctor to choose a treatment (the "indication") is a cause of the observed outcome, not just the treatment itself. For example, patients may be offered a new surgical procedure because they are a good surgical risk or have less aggressive disease and, therefore, seem especially likely to benefit from the procedure. To the extent that the reasons for treatment choice are known, they can be taken into account like any other confounders.

Example

Influenza can cause worsening of bronchospasm in children with asthma. Influenza vaccine is recommended, but many children with asthma were not getting vaccinated, perhaps because of concern that vaccination might cause an exacerbation of asthma, which was suggested by observational studies. The association might have been the result of confounding by indication, whereby children with worse asthma were both more likely to be vaccinated and more likely to experience exacerbations. To test this possibility, investigators did a population-based cohort study of the influenza vaccine and asthma exacerbations in children 1 to 6 years of age in four large health maintenance organizations during three influenza seasons (13). In crude (unadjusted) analyses, asthma exacerbation rates were two to three times higher in vaccinated children compared with those not vaccinated. Risk was smaller, but still elevated, after adjusting for age, sex, health care organization, calendar time, asthma severity (based on the use of drugs and medical visits for asthma), and preventive care practices. To achieve more precise control for severity of asthma, rates in the 2 weeks after vaccination were compared with rates in the same children in periods outside this interval. In this analysis, each child served as his or her own control. The resulting relative risks indicated protection with vaccination: 0.58, 0.74, and 0.98 in the three seasons. A summary of randomized controlled trials suggests that the vaccine is unlikely to precipitate asthma attacks (14).

Clinical Databases

Sometimes, databases are available that include baseline characteristics and outcomes for a large number of patients. Clinicians can match characteristic of a specific patient to similar patients in the database and see what their outcomes were. When use of the database is not part of formal research, there is no accounting for confounding and effect modification, but the predictions do have the advantage of being about real-world patients, not those as highly selected as in most clinical trials.

Randomized versus Observational Studies?

Are observational studies a reliable substitute for randomized controlled trials? With controlled trials as the gold standard, most observational studies of most questions get the right answer. However, there are dramatic exceptions. For example, observational studies have consistently shown that antioxidant vitamins are associated with lower cardiovascular risk, but large randomized controlled trials have found no such effect. Therefore, clinicians can be guided by observational studies of treatment effects when there are no randomized trials to rely on, but they should maintain a healthy skepticism.

Well-designed observational studies of interventions have some strengths that complement the limitations of usual randomized trials. They count the effects of actual treatment, not just of offering treatment, which is a legitimate question in its own right. They commonly include most people as they exist in naturally occurring populations, in either clinical or community settings, without severe inclusion and exclusion criteria. They can often accomplish longer follow-up than trials, matching the time it takes for disease and outcomes to develop. By taking advantage of treatments and outcomes as they happen, observational studies (especially case-control studies and historical cohort studies using health records) can answer clinical questions more quickly than it takes to complete a randomized trial. Of course, they are also less expensive.

Because an ideal randomized controlled trial is the standard of excellence, it has been suggested that observational studies of treatment be designed to resemble, as closely as possible, a randomized trial of the same question (15). One might ask, if the study had been a randomized trial what would be the inclusion and exclusion criteria (e.g., excluding patients with contraindications to either intervention), how would exposure be precisely defined and how should drop-outs and cross-overs be managed? The resulting observational study cannot be expected to avoid all vulnerabilities, but at least it would be stronger.

PHASES OF CLINICAL TRIALS

For studies of drugs, it is customary to define three phases of trials in the order they are undertaken.

Phase I trials are intended to identify a dose range that is well tolerated and safe (at least for high-frequency, severe side effects) and include very small numbers of patients (perhaps a dozen) without a control group. Phase II trials provide preliminary information on whether the drug is efficacious and the relationship between dose and efficacy. These trials may be controlled but include too few patients in treatment groups to detect any but the largest treatment effects. Phase III trials are randomized trials and can provide definitive evidence of efficacy and

rates of common side effects. They include enough patients, sometimes thousands, to detect clinically important treatment effects and are usually published in biomedical journals.

Phase III trials are not large enough to detect differences in the rate, or even the existence, of uncommon side effects (see discussion of statistical power in Chapter 11). Therefore, it is necessary to follow up very large numbers of patients after a drug is in general use, a process called postmarketing surveillance.

Review Questions

Read the following and select the best response.

9.1. A randomized controlled trial compares two drugs in common use for the treatment of asthma. Three hundred patients were entered into the trial, and eligibility criteria were broad. No effort was made to blind patients to their treatment group after enrollment. Except for the study drugs, care was decided by each individual physician and patient. The outcome measure was a brief questionnaire assessing asthma-related quality of life. Which of the following best describes this trial?

A. Practical clinical trial
B. Large simple trial
C. Efficacy trial
D. Equivalence trial
E. Non-inferiority trial

9.2. A randomized controlled trial compared angioplasty with fibrinolysis for the treatment of acute myocardial infarction. The authors state that "analysis was by intention to treat." Which of the following is an advantage of this approach?

A. It describes the effects of treatments that patients have actually received.
B. It is unlikely to underestimate treatment effect.
C. It is not affected by patients dropping out of the study.
D. It describes the consequences of offering treatments regardless of whether they are actually taken.
E. It describes whether treatment can work under ideal circumstances.

9.3. In a randomized trial, patients with meningitis who were treated with corticosteroids had lower rates of death, hearing loss, and neurologic sequelae. Which of the following is a randomized comparison?

A. The subset of patients who, at the time of randomization, were severely affected by the disease
B. Patients who experienced other treatments versus those who did not
C. Patients who remained in the trial versus those who dropped out after randomization
D. Patients who responded to the drug versus those who did not
E. Patients who took the drug compared with those who did not

9.4. A patient asks for your advice about whether to begin an exercise program to reduce his risk of sudden death. You look for randomized controlled trials but find only observational studies of this question. Some are cohort studies comparing sudden death rates in exercisers with rates of sudden death in sedentary people; others are case-control studies comparing exercise patterns in people who had experienced sudden death and matched controls. Which of the following is *not* an advantage of observational studies of treatments like these over randomized controlled trials?

A. Reported effects are for patients who have actually experienced the intervention.
B. It may be possible to carry out these studies by using existing data that was collected for other purposes.

C. The results can be generalized to more ordinary, real world settings.
D. Treatment groups would have had a similar prognosis except for treatment itself.
E. A large sample size is easier to achieve.

9.5. In a randomized controlled trial of a program to reduce lower extremity problems in patients with diabetes mellitus, patients were excluded if they were younger than age 40, were diagnosed before becoming 30 years old, took specific medication for hyperglycemia, had other serious illness or disability, or were not compliant with prescribed treatment during a run-in period. Which of the following is an advantage of this approach?

A. It makes it possible to do an intention-to-treat analysis.
B. It avoids selection bias.
C. It improves the generalizability of the study.
D. It makes an effectiveness trial possible.
E. It improves the internal validity of the study.

9.6. Which of the following is *not* accomplished by an intention-to-treat analysis?

A. A comparison of the effects of actually taking the experimental treatments
B. A comparison of the effects of offering the experimental treatments
C. A randomized comparison of treatment effects

9.7. You are reading a report of a randomized controlled trial and wonder whether stratified randomization, which the trial used, was likely to improve internal validity. For which of the following is stratified randomization particularly helpful?

A. The study includes many patients.
B. One of the baseline variables is strongly related to prognosis.
C. Assignment to treatment group is not blinded.
D. Many patients are expected to drop out.
E. An intention-to-treat analysis is planned.

9.8. A randomized controlled trial is analyzed according the treatment each patient actually received. Which of the following best describes this approach to analysis?

A. Superiority
B. Intention-to-treat
C. Explanatory
D. Phase I
E. Open-label

9.9. In a randomized controlled trial, a beta-blocking drug is found to be more effective than placebo for stage fright. Patients taking the beta-blocker tended to have a lower pulse rate and to feel more lethargic, which are known effects of this drug. For which of the following is blinding possible?

A. The patients' physicians
B. The investigators who assigned patients to treatment groups
C. The patients in the trial
D. The investigators who assess outcome

9.10. Which of the following best describes "equipoise" as the rationale for a randomized trial of two drugs?

A. The drugs are known to be equally effective.
B. One of the drugs is known to be more toxic.
C. Neither drug is known to be more effective than the other.
D. Although one drug is more effective, the other drug is easier to take with fewer side effects.

9.11. Antibiotic A is the established treatment for community-acquired pneumonia, but it is expensive and has many side effects. A new drug, antibiotic B, has just been developed for community-acquired pneumonia and is less expensive and has fewer side effects, but its efficacy, relative to drug A, is not well established. Which of the following would be the best kind of trial for evaluating drug B?

A. Superiority
B. Cross-over
C. Cluster
D. Non-inferiority
E. Equivalence

9.12. In a randomized controlled trial of two drugs for coronary artery disease, the primary outcome is a composite of acute myocardial infarction, severe angina pectoris, and cardiac death. Which of the following is the main advantage of this approach?

A. There are more outcomes events than there would be for any of the individual outcomes.
B. All outcomes are equally affected by the interventions.
C. The trial has more generalizability.
D. Each of the individual outcomes is important in its own right.
E. If one outcome is infrequent, others make up for it.

9.13. In a randomized controlled trial comparing two approaches to managing children with bronchiolitis, baseline characteristics of the 200 children in the trial are somewhat different in the two randomly allocated groups. Which of the following might explain this finding?

A. "Bad luck" in randomization
B. A breakdown in allocation concealment
C. Both
D. Neither

9.14. Which of the following is usually learned from a Phase III drug trial?

A. The relationship between dose and efficacy
B. Rates of uncommon side effects
C. Efficacy or effectiveness
D. The dose range that is well tolerated

9.15. Which of the following is the main advantage of randomized controlled trials over observational studies of treatment effects?

A. Fewer ethical challenges
B. Prevention of confounding
C. Resemble usual care
D. Quicker answer
E. Less expensive

Answers are in Appendix A.

REFERENCES

1. Action to Control Cardiovascular Risk in Diabetes Study Group, Gerstein HC, Miller ME, et al. Effects of intensive glucose lowering in type 2 diabetes. N Engl J Med 2008; 358:2545–2559.
2. Allen C, Glasziou P, Del Mar C. Bed rest: a potentially harmful treatment needing more careful evaluation. Lancet 1999;354:1229–1233.
3. Hawkins G, McMahon AD, Twaddle S, et al. Stepping down inhaled corticosteroids in asthma: randomized controlled trial. BMJ 2003;326:1115–1121.
4. Lamb SE, Marsh JL, Hutton JL, et al. Mechanical supports for acute, severe ankle sprain: a pragmatic, multicentre, randomized controlled trial. Lancet 2009;373:575–581.
5. Dykes PC, Carroll DL, Hurley A, et al. Fall prevention in acute care hospitals. A randomized trial. JAMA 2010;304:1912–1918.
6. Carson JL, Terrin ML, Noveck H, et al. Liberal or restrictive transfusion in high-risk patients after hip surgery. N Engl J Med 2011;365:2453–2462.
7. Sprung CL, Annane D, Keh D, et al. Hydrocortisone therapy for patients with septic shock. N Engl J Med 2008;358:111–124.
8. Avins AL, Pressman A, Ackerson L, et al. Placebo adherence and its association with morbidity and mortality in the studies of left ventricular dysfunction. J Gen Intern Med 2010;25: 1275–1281.
9. The AIM-HIGH Investigators. Niacin in patients with low HDL cholesterol levels receiving intensive statin therapy. N Engl J Med 2011;365:2255–2267.
10. Feldman T, Foster E, Glower DG, et al. Percutaneous repair or surgery for mitral regurgitation. N Engl J Med 2011;364: 1395–1406.
11. Mitja O, Hayes R, Ipai A, et al. Single-dose azithromycin versus benzathine benzylpenicillin for treatment of yaws in children in Papua New Guinea: an open-label, non-inferiority, randomized trial. Lancet 2012;379:342–347.
12. Chrischilles EA, Pendergast JF, Kahn KL, et al. Adverse events among the elderly receiving chemotherapy for advanced non-small cell lung cancer. J Clin Oncol 2010;28:620–627.
13. Kramarz P, DeStefano F, Gargiullo PM, et al. Does influenza vaccination exacerbate asthma. Analysis of a large cohort of children with asthma. Vaccine Safety Datalink Team. Arch Fam Med 2000;9:617–623.
14. Cates CJ, Jefferson T, Rowe BH. Vaccines for preventing influenza in people with asthma. Available at http://summaries. cochrane.org/CD000364/vaccines-for-preventing-influenza-in-people-with-asthma. Accessed July 26, 2012.
15. Feinstein AR, Horwitz RI. Double standards, scientific methods, and epidemiologic research. N Engl J Med 1982;307: 1611–1617.

Chapter 10

Prevention

If a patient asks a medical practitioner for help, the doctor does the best he can. He is not responsible for defects in medical knowledge. If, however, the practitioner initiates screening procedures, he is in a very different situation. He should have conclusive evidence that screening can alter the natural history of disease in a significant proportion of those screened.

—*Archie Cochrane and Walter Holland*
1971

KEY WORDS

Preventive care	Placebo adherence
Immunizations	Interval cancer
Screening	Detection Method
Behavioral counseling	Incidence method
Chemoprevention	False-positive
Primary prevention	screening test result
Secondary prevention	Labeling effect
Tertiary prevention	Overdiagnosis
Surveillance	Predisease
Prevalence screen	Incidentaloma
Incidence screen	Quality adjusted life
Lead-time bias	year (QALY)
Length-time bias	Cost-effectiveness
Compliance bias	analysis

Most doctors are attracted to medicine because they look forward to curing disease. But all things considered, most people would prefer never to contract a disease in the first place—or, if they cannot avoid an illness, they prefer that it be caught early and stamped out before it causes them any harm. To accomplish this, people without specific complaints undergo interventions to identify and modify risk factors to avoid the onset of disease or to find disease early in its course so that early treatment prevents illness. When these interventions take place in clinical practice, the activity is referred to as preventive care.

Preventive care constitutes a large portion of clinical practice (1). Physicians should understand

its conceptual basis and content. They should be prepared to answer questions from patients such as, "How much exercise do I need, Doctor?" or "I heard that a study showed antioxidants were not helpful in preventing heart disease. What do you think?" or "There was a newspaper ad for a calcium scan. Do you think I should get one?"

Much of the scientific approach to prevention in clinical medicine has already been covered in this book, particularly the principles underlying risk, the use of diagnostic tests, disease prognosis, and effectiveness of interventions. This chapter expands on those principles and strategies as they specifically relate to prevention.

PREVENTIVE ACTIVITIES IN CLINICAL SETTINGS

In the clinical setting, preventive care activities often can be incorporated into the ongoing care of patients, such as when a doctor checks the blood pressure of a patient complaining of a sore throat or orders pneumococcal vaccination in an older person after dealing with a skin rash. At other times, a special visit just for preventive care is scheduled; thus the terms annual physical, periodic checkup, or preventive health examination.

Types of Clinical Prevention

There are four major types of clinical preventive care: immunizations, screening, behavioral counseling (sometimes referred to as lifestyle changes), and chemoprevention. All four apply throughout the life span.

Immunization

Childhood immunizations to prevent 15 different diseases largely determine visit schedules to the pediatrician in the early months of life. Human papillomavirus (HPV) vaccinations of adolescent girls has recently been added for prevention of cervical cancer. Adult immunizations include diphtheria, pertussis, and tetanus (DPT) boosters and well as vaccinations to prevent influenza, pneumococcal pneumonia, and hepatitis A and B.

Screening

Screening is the identification of asymptomatic disease or risk factors. Screening tests start in the prenatal period (such as testing for Down syndrome in the fetuses of older pregnant women) and continue throughout life (e.g., when inquiring about hearing in the elderly). The latter half of this chapter discusses scientific principles of screening.

Behavioral Counseling (Lifestyle Changes)

Clinicians can give effective behavioral counseling to motivate lifestyle changes. Clinicians counsel patients to stop smoking, eat a prudent diet, drink alcohol moderately, exercise, and engage in safe sexual practices. It is important to have evidence that (i) behavior change decreases the risk for the condition of interest, and (ii) counseling leads to behavior change before spending time and effort on this approach to prevention (see Levels of Prevention later in the chapter).

Chemoprevention

Chemoprevention is the use of drugs to prevent disease. It is used to prevent disease early in life (e.g., folate during pregnancy to prevent neural tube defects and ocular antibiotic prophylaxis in all newborns to prevent gonococcal ophthalmia neonatorum) but is also common in adults (e.g., low-dose aspirin prophylaxis for myocardial infarction, and statin treatment for hypercholesterolemia).

LEVELS OF PREVENTION

Merriam-Webster's dictionary defines prevention as "the act of preventing or hindering" and "the act or practice of keeping something from happening" (2). With these definitions in mind, almost all activities in medicine could be defined as prevention. After

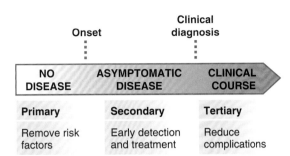

Figure 10.1 ■ Levels of prevention. Primary prevention prevents disease from occurring. Secondary prevention detects and cures disease in the asymptomatic phase. Tertiary prevention reduces complications of disease.

all, clinicians' efforts are aimed at preventing the untimely occurrences of the 5 Ds: death, disease, disability, discomfort, and dissatisfaction (discussed in Chapter 1). However, in clinical medicine, the definition of prevention has traditionally been restricted to interventions in people who are not known to have the particular condition of interest. Three levels of prevention have been defined: primary, secondary, and tertiary prevention (Fig. 10.1).

Primary Prevention

Primary prevention keeps disease from occurring at all by removing its causes. The most common clinical primary care preventive activities involve immunizations to prevent communicable diseases, drugs, and behavioral counseling. Recently, prophylactic surgery has become more common, with bariatric surgery to prevent complications of obesity, and ovariectomy and mastectomy to prevent ovarian and breast cancer in women with certain genetic mutations.

Primary prevention has eliminated many infectious diseases from childhood. In American men, primary prevention has prevented many deaths from two major killers: lung cancer and cardiovascular disease. Lung cancer mortality in men decreased by 25% from 1991 to 2007, with an estimated 250,000 deaths prevented (3). This decrease followed smoking cessation trends among adults, without organized screening and without much improvement in survival after treatment for lung cancer. Heart disease mortality rates in men have decreased by half over the past several decades (4) not only because medical care has improved, but also because of primary prevention efforts such as smoking cessation and use of antihypertensive and statin medications. Primary prevention is now possible for cervical, hepatocellular, skin and breast cancer, bone fractures, and alcoholism.

A special attribute of primary prevention involving efforts to help patients adopt healthy lifestyles is that a single intervention may prevent multiple diseases. Smoking cessation decreases not only lung cancer but also many other pulmonary diseases, other cancers, and, most of all, cardiovascular disease. Maintaining an appropriate weight prevents diabetes and osteoarthritis, as well as cardiovascular disease and some cancers.

Primary prevention at the community level can also be effective. Examples include immunization requirements for students, no-smoking regulations in public buildings, chlorination and fluoridation of the water supply, and laws mandating seatbelt use in automobiles and helmet use on motorcycles and bicycles. Certain primary prevention activities occur in specific occupational settings (use of earplugs or dust masks), in schools (immunizations), or in specialized health care settings (use of tests to detect hepatitis B and C or HIV in blood banks).

For some problems, such as injuries from automobile accidents, community prevention works best. For others, such as prophylaxis in newborns to prevent gonococcal ophthalmia neonatorum, clinical settings work best. For still others, clinical efforts can complement community-wide activities. In smoking prevention efforts, clinicians help individual patients stop smoking and public education, regulations, and taxes prevent teenagers from starting to smoke.

Secondary Prevention

Secondary prevention detects early disease when it is asymptomatic and when treatment can stop it from progressing. Secondary prevention is a two-step process, involving a screening test and follow-up diagnosis and treatment for those with the condition of interest. Testing asymptomatic patients for HIV and routine Pap smears are examples. Most secondary prevention is done in clinical settings.

As indicated earlier, screening is the identification of an unrecognized disease or risk factor by history taking (e.g., asking if the patient smokes), physical examination (e.g., a blood pressure measurement), laboratory test (e.g., checking for proteinuria in a diabetic), or other procedure (e.g., a bone mineral density examination) that can be applied reasonably rapidly to asymptomatic people. Screening tests sort out apparently well persons (for the condition of interest) who have an increased likelihood of disease or a risk factor for a disease from people who have a low likelihood. Screening tests are part of all secondary and some primary and tertiary preventive activities.

A screening test is usually not intended to be diagnostic. If the clinician and/or patient are not committed to further investigation of abnormal results and treatment, if necessary, the screening test should not be performed at all.

Tertiary Prevention

Tertiary prevention describes clinical activities that prevent deterioration or reduce complications after a disease has declared itself. An example is the use of beta-blocking drugs to decrease the risk of death in patients who have recovered from myocardial infarction. Tertiary prevention is really just another term for treatment, but treatment focused on health effects occurring not so much in hours and days but months and years. For example, in diabetic patients, good treatment requires not just control of blood glucose. Searches for and successful treatment of other cardiovascular risk factors (e.g., hypertension, hypercholesterolemia, obesity, and smoking) help prevent cardiovascular disease in diabetic patients as much, and even more, than good control of blood glucose. In addition, diabetic patients need regular ophthalmologic examinations for detecting early diabetic retinopathy, routine foot care, and monitoring for urinary protein to guide use of angiotensin-converting enzyme inhibitors to prevent renal failure. All these preventive activities are tertiary in the sense that they prevent and reduce complications of a disease that is already present.

Confusion about Primary, Secondary, and Tertiary Prevention

Over the years, as more and more of clinical practice has involved prevention, the distinctions among primary, secondary, and tertiary prevention have become blurred. Historically, primary prevention was thought of as primarily vaccinations for infectious disease and counseling for healthy lifestyle behaviors, but primary prevention now includes prescribing antihypertensive medication and statins to prevent cardiovascular diseases, and performing prophylactic surgery to prevent ovarian cancer in women with certain genetic abnormalities. Increasingly, risk factors are treated as if they are diseases, even at a time when they have not caused any of the 5 Ds. This is true for a growing number of health risks, for example, low bone mineral density, hypertension, hyperlipidemia, obesity, and certain genetic abnormalities. Treating risk factors as disease broadens the definition of secondary prevention into the domain of traditional primary prevention.

In some disciplines, such as cardiology, the term secondary prevention is used when discussing tertiary prevention. "A new era of secondary prevention" was declared when treating patients with acute coronary syndrome (myocardial infarction or unstable angina) with a combination of antiplatelet and anticoagulant therapies to prevent cardiovascular death (5). Similarly, "secondary prevention" of stroke is used to describe interventions to prevent stroke in patients with transient ischemia attacks.

Tests used for primary, secondary, and tertiary prevention, as well as for diagnosis, are often identical, another reason for confusing the levels of prevention (and confusing prevention with diagnosis). Colonoscopy may be used to find a cancer in a patient with blood in his stool (diagnosis); to find an early asymptomatic colon cancer (secondary prevention); remove an adenomatous polyp, which is a risk factor for colon cancer (primary prevention); or to check for cancer recurrence in a patient treated for colon cancer (a tertiary preventive activity referred to as surveillance).

Regardless of the terms used, an underlying reason to differentiate levels among preventive activities is that there is a spectrum of probabilities of disease and adverse health effects from the condition(s) being sought and treated during preventive activities, as well as different probabilities of adverse health effects from interventions that are used for prevention at the various levels. The underlying risk of certain health problems is usually much higher in diseased than healthy people. For example, the risk of cardiovascular disease in diabetics is much greater than in asymptomatic non-diabetics. Identical tests perform differently depending on the level of prevention. Furthermore, the trade-offs between effectiveness and harms can be quite different for patients in different parts of the spectrum. False-positive test results and overdiagnosis (both discussed later in this chapter) among people without the disease being sought are important issues in secondary prevention, but they are less important in treatment of patients already known to have the disease in question. The terms primary, secondary, and tertiary prevention are ways to consider these differences conceptually.

SCIENTIFIC APPROACH TO CLINICAL PREVENTION

When considering what preventive activities to perform, the clinician must first decide with the patient which medical problems or diseases they should try to prevent. This statement is so clear and obvious that it would seem unnecessary to mention, but the fact is that many preventive procedures, especially screening tests, are performed without a clear understanding of what is being sought or prevented. For instance, physicians performing routine check-ups on their patients may order a urinalysis. However, a urinalysis might be used to search for any number of medical problems, including diabetes, asymptomatic urinary tract infections, renal cancer, or renal failure. It is necessary to decide which, if any, of these conditions is worth screening for before undertaking the test. One of the most important scientific advances in clinical prevention has been the development of methods for deciding whether a proposed preventive activity should be undertaken (6). The remainder of this chapter describes these methods and concepts.

Three criteria are important when judging whether a condition should be included in preventive care (Table 10.1):

1. The burden of suffering caused by the condition.
2. The effectiveness, safety, and cost of the preventive intervention or treatment.
3. The performance of the screening test.

Table 10.1

Criteria for Deciding Whether a Medical Condition Should Be Included in Preventive Care

1. How great is the burden of suffering caused by the condition in terms of:

   Death   Discomfort
   Disease   Dissatisfaction
   Disability   Destitution

2. How good is the screening test, if one is to be performed, in terms of:

   Sensitivity   Safety
   Specificity   Acceptability
   Simplicity
   Cost

3. A. For primary and tertiary prevention, how good is the therapeutic intervention in terms of:

   Effectiveness
   Safety
   Cost-effectiveness

   Or

   B. For secondary prevention, if the condition is found, how good is the ensuing treatment in terms of:

   Effectiveness
   Safety
   Early treatment after screening being more effective than later treatment without screening, when the patient becomes symptomatic
   Cost-effectiveness

BURDEN OF SUFFERING

Only conditions posing threats to life or health (the 5 Ds in Chapter 1) should be included in preventive care. The burden of suffering of a medical condition is determined primarily by (i) how much suffering (in terms of the 5 Ds) it causes those afflicted with the condition, and (ii) its frequency.

How does one measure suffering? Most often, it is measured by mortality rates and frequency of hospitalizations and amount of health care utilization caused by the condition. Information about how much disability, pain, nausea, or dissatisfaction a given disease causes is much less available.

The frequency of a condition is also important in deciding about prevention. A disease may cause great suffering for individuals who are unfortunate enough to get it, but it may occur too rarely—especially in the individual's particular age group—for screening to be considered. Breast cancer is an example. Although it can occur in much younger women, most breast cancers occur in women older than 50 years of age. For 20-year-old women, annual breast cancer incidence is 1.6 in 100,000 (about one-fifth the rate for men in their later 70s) (7). Although breast cancer should be sought in preventive care for older women, it is too uncommon in average 20-year-old women and 70-year-old men for screening. Screening for very rare diseases means not only that, at most, very few people will benefit, but screening also results in false-positive tests in some people who are subject to complications from further diagnostic evaluation.

The incidence of what is to be prevented is especially important in primary and secondary prevention because, regardless of the disease, the risk is low for most individuals. Stratifying populations according to risk and targeting the higher-risk groups can help overcome this problem, a practice frequently done by concentrating specific preventive activities on certain age groups.

EFFECTIVENESS OF TREATMENT

As pointed out in Chapter 9, randomized controlled trials are the strongest scientific evidence for establishing the effectiveness of treatments. It is usual practice to meet this standard for tertiary prevention (treatments). On the other hand, to conduct randomized trials when evaluating primary or secondary prevention requires very large studies on thousands, often tens of thousands, of patients, carried out over many years, sometimes decades, because the outcome of interest is rare and often takes years to occur. The task is daunting; all the difficulties of randomized

controlled trials laid out in Chapter 9 on Treatment are magnified many-fold.

Other challenges in evaluating treatments in prevention are outlined in the following text for each level of prevention.

Treatment in Primary Prevention

Whatever the primary intervention (immunizations, drugs, behavioral counseling, or prophylactic surgery), it should be efficacious (able to produce a beneficial result in ideal situations) and effective (able to produce a beneficial net result under usual conditions, taking into account patient compliance). Because interventions for primary prevention are usually given to large numbers of healthy people, they also must be very safe.

Randomized Trials

Virtually all recommended immunizations are backed by evidence from randomized trials, sometimes relatively quickly when the outcomes occur within weeks or months, as in childhood infections. Because pharmaceuticals are regulated, primary and secondary preventive activities involving drugs (e.g., treatment of hypertension and hyperlipidemia in adults) also usually have been evaluated by randomized trials. Randomized trials are less common when the proposed prevention is not regulated, as is true with vitamins, minerals, and food supplements, or when the intervention is behavioral counseling.

Observational Studies

Observational studies can help clarify the effectiveness of primary prevention when randomization is not possible.

Example

Randomized trials have found hepatitis B virus (HBV) vaccines highly effective in preventing hepatitis B. Because HBV is a strong risk factor for hepatocellular cancer, one of the most common and deadly cancers globally, it was thought that HBV vaccination would be useful in preventing liver cancer. However, the usual interval between HBV infection and development of hepatocellular cancer is two to three decades. It would not be ethical to withhold from a control group a highly effective intervention against an infectious disease to determine if decades later it also was effective against cancer. A study was done in Taiwan, where nationwide HBV vaccination was begun in 1984. The rates of hepatocellular cancer rates were compared among people who were immunized at birth between 1984 and 2004 to those born between 1979 and 1984 when no vaccination program existed. (The comparison was made possible by thorough national health databases on the island.) Hepatocellular cancer incidence decreased almost 70% among young people in the 20 years after the introduction of HBV vaccination (8).

As pointed out in Chapter 5, observational studies are vulnerable to bias. The conclusion that HBV vaccine prevents hepatocellular carcinoma is reasonable from a biologic perspective and from the dramatic result. It will be on even firmer ground if studies of other populations who undergo vaccination confirm the results from the Taiwan study. Building the case for causation in the absence of randomized trials is covered in Chapter 12.

Safety

With immunizations, the occurrence of adverse effects may be so rare that randomized trials would be unlikely to uncover them. One way to study this question is to track illnesses in large datasets of millions of patients and to compare the frequency of an adverse effect linked temporally to the vaccination among groups at different time periods.

Example

Guillain-Barré syndrome (GBS) is a rare, serious immune-mediated neurological disorder characterized by ascending paralysis that can temporarily involve respiratory muscles so that intubation and ventilator support are required. A vaccine developed against swine flu in the 1970s was associated with an unexpected sharp rise in the number of cases of GBS and contributed to suspension of the vaccination program. In 2009, a vaccine was developed to protect against a novel influenza A (H1N1) virus of swine origin, and a method was needed to track GBS incidence. One way this was done was to utilize a surveillance system of the electronic health databases of more than 9 million persons. Comparing the incidence of GBS occurring up to 6 weeks after vaccination to that of later (background) GBS occurrence in the same group of vaccinated individuals, the attributable risk of the 2009 vaccine was estimated to be an additional five cases of GBS per million vaccinations. Although GBS incidence increased after vaccination, the effect in 2009 was about half that seen in the 1970s (9). The very low estimated attributable risk in 2009 is reassuring. If rare events, occurring in only a few people per million are to be detected in near real time, population-based surveillance systems are required. Even so, associations found in surveillance systems are weak evidence for a causal relationship because they are observational in nature and electronic databases often do not have information on all important possible confounding variables.

Counseling

U.S. laws do not require rigorous evidence of effectiveness of behavioral counseling methods. Nevertheless, clinicians should require scientific evidence before incorporating routine counseling into preventive care; counseling that does not work wastes time, costs money, and may harm patients. Research has demonstrated that certain counseling methods can help patients change some health behaviors. Smoking cessation efforts have led the way with many randomized trials evaluating different approaches.

Example

Smoking kills approximately 450,000 Americans each year. But, what is the evidence that advising patients to quit smoking gets them to stop? Are some approaches better than others? These questions were addressed by a panel that reviewed all studies done on smoking cessation, focusing on randomized trials (10). They found 43 trials that assessed amounts of counseling contact and found a dose-response—the more contact time the better the abstinence rate (Fig. 10.2). In addition, the panel found that randomized trials demonstrated that pharmacotherapy with bupropion (a centrally acting drug that decreases craving), varenicline (a nicotine

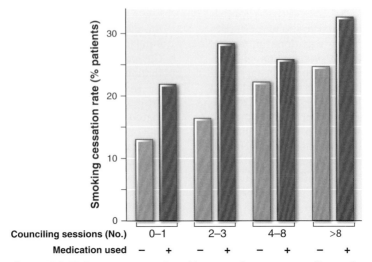

Figure 10.2 ■ **Dose response of smoking cessation rates according to the number of counseling sessions clinicians have with patients and use of medication.** (Data from Fiore MC, Jaén CR, Baker TB, et al. Treating tobacco use and dependence: 2008 Update. Clinical Practice Guideline. Rockville, MD: U.S. Department of Health and Human Services. Public Health Service. May 2008.)

receptor agonist), nicotine gum, nasal spray, or patches were effective. Combining counseling and medication (evaluated in 18 trials) increased the smoking cessation rate still further. On the other hand, there was no effect of anxiolytics, beta-blockers, or acupuncture.

Treatment in Secondary Prevention

Treatments in secondary prevention are generally the same as treatments for curative medicine. Like interventions for symptomatic disease, they should be both efficacious and effective. Unlike usual interventions for disease, however, it typically takes years to establish that a secondary preventive intervention is effective, and it requires large numbers of people to be studied. For example, early treatment after colorectal cancer screening can decrease colorectal cancer deaths by approximately one-third, but to show this effect, a study of 45,000 people with 13 years of follow-up was required (11).

A unique requirement for treatment in secondary prevention is that treatment of *early, asymptomatic* disease must be superior to treatment of the disease when it would have been diagnosed in the usual course of events, when a patient seeks medical care for symptoms. If outcome in the two situations is the same, screening does not add value.

Example

Lung cancer is the leading cause of cancer-related death in the United States. Why, then, did no major professional medical group recommend screening for lung cancer throughout the first decade of the 21st century? Several randomized trials begun in the 1970s and 1980s found screening was not protective. In one study of the use of chest x-rays and sputum cytology to screen for lung cancer, male cigarette smokers who were screened every 4 months and treated promptly when cancer was found did no better than those not offered screening and treated only when they presented with symptoms. Twenty years later, death rates from lung cancer were similar in the two groups—4.4 per 1,000 person-years in the screened men versus 3.9 per 1,000 persons-years in men not offered screening (12). However, in 2011, a randomized controlled trial of low-dose computed tomography (CT) screening reported a 20% reduction in lung cancer mortality after a median of 6.5 years (13). This trial convincingly demonstrated for the first time that treatment of asymptomatic lung cancer found on screening decreased mortality.

Treatment in Tertiary Prevention

All new pharmaceutical treatments in the United States are regulated by the U.S. Food and Drug Administration, which almost always requires evidence of efficacy from randomized clinical trials. It is easy to assume, therefore, that tertiary preventive treatments have been carefully evaluated. However, after a drug has been approved, it may be used for new, unevaluated, indications. Patients with some diseases are at increased risk for other diseases; thus, some drugs are used not only to treat the condition for which they are approved but also to prevent other diseases for which patients are at increased risk. The distinction between proven therapeutic effects of a medicine for a given disease and its effect in preventing other diseases is a subtle challenge facing clinicians when considering tertiary preventive interventions that have not been evaluated for that purpose. Sometimes, careful evaluations have led to surprising results.

Example

In Chapter 9, we presented an example of a study of treatment for patients with type 2 diabetes. It showed the surprising result that tight control of blood sugar (bringing the level down to normal range) did not prevent cardiovascular disease and mortality any better than looser control. The diabetic medications used in this and other studies finding similar results were approved after randomized controlled studies. However, the outcomes leading to approval of the drugs was not prevention of long-term cardiovascular disease (tertiary prevention) among diabetics, but rather the effect of the medications on blood sugar levels. The assumption was made that these medications would also decrease cardiovascular disease because observational studies had shown blood sugar levels correlated with cardiovascular disease risk. Putting this assumption to the test in rigorous randomized trials produced surprising and important results. As a result, tertiary prevention in diabetes has shifted toward including aggressive treatment of other risk factors for cardiovascular disease. With such an approach, a randomized trial showed that cardiovascular disease and death in diabetics were reduced about 50% over a 13-year period, compared to a group receiving conventional therapy aimed at controlling blood sugar levels (14).

METHODOLOGIC ISSUES IN EVALUATING SCREENING PROGRAMS

Several problems arise in the evaluation of screening programs, some of which can make it appear that early treatment is effective after screening when it is not. These issues include the difference between prevalence and incidence screens and three biases that can occur in screening studies: lead-time, length-time, and compliance biases.

Prevalence and Incidence Screens

The yield of screening decreases as screening is repeated over time. Figure 10.3 demonstrates why this is so. The first time that screening is carried out—the prevalence screen—cases of the medical condition will have been present for varying lengths of time. During the second round of screening, most cases found will have had their onset between the first and second screening. (A few will have been missed by the first screen.) Therefore, the second (and subsequent) screenings are called incidence screens. Thus, when a group of people are periodically rescreened, the number of cases of disease

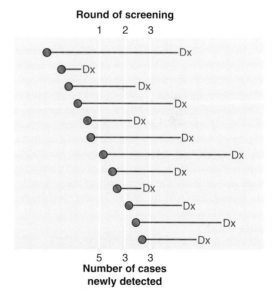

Figure 10.3 ■ The decreasing yield of a screening test after the first round of screening. The first round (prevalence screening) detects prevalent cases. The second and third rounds (incidence screenings) detect incident cases. In this figure, it is assumed that the test detects all cases and that all people in the population are screened. When this is not so, cases missed in the first round are available for detection in subsequent rounds—and the yield would be higher. O = onset of disease; Dx = diagnosis time, if screening were not carried out.

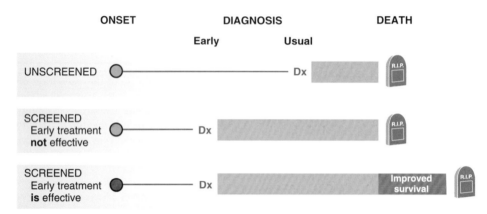

Figure 10.4 ■ **How lead time affects survival time after screening; O = onset of disease.** Pink-shaded areas indicate length of survival after diagnosis (Dx).

in the group drops after the prevalence screen. This means that the positive predictive value for test results will decrease after the first round of screening.

Special Biases

The following biases are most likely to be a problem in observational studies of screening.

Lead-Time Bias

Lead time is the period of time between the detection of a medical condition by screening and when it ordinarily would have been diagnosed because a patient experienced symptoms and sought medical care (Fig. 10.4). The amount of lead time for a given disease depends on the biologic rate of progression of the disease and how early the screening test can detect the disease. When lead time is very short, as is true with lung cancer, it is difficult to demonstrate that treatment of medical conditions picked up on screening is more effective than treatment after symptoms appear. On the other hand, when lead time is long, as is true for cervical cancer (on average,

it takes 20 to 30 years for it to progress from carcinoma in situ into a clinically invasive disease), treatment of the medical condition found on screening can be very effective.

How can lead time cause biased results in a study of the efficacy of early treatment? As Figure 10.4 shows, because of screening, a disease is found earlier than it would have been after the patient developed symptoms. As a result, people who are diagnosed by screening for a deadly disease will, on average, survive longer from the time of diagnosis than people who are diagnosed after they develop symptoms, even if early treatment is no more effective than treatment at the time of clinical presentation. In such a situation, screening would appear to help people live longer, spuriously improving survival rates when, in reality, they would have been given not more "survival time" but more "disease time."

An appropriate method of analysis to avoid lead-time bias is to compare age-specific mortality rates rather than survival rates in a screened group of people and a control group of similar people who do not get screened, as in a randomized trial (Table 10.2). Screening for breast, lung, and colorectal cancers are

Table 10.2

Avoiding Bias in Screening		
Bias	**Effect**	**How to Avoid**
Lead time	Appears to improve survival time but actually increases "disease time" after disease detection.	Use mortality rather than survival rates.
Length time	Outcome appears better in screened group because more cancers with a good prognosis are detected.	Compare outcomes in randomized controlled trial with control group and one offered screening. Count *all* outcomes regardless of method of detection.
Compliance	Outcome in screened group appears better due to compliance, not screening.	Compare outcomes in randomized controlled trial with control group and one offered screening. Count *all* outcomes regardless of compliance.

known to be effective because studies have shown that *mortality rates* of screened persons are lower than those of a comparable group of unscreened people.

Length-Time Bias

Length-time bias occurs because the proportion of slow-growing lesions diagnosed during screening is greater than the proportion of those diagnosed during usual medical care. As a result, length-time bias makes it seem that screening and early treatment are more effective than usual care.

Length-time bias occurs in the following way. Screening works best when a medical condition develops slowly. Most types of cancers, however, demonstrate a wide range of growth rates. Some of them grow slowly, some very fast. Screening tests are likely to find mostly slow-growing tumors because they are present for a longer period of time before they cause symptoms. Fast-growing tumors are more likely to cause symptoms that lead to diagnosis in the interval between screening examinations, as illustrated in Figures 10.5 and 10.6. Screening, therefore, tends to find tumors with inherently better prognoses. As a result, the mortality rates of cancers found through screening may be better than those not found through screening, but screening is not protective in this situation.

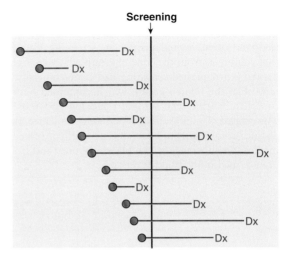

Figure 10.5 ■ Length-time bias. Cases that progress rapidly from onset (O) to symptoms and diagnosis (Dx) are less likely to be detected during a screening examination.

Compliance Bias

The third major bias that can occur in prevention studies is compliance bias. Compliant patients tend to have better prognoses regardless of preventive activities. The reasons for this are not completely clear, but on average, compliant patients are more

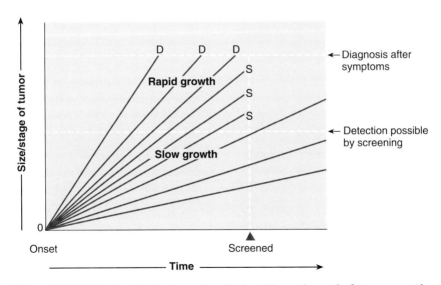

Figure 10.6 ■ Relationship between length-time bias and speed of tumor growth. Rapidly growing tumors come to medical attention before screening is performed, whereas more slowly growing tumors allow time for detection. *D* = diagnosis after symptoms; *S* = detection after screening.

interested in their health and are generally healthier than non-compliant ones. For example, a randomized study that invited people for screening found that volunteers from the control group who were not invited but requested screening had better mortality rates than the invited group, which contained both compliant people who wanted screening and those who refused (15). The effect of patient compliance, as distinct from treatment effect, has primarily involved medication adherence in the placebo group, and has been termed placebo adherence.

be made up of similar populations, the control population should not have access to screening, and both populations must have careful follow-up to document all cases of the outcome being studied.

Because randomized controlled trials and prospective population-based studies are difficult to conduct, take a long time, and are expensive, investigators sometimes try to use other kinds of studies, such as historical cohort studies (Chapter 5) or case control studies (Chapter 6), to investigate preventive maneuvers.

Example

An analysis was done to determine if health outcomes differed in the placebo arm of a randomized trial among patients who demonstrated different degrees of placebo adherence (16). The original study was a tertiary prevention trial that randomized asymptomatic patients with left ventricular dysfunction (cardiac ejection fraction <35%) to active treatment (enalapril) or placebo. The analysis showed that after 3 years, patients randomized to placebo who took at least 75% of the placebo medication ("highly adherent" patients) had half the mortality rate of "lower adherent" patients randomized to placebo. Explanations for this strange result were sought. The difference in mortality was not changed after adjusting for several risk factors, including serious illness. The placebo medication itself was chemically inert. Placebo adherence appears to be a marker of healthier people even though the underlying mechanism remains to be determined.

Biases from length time and patient compliance can be avoided by relying on studies that have concurrent screened and control groups that are comparable. In each group, all people experiencing the outcomes of interest must be counted, regardless of the method of diagnosis or degree of participation (Table 10.2). Randomized trials are the strongest design because patients who are randomly allocated will have comparable numbers of slow- and fast-growing tumors and, on average, comparable levels of compliance. These groups then can be followed over time with mortality rates, rather than survival rates, to avoid lead-time bias. If a randomized trial is not possible, results of population-based observational studies can be valid. In such cases, the screened and control groups must

Example

To test whether periodic screening with sigmoidoscopy reduces mortality from colorectal cancer within the reach of the sigmoidoscope, researchers investigated the frequency of screening sigmoidoscopy over the previous 10 years among patients dying of colorectal cancer and among well patients, matched for age and sex (17). To deal with lead-time and length-time biases, they investigated screening only in people who were known to have died (case group) or not to have died (control group) from colorectal cancer. To deal with compliance bias, they adjusted their results for the number of general periodic health examinations each person had. They also adjusted the results for the presence of medical conditions that could have led to both increased screening and increased likelihood of colorectal cancer. Patients dying of colorectal cancer in the rectum or distal sigmoid (where tumors could have been detected by sigmoidoscopy) were less likely to have undergone a screening sigmoidoscopy in the previous 10 years (8.8%) than those in the control group (24.2%). The investigators found that sigmoidoscopy followed by early therapy prevented almost 60% of deaths resulting from colorectal cancer arising in the distal colon or rectum, equivalent to about a 30% reduction in mortality from cancer of the colon and rectum as a whole. Also, by showing that there was no protection for colorectal cancers above the level reached by the sigmoidoscope, the authors suggested that "it is difficult to conceive of how such anatomical specificity of effect could be explained by confounding." The findings of this study have been corroborated by two subsequent randomized trials of sigmoidoscopy.

PERFORMANCE OF SCREENING TESTS

Tests used for screening should meet the criteria for diagnostic tests laid out in Chapter 8.

The following criteria for a good screening test apply to all types of screening tests, whether they are history, physical examination or laboratory tests.

High Sensitivity and Specificity

The very nature of searching for a disease in people without symptoms means that prevalence is usually very low, even among high-risk groups who were selected because of age, sex, and other risk characteristics. A good screening test must, therefore, have a high sensitivity so that it does not miss the few cases of disease present. It must also be sensitive early in the disease, when the subsequent course can still be altered. If a screening test is sensitive only for late-stage disease, which has progressed too far for effective treatment, the test would be useless. A screening test should also have a high specificity to reduce the number of people with false-positive results who require diagnostic evaluation.

Sensitivity and specificity are determined for screening tests much as they are for diagnostic tests, with one major difference. As discussed in Chapter 8, the sensitivity and specificity of a diagnostic test are determined by comparing the results to another test (the gold standard). In screening, the gold standard for the presence of disease often is not only another, more accurate, test but also *a period of time for follow-up*. The gold standard test is routinely applied only to people with positive screening test results, to differentiate between true- and false-positive results. A period of follow-up is applied to all people who have a negative screening test result, in order to differentiate between true- and false-negative test results.

Follow-up is particularly important in cancer screening, where interval cancers, cancers not detected during screening but subsequently discovered over the follow-up period, occur. When interval cancers occur, the calculated test sensitivity is lowered.

Example

In Chapter 8, we presented a study in which prostate-specific antigen (PSA) levels were measured in stored blood samples collected from a cohort of healthy men (physicians) who later were or were not diagnosed with prostate cancer (18). Thirteen of 18 men who were diagnosed with prostate cancer within a year after the blood sample had elevated PSA levels (>4.0 ng/mL) and would have been diagnosed after an abnormal PSA result; the other five had normal PSA results and developed interval cancers during the first year after a normal PSA test. Thus, sensitivity of PSA was calculated as 13 divided by (13 + 5), or 72%.

A key challenge is to choose a correct period of follow-up. If the follow-up period is too short, disease missed by the screening test might not have a chance to make itself obvious, so the test's sensitivity may be overestimated. On the other hand, if the follow-up period is too long, disease not present at the time of screening might be found, resulting in a falsely low estimation of the test's sensitivity.

Detection and Incidence Methods for Calculating Sensitivity

Calculating sensitivity by counting cancers detected during screening as true positives and interval cancers as false negatives is sometimes referred to as the detection method (Table 10.3). The method works well for many screening tests, but there are two difficulties with it for some cancer screening tests. First, as already pointed out, it requires that the appropriate amount of follow-up time for interval cancers be known; often, it is not known and must be guessed. The detection method also assumes that the abnormalities detected by the screening test would go on to cause trouble if left alone. This is not necessarily so for several cancers, particularly prostate cancer.

Example

Histologic prostate cancer is common in men, especially older men. A review of autopsy studies showed that in the United States, prevalence rates of prostate cancer ranged from 8% among men in their 20s to 83% among men in their 70s (19). Screening tests can find such cancers in many men, but for most, the cancer will never become invasive. Thus, when the sensitivity of prostate cancer tests such as PSA is determined by the detection method, the test may look quite good because the numerator includes all cancers found, not just those with malignant potential.

Table 10.3

Calculating Sensitivity of a Cancer Screening Test According to the Detection Method and the Incidence Method

Theoretical Example

A new screening test is introduced for pancreatic cancer. In a screening group, cancer is detected in 200 people; over the ensuing year, another 50 who had negative screening tests are diagnosed with pancreatic cancer. In a concurrent control group with the same characteristics and the same size, members did not undergo screening; 100 people were diagnosed with pancreatic cancer during the year.

Sensitivity of the Test Using the Detection Method

$$\text{Sensitivity} = \frac{\text{Number of screen-detected cancers}}{\text{Number of screen-detected cancers plus number of interval cancers}}$$

$$= \frac{200}{(200 + 50)}$$

$$= .80 \text{ or } 80\%$$

Sensitivity of the Test Using the Incidence Method

$$\text{Sensitivity} = 1 - (\text{interval rate in the screening group/incidence rate in the control group})$$

$$= 1 - \left(\frac{50}{100}\right) = 0.50 \text{ or } 50\%$$

The incidence method calculates sensitivity by using the incidence in persons not undergoing screening and the interval cancer rate in persons who are screened (Table 10.3). The rationale for this approach is that the sensitivity of a test should affect interval cancer rates, not disease incidence. For prostate cancer, the incidence method defines sensitivity of the test as 1 minus the ratio of the interval prostate cancer rate in a group of men undergoing periodic screening to the incidence of prostate cancer in a group of men not undergoing screening (control group). The incidence method of calculating sensitivity gets around the problem of counting "benign" prostate cancers, but it may underestimate sensitivity because it excludes cancers with long lead times. True sensitivity of a test is, therefore, probably between the estimates of the two methods.

Low Positive Predictive Value

Because of the low prevalence of most diseases in asymptomatic people, the positive predictive value of most screening tests is low, even for tests with high specificity. (The reverse is true for negative predictive value, because when prevalence is low, the negative predictive value is likely to be high.) Clinicians who perform screening tests on their patients must accept the fact that they will have to work up many patients who have positive screening test results but do not have disease. However, they can minimize the problem by concentrating their screening efforts on people with a higher prevalence for disease.

Example

The incidence of breast cancer increases with age, from approximately 1 in 100,000/year at age 20 to 1 in 200/year over age 70. Also, sensitivity and specificity of mammography are better in older women. Therefore, a lump found during screening in a young woman's breast is more likely to be non-malignant than a lump in an older woman. In a large study of breast cancer screening, finding cancer after an abnormal mammogram varied markedly according to the age of women; in women in their early 40s, about 57 women without cancer experienced further workup for every woman who was found to have a malignancy (Fig. 10.7) with a positive predictive value of 1.7% (20). However, for women in their 80s, the number dropped to about 10, with a positive predictive value of 9.5%.

Simplicity and Low Cost

An ideal screening test should take only a few minutes to perform, require minimum preparation by the patient, depend on no special appointments, and be inexpensive.

Simple, quick examinations such as blood pressure determinations are ideal screening tests. Conversely, tests such as colonoscopy, which are expensive and

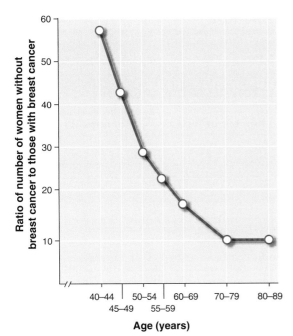

Figure 10.7 ■ Yield of abnormal screening mammograms according to patient age. Number of women without breast cancer for each woman diagnosed with breast cancer among women having an abnormal mammogram when screened for breast cancer. (Data from Carney PA, Miglioretti DL, Yankaskas BC, et al. Individual and combined effects of age, breast density, and hormone replacement therapy use on the accuracy of screening mammography. Ann Intern Med 2003;138:168–175.)

require an appointment and bowel preparation, are best suited for diagnostic testing in patients with symptoms and clinical indications. Nevertheless, screening colonoscopy has been found to be highly effective in decreasing colorectal mortality, and a negative test does not have to be repeated for several years. Other tests, such as visual field testing for the detection of glaucoma and audiograms for the detection of hearing loss, fall between these two extremes.

The financial "cost" of the test depends not only on the cost of (or charge for) the procedure itself but also on the cost of subsequent evaluations performed on patients with positive test results. Thus sensitivity, specificity, and predictive value affect cost. Cost is also affected by whether the test requires a special visit to the physician. Screening tests performed while the patient is seeing his or her physician for other reasons (as is frequently the case with blood pressure measurements) are much cheaper for patients than tests requiring special visits, extra time off work, and additional transportation. Cost also is determined by how often a screening test must be repeated.

Taking all these issues into account sometimes leads to surprising conclusions.

Example

Several different tests can be used to screen for colorectal cancer. They include annual fecal occult blood tests, sigmoidoscopy every 5 years, and colonoscopy every 10 years. The tests vary greatly in their upfront costs, ranging from $20 for fecal occult blood tests to more than a $1,000 for screening colonoscopy. However, the cost per year of life saved by screening is not very different for these tests; all were in an acceptable range by U.S. standards in 2011 (21). This is true for several reasons. First, the simpler, cheaper tests have to be done more often. Fecal occult blood tests are recommended yearly, whereas colonoscopy is recommended every 10 years. The cheaper tests also produce more false-positive results that lead to more testing (and, therefore, more costs). Finally, they produce more false-negative results and miss patients who actually have cancer. This leads to increased costs for care of patients with more advanced cancer.

Safety

It is reasonable and ethical to accept a certain risk for diagnostic tests applied to sick patients seeking help for specific complaints. The physician cannot avoid action when the patient is severely ill, and does his or her best. It is quite another matter to subject presumably well people to risks. In such circumstances, the procedure should be especially safe. This is partly because the chances of finding disease in healthy people are so low. Thus, although colonoscopy is hardly thought of as a dangerous procedure when used on patients with gastrointestinal complaints, it can cause bowel perforation. In fact, when colonoscopy, with a rate of two perforations per 1,000 examinations, is used to screen for colorectal cancer in people in their 50s, perforations occur more often than cancers are found.

Concerns have been raised about possible long-term risks with the increasing use of CT scans to screen for coronary artery disease or, in the case of whole-body scans, a variety of abnormalities. The radiation dose of CT scans varies by type, with a CT scan for coronary calcium on average being the equivalent of about 30, and a whole-body scan about 120, chest x-rays. One estimate of risk projected 29,000 excess cancers as a result of 70 million CT scans performed in the United States in 2007 (22). If these concerns are correct, CT scans used to screen for early cancer could themselves cause cancer over subsequent decades.

Acceptable to Patients and Clinicians

If a screening test is associated with discomfort, it usually takes several years to convince large percentages of patients to obtain the test. This has been true for Pap smears, mammograms, sigmoidoscopies, and colonoscopies. By and large, however, the American public supports screening.

The acceptability of the test to clinicians may be overlooked by all but the ones performing it. Clinician acceptance is especially relevant for screening tests that involve clinical skill, such as mammography, sigmoidoscopy, or colonoscopy. In a survey of 53 mammography facilities, 44% indicated shortages of mammographers. The authors speculated that low reimbursement for screening mammograms, high levels of malpractice litigation in breast imaging, and administrative regulations all may be reasons (23).

UNINTENDED CONSEQUENCES OF SCREENING

Adverse effects of screening tests include discomfort during the test procedure (the majority of women undergoing mammography say that the procedure is painful, although usually not so severe that patients refuse the test), long-term radiation effects after exposure to radiographic procedures, false-positive test results (with resulting needless workups and negative labeling effects), overdiagnosis, and incidentalomas. The last three will be discussed in this section.

Risk of False-Positive Result

A false-positive screening test result is an abnormal result in a person without disease. As already mentioned, tests with low positive predictive values (resulting from low prevalence of disease, poor specificity of the test, or both) are likely to lead to a higher frequency of false positives. False-positive results, in turn, can lead to negative labeling effects, inconvenience, and expense in obtaining follow-up procedures. In certain situations, false-positive results can lead to major surgery. In a study of ovarian cancer screening, 8.4% (3,285) of 39,000 women had a false-positive result and one-third of those underwent surgery as part of the diagnostic evaluation of the test result. Because of false-positive screening tests, five

Table 10.4

Relation between Number of Different Screening Tests Ordered and Percentage of Normal People with at Least One Abnormal Test Result

Number of Tests	People With at Least One Abnormality (%)
1	5
5	23
20	64
100	99.4

Data from Sackett DL. Clinical diagnosis and the clinical laboratory. Clin Invest Med 1978;1:37–43.

times more women without ovarian cancer had surgery than those with ovarian cancer (24).

False-positive results account for only a minority of screening test results (only about 10% of screening mammograms are false positives). Even so, they can affect large percentages of people who get screened. This happens in two ways. Most clinicians do not perform only one or two tests on patients presenting for routine checkups. Modern technology, and perhaps the threat of lawsuits, has fueled the propensity to "cover all the bases." Automated tests allow physicians to order several dozen tests with a few checks in the appropriate boxes.

When the measurements of screening tests are expressed on interval scales (as most blood tests are), and when *normal* is defined by the range covered by 95% of the results (as is usual), the more tests the clinician orders, the greater the risk of a false-positive result. In fact, as Table 10.4 shows, if the physician orders enough tests, "abnormalities" will be discovered in virtually all healthy patients. A spoof entitled "The Last Well Person" commented on this phenomenon (25).

Another reason that many people may experience a false-positive screening test result is that most screening tests are repeated at regular intervals. With each repeat screen, the patient is at risk for a false-positive result.

Example

In a clinical trial of lung cancer screening with low-dose spiral CT or chest x-ray, the first round of screening produced false-positive results in 21% of people screened with CT and 9% of people screened with chest x-ray; after the second round, the total proportion of people experiencing a false-positive had increased to 33% in the CT group and 15% in the chest x-ray group (26). In a related study, participants received screening tests for prostate, ovarian, and colorectal cancer as well as chest x-rays for lung cancer, for a total of 14 tests over 3 years. The cumulative risk of having at least one false-positive screening test result was 60.4% for men and 48.8% for women. The risk for undergoing an invasive diagnostic procedure prompted by a false-positive test result was 28.5% for men and 22.1% for women (27).

Risk of Negative Labeling Effect

Test results can sometimes have important psychological effects on patients, called a labeling effect. A good screening test result produces either no labeling effect or a positive labeling effect.

A positive labeling effect may occur when a patient is told that all the screening test results were normal. Most clinicians have heard such responses as, "Great, that means I can keep working for another year." On the other hand, being told that the screening test result is abnormal and more testing is necessary may have an adverse psychological effect, particularly in cancer screening. Some people with false-positive tests continue to worry even after being told everything was normal on follow-up tests. Because this is a group of people *without* disease, negative labeling effects are particularly worrisome ethically. In such situations, screening efforts might promote a sense of vulnerability instead of health and might do more harm than good.

Example

A study of men with abnormal PSA screening test results who subsequently were declared to be free of cancer after workup found that, 1 year after screening, 26% reported worry about prostate cancer, compared to 6% among men with normal PSA results, and 46% reported their wives or significant others were concerned about prostate cancer versus 14% of those with normal results (28). Anxiety has also been reported after false-positive results for other cancers as well as in blood pressure screening. In summary, people do not respond well when told, "Your screening test result was not quite normal, and we need to do more tests."

Labeling effects are sometimes unpredictable, especially among people who know they are at high risk for a genetic disease because of a family history. Studies of relatives of patients with Huntington disease—a neurological condition with onset in middle age causing mental deterioration leading to dementia, movement disorders, and death—have found psychological health after genetic testing did not deteriorate in those testing positive, perhaps because they were no longer dealing with uncertainty. Studies of women being tested for genetic mutations that increase their risk for breast and ovarian cancer have also found that women testing positive for the mutation experience little or no psychological deterioration.

Risk of Overdiagnosis (Pseudodisease) in Cancer Screening

The rationale for cancer screening is that the earlier a cancer is found, the better the chance of cure. Therefore, the thinking goes, it is always better to find cancer as early as possible. This thesis is being challenged by the observation that incidence often increases after the introduction of widespread screening for a particular cancer. A temporary increase in incidence is to be expected because screening moves the time of diagnosis forward, adding early cases to the usual number of prevalent cancers being diagnosed without screening, but the temporary bump in incidence should come down to the baseline level after a few years. With several cancers, however, incidence has remained at a higher level, as illustrated for prostate cancer in Figure 2.5 in Chapter 2. It is as if screening caused more cancers. How could this be?

Some cancers are so slow growing (some even regress) that they do not cause any trouble for the patient. If such cancers are found through screening, they are called pseudodisease; the process leading to their detection is called overdiagnosis because finding them does not help the patient. Overdiagnosis is an extreme example of length-time bias (Fig. 10.8). The cancers found have such a good prognosis that they would never become evident without screening technology. Some estimates are that as many as 50% of prostate cancers diagnosed by screening are due to overdiagnosis.

As research unravels the development of cancer, it appears that a sequence of genetic and other changes accompany pathogenesis from normal tissue to malignant disease. At each step, only some lesions go on to the next stage of carcinogenesis. It is likely that overdiagnosis occurs because cancers early in the chain are being picked up by screening tests. The challenge is

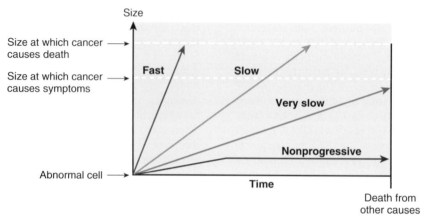

Figure 10.8 ■ Mechanism of overdiagnosis in cancer screening. Note that non-progressive, as well as some very slow-growing, cancers will never cause clinical harm. When these cancers are found on screening, overdiagnosis has occurred. Overdiagnosis is an extreme form of length-time bias. (Redrawn with permission from Welsh HG. Should I Be Tested for Cancer? Maybe Not and Here's Why. Berkeley, CA: University of California Press; 2004.)

to differentiate those early cancers that will go on to cause morbidity and mortality from those that will lie dormant throughout life, even though pathologically they appear the same. Currently, screening technology is not able to do this.

To determine if and to what degree overdiagnosis occurs, it is necessary to compare a screened group with a similar unscreened group and determine incidence and disease-specific mortality rates (not survival rates). This can be done by long-term randomized trials or by careful population-based observational studies.

Example

Neuroblastoma, a tumor of neurologic tissue near the kidney, is the second most common tumor occurring in children. Prognosis depends on the stage of the disease and is better when the tumor is diagnosed during infancy. Treatment involves surgery and chemotherapy. A simple urine test for catecholamine metabolites can be used to screen for the tumor. Japanese studies showed improved survival rates after screening, but lead time and a historical control group could have biased the results. Also, there was no population-based registry of childhood cancers in Japan to ensure ascertainment of all neuroblastoma cases. Finally, at least some cases of neuroblastomas regress without treatment, which raised the possibility of overdiagnosis.

Two population-based studies were, therefore, undertaken in Germany (29) and Quebec (30), in which screening was offered for all infants in certain areas, while infants in other areas were not screened and acted as concurrent controls. Existing tumor registries were used to track all cases of and deaths due to neuroblastoma. In both studies, the incidence of neuroblastoma doubled in the screened group, but mortality rates from neuroblastoma over the subsequent 5 years were equivalent in the screened groups and the unscreened groups. It appeared that the screening test primarily detected tumors with a favorable prognosis, many of which would have regressed if left undetected. Meanwhile, highly invasive disease was often missed. Investigators of both studies concluded that screening infants for neuroblastoma leads to overdiagnosis but does not reduce mortality from neuroblastoma.

Overdiagnosis has been shown in randomized trials of screening for lung and breast cancer. It also can occur when detecting precancerous abnormalities in cervical, colorectal, and breast cancer screening, that is, with cervical dysplasia, adenomatous polyps, and ductal carcinoma in situ (abnormalities sometimes termed predisease). It is important to understand that overdiagnosis can coexist with effective screening and that although randomized trials and population studies can help determine the amount of overdiagnosis, it is impossible to identify it in an individual patient.

Incidentalomas

Over the past couple of decades, using CT as a screening test has become more common. CT has been evaluated rigorously as "virtual colonoscopy" for colorectal cancer screening and also for lung cancer screening. It has been advocated as a screening test for coronary heart disease (with calcium scores) and for screening in general with full-body CT scans. Unlike most screening tests, CT often visualizes much more than the targeted area of interest. For example, CT colonography visualizes the abdomen and lower thorax. In the process, abnormalities are sometimes detected outside the colon. Masses or lesions detected incidentally by an imaging examination are called incidentalomas.

Example

A systematic review of 17 studies found that incidentalomas were common in CT colonography; 40% of 3,488 patients had at least one incidental finding, and 14% had further evaluation (31). Workups uncovered early stage noncolonic cancers in about 1% of patients and abdominal aortic aneurysms >5.5 cm in size in about 0.1%. Therefore, incidentalomas were very common but included some potentially important conditions. There was no information about how many patients who did not receive further evaluation went on to suffer serious consequences. Also, most of the detected cancers were ones for which screening is not recommended. With inadequate evidence about benefits and likelihood of increased costs in pursuit of extracolonic findings, the Center for Medicare and Medicaid Services declined to cover screening CT colonography in the Medicare population.

CHANGES IN SCREENING TESTS AND TREATMENTS OVER TIME

Careful evaluation of screening has been particularly difficult when tests approved for diagnostic purposes are then used as screening tests before evaluation in a screening study, a problem analogous to using therapeutic interventions for prevention without evaluating

them in prevention. For example, CT scans and magnetic resonance imaging were developed for diagnostic purposes in patients with serious complaints or known disease and PSA was developed to determine whether treatment for prostate cancer was successful. All of these tests are now commonly used as screening tests, but most became common in practice without careful evaluation. Only low-dose CT scans for lung cancer screening underwent careful evaluation prior to widespread use. PSA screening became so common in the United States that when it was subjected to a careful randomized trial, more than half the men assigned to the control arm had a PSA test during the course of a trial. When tests are so commonly used, it is difficult to determine rigorously whether they are effective.

Over time, improvements in screening tests, treatments, and vaccinations may change the need for screening. As indicated earlier, effective secondary prevention is a two-step process; a good screening test followed by a good treatment for those found to have disease. Changes in either one may affect how well screening works in preventing disease. At one extreme, a highly accurate screening test will not help prevent adverse outcomes of a disease if there is no effective therapy. Screening tests for HIV preceded the development of effective HIV therapy; therefore, early in the history of HIV, screening could not prevent disease progression in people with HIV. With the development of increasingly effective treatments, screening for HIV has increased. At the other extreme, a highly effective treatment may make screening unnecessary. With modern therapy the 10-year survival rate of testicular cancer is about 85%, so high that it would be difficult to show improvement with screening for this rare cancer. As HPV vaccination for prevention of cervical cancer becomes more widespread and if it is able to cover all carcinogenic types of HPV, the need for cervical cancer screening should decrease over time. Some recent studies of mammography screening have not found the anticipated mortality benefits seen in earlier studies, partly because breast cancer mortality among women not screened was lower than in the past, probably due to improved treatments. Thus, with the introduction of new therapies and screening tests, effectiveness of screening will change and on-going re-evaluation is necessary.

WEIGHING BENEFITS AGAINST HARMS OF PREVENTION

How can the many aspects of prevention covered in this chapter be combined to make a decision whether to include a preventive intervention in clinical practice?

Conceptually, the decision should be based on the weighing the *magnitude of benefits against the magnitude of harms* that will occur as a result of the action. This approach has become common when making treatment decisions; reports of randomized trials routinely include harms as well as benefits.

A straightforward approach is to present the benefits and harms for a particular preventive activity in some orderly and understandable way. Whenever possible, these should be presented using absolute, not relative risks. Figure 10.9 summarizes the estimated key benefits and harms of annual mammography for women in their 40s, 50s, and 60s (7,32,33). Such an approach can help clinicians and patients understand what is involved when making the decision to screen. It can also help clarify why different individuals and expert groups come to different decisions about a preventive activity, even when looking at the same set of information. Different people put different values on benefits and harms (34).

Another approach to weighing benefits and harms is a modeling process that expresses both benefits and harms in a single metric and then subtracts harms from benefits. (The most common metric used is the quality adjusted life year [QALY]). The advantage of this approach is that different types of prevention (e.g., vaccinations, colorectal cancer screening, and tertiary treatment of diabetes) can all be compared to each other, which is important for policymakers with limited resources. The disadvantage is that for most clinicians and policymakers, it is difficult to understand the process by which benefits and harms are handled.

Regardless of the method used in weighing the benefits and harms of preventive activities, the quality of the evidence for each benefit and harm must be evaluated to prevent the problem of "garbage in, garbage out." Several groups making recommendations for clinical prevention have developed explicit methods to evaluate the evidence and take into account the strength of evidence when making their recommendations (see Chapter 14).

If the benefits of a preventive activity outweigh the harms, the final step is to determine the economic effect of using it. Some commentators like to claim that "prevention saves money," but it does so only rarely. (One possible exception is screening for colorectal cancer. Chemotherapy for the disease has become so expensive that some analyses now find screening for this cancer saves money.) Even so, most preventive services recommended by groups who have carefully evaluated the data are as cost-effective as other clinical activities.

Cost-effectiveness analysis is a method for assessing the costs and health benefits of an intervention. All costs related to disease occurrence and treatment should be counted, both with and without the preventive activity, as well as all costs related to the preventive activity itself. The health benefits of the activity are then calculated, and the incremental cost for each unit of benefit is determined.

Example

Cervical cancer is caused by persistent infection of epithelial cells with certain HPV genotypes. Vaccines have been developed against carcinogenic HPV genotypes that cause approximately 70% of all cervical cancers. A randomized trial found the vaccine highly effective in preventing precursors of and early cervical cancer in women without evidence of prior HPV infection. A cost-effectiveness analysis was performed to assess the benefits and costs of vaccinating girls at age 12 who would then go on to be screened for cervical cancer beginning in early adulthood (35). The investigators estimated medical costs from a societal perspective that includes costs of medical care (e.g., vaccine and screening costs as well as diagnostic and treatment costs for cervical cancer) and indirect costs (e.g., work time taken off by patients for office visits). They expressed the benefit in terms of QALYs gained by the combination of vaccine plus screening versus no screening or vaccine. In the analysis, they varied the age and intervals at which screening would occur as well as the effectiveness of vaccine over time. Assuming a vaccine efficacy of 90%, the analysis estimated that starting conventional Pap smear screening at age 25 and repeating screening at a 3-year interval would reduce the lifetime cervical cancer risk by 94%, at a cost of $58,500 per QALY. (Upper limits of acceptable cost-effectiveness ratios in the United States are usually set at about $50,000 per QALY gained.) Screening begun at age 21 and repeated every 5 years would reduce the lifetime cancer risk by 90% at a cost of $57,400 per QALY. In summary, the results suggested that the combination of HPV vaccine and screening for cervical cancer can decrease the risk of cancer, is cost-effective, and permits delayed onset of screening and/or decreased frequency.

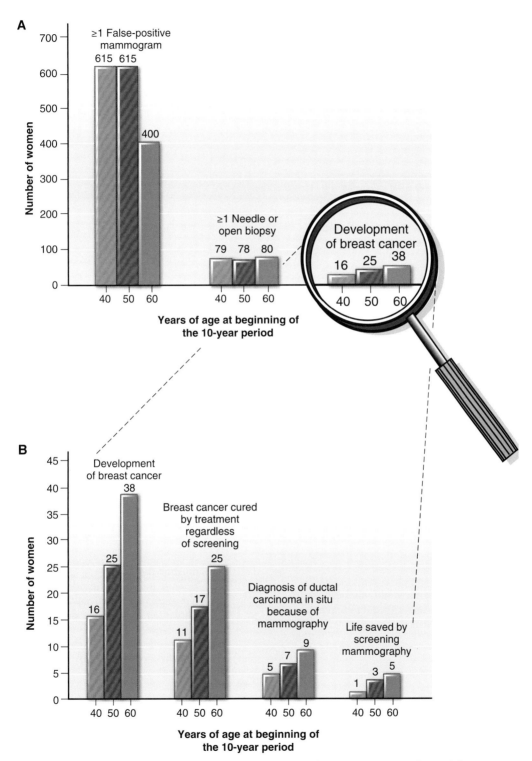

Figure 10.9 ■ **Weighing the benefits and harms when deciding about a preventive activity: comparing estimated benefits and harms of screening mammography.** Chances among 1,000 women ages 40, 50, or 60 who undergo annual screening mammography for 10 years: **(A)** of experiencing a false-positive mammogram, undergoing a breast biopsy, and developing breast cancer, and **(B)** being cured of breast cancer regardless of screening, being diagnosed with non-invasive ductal carcinoma in situ, and averting death from breast cancer because of screening mammography. (Estimates calculated from references 7, 32, and 33.)

The effort to gather all the information needed to make a decision whether to conduct a preventive activity in clinical practice is not something a single clinician can accomplish, but when reviewing recommendations about prevention, individual clinicians can determine if the benefits and harms of the activity are presented in an understandable way and if the recommendation has taken into account the strength of the evidence. They can also look for estimates of cost-effectiveness. With these facts, they should be able to share with their patients the information they need. Patients can then make an informed decision about preventive activities that takes into account the scientific information and their individual values.

Review Questions

For questions 10.1–10.6, read the related scenarios and select the best answer.

A study was conducted to determine whether a fecal occult blood screening test reduced mortality from colorectal cancer (11). People ages 50 to 60 years were randomized to the screening test or to a control group and followed for 13 years. Over this time, there were 323 cancer cases and 82 colorectal cancer deaths in the 15,570 people randomized to annual screening; there were 356 cancers and 121 colorectal cancer deaths in the 15,394 people randomized to the control group. Investigations of positive tests found that about 30% of the screened group had colon polyps. The sensitivity and specificity of the test for colon cancer were both about 90%.

10.1. What is the relative risk reduction of colorectal mortality in the screened group?

   A. 33%
   B. 39%
   C. 48%

10.2. How many patients would you need to screen over the next 13 years to prevent one death from colorectal cancer?

   A. 43
   B. 194
   C. 385

10.3. The fact that 30% of the screened group had colon polyps suggests all of the following *except:*

   A. At least 30% of the screened group was investigated for positive fecal occult blood tests.

   B. The positive predictive value of the test was low.
   C. The negative predictive value of the test was low.

In a randomized controlled trial of screening chest x-rays and sputum cytology for lung cancer, approximately 9,000 men were randomized to screening for 6 years or a control group (16). After 20 years, the lung cancer mortality was the same in both groups (4.4/1,000 person-years in the screened group and 3.9/1,000 person-years in the control group). However, the median survival for patients diagnosed with lung cancer was 1.3 years in the screened group and 0.9 years in the control group. Also, screening found more lung cancer—206 cancers were diagnosed in the screened group and 160 in the control group.

10.4. What is the best conclusion after reading such a study?

   A. Finding a better survival rate but not a change in the mortality rate of lung cancer makes no sense and the study must be flawed.

   B. Because mortality did not change, screening may have resulted in more "disease time" for those diagnosed with lung cancer.
   C. Improved survival demonstrates screening was effective in the study.

10.5. What bias is the best explanation for the improved survival in the face of no improvement in the mortality rate in this study?

   A. Lead-time bias
   B. Survival bias
   C. Compliance bias
   D. Length-time bias

10.6. What is the most likely reason for the fact that 206 lung cancers were found in the screened group and only 160 in the control group?

    A. There were more smokers in the screened group.

    B. Screening found cancers earlier and the number of cancers in the control group will catch up over time.

    C. Screening picked up some cancers that would not have come to medical attention without screening.

For questions 10.7–10.11, choose the best answer.

10.7. When assessing a new vaccine, which of the following is least important:

    A. Efficacy in preventing the disease
    B. Safety of the vaccine
    C. Danger of the disease
    D. Cost of giving the vaccine

10.8. When the same test is used in diagnostic and screening situations, which of the following statements is most likely correct?

    A. The sensitivity and specificity will likely be the same in both situations.

    B. The positive predictive value will be higher in a screening situation.

    C. Disease prevalence will be higher in the diagnostic situation.

    D. Overdiagnosis is equally likely in both situations.

10.9. A study found that volunteers for a new screening test had better health outcomes than people who refused testing. Which of the following statements most likely explains the finding?

    A. People who refuse screening are usually healthier than those who accept.

    B. Volunteers for screening are more likely to need screening than those who refuse.

    C. Volunteers tend to be more interested in their health than those who do not participate in preventive activities.

10.10. All of the following statements are correct *except:*

    A. The gold standard for a test used for diagnosis may be different than that for the same test when used for screening.

    B. The incidence method cannot be used to calculate sensitivity for cancer screening tests.

    C. When a screening program is begun, more people with disease are found on the first round of screening than on later rounds.

10.11. For a cost-effectiveness analysis of a preventive activity, which kinds of costs should be included?

    A. Medical costs, such as those associated with delivering the preventive intervention

    B. All medical costs, including diagnostic follow up of positive tests and treatment for persons diagnosed with disease, with and without the preventive activity

    C. Indirect costs, such as loss of income due to time off from work, among patients receiving the prevention and those who develop the disease

    D. Indirect costs for both patients and care givers

    E. All of the above

Answers are in Appendix A.

REFERENCES

1. Schappert SM, Rechtsteiner EA. Ambulatory medical care utilization estimates for 2007. National Center for Health Statistics. Vital Health Stat 2011;13(169). Available at http://www.cdc.gov/nchs/data/series/sr_13/sr13_169.pdf. Accessed January 11, 2012.

2. Prevention. 2011. In Meriam-webster.com. Available at http://www.merriam-webster.com/dictionary/prevention. Accessed January 13, 2012.

3. Siegel R, Ward E, Brawley O, et al. Cancer statistics, 2011. The impact of eliminating socioeconomic and racial disparities on premature cancer deaths. CA Cancer J Clin 2011;61: 212–236.

4. National Center for Health Statistics. Health. United States. 2010; With special feature on death and dying. Hyattsville, MD. 2011.

5. Roe MT, Ohman EM. A new era in secondary prevention after acute coronary syndrome. N Engl J Med 2012;366:85–87.

6. Harris R, Sawaya GF, Moyer VA, et al. Reconsidering the criteria for evaluating proposed screening programs: reflections from 4 current and former members of the U.S. Preventive Services Task Force. Epidemiol Rev 2011;33:20–35.

7. Howlader N, Noone AM, Krapcho M, et al. (eds). SEER Cancer Statistics Review, 1975-2008, National Cancer Institute. Bethesda,

MD. Available at http://seer.cancer.gov/csr/1975_2008/, based on November 2010 SEER data submission, posted to the SEER Web site, 2011. Accessed January 13, 2012.

8. Chang MH, You SL, Chen CJ, et al. Decreased incidence of hepatocellular carcinoma in hepatitis B vaccinees: a 20 year follow-up study. J Natl Cancer Inst 2009;101:1348–1355.

9. Greene SK, Rett M, Weintraub ES, et al. Risk of confirmed Guillain-Barré Syndrome following receipt of monovalent inactivated influenza A (H1N1) and seasonal influenza vaccines in the Vaccine Safety Datalink Project, 2009-2010. Am J Epidemiol 2012;175:1100–1109.

10. Fiore MC, Jaén CR, Baker TB, et al. Treating tobacco use and dependence: 2008 Update. Clinical Practice Guideline. Rockville, MD: U.S. Department of Health and Human Services. Public Health Service. May 2008.

11. Mandel JS, Bond JH, Church TR, et al. (for the Minnesota Colon Cancer Control Study). Reducing mortality from colorectal cancer by screening for fecal occult blood. N Engl J Med 1993;328:1365–1371.

12. Marcus PM, Bergstralh EJ, Fagerstrom RM, et al. Lung cancer mortality in the Mayo Lung Project: impact of extended follow-up. J Natl Cancer Inst. 2000;92:1308–1316.

13. The National Lung Screening Trial Research Team. Reduced lung-cancer mortality with low-dose computed tomographic screening. N Engl J Med 2011;365:395–409.

14. Gǽde P, Lund-Andersen H, Hans-Henrik P, et al. Effect of a multifactorial intervention on mortality in type 2 diabetes. N Engl J Med 2008;358:580–591.

15. Friedman GD, Collen MF, Fireman BH. Multiphasic health checkup evaluation: a 16-year follow-up. J Chron Dis 1986;39:453–463.

16. Avins AL, Pressman A, Ackerson L, et al. Placebo adherence and its association with morbidity and mortality in the studies of left ventricular dysfunction. J Gen Intern Med 2010;25:1275–1281.

17. Selby JV, Friedman GD, Quesenberry CP, et al. A case-control study of screening sigmoidoscopy and mortality from colorectal cancer. N Eng J Med 1992;326:653–657.

18. Gann PH, Hennekens CH, Stampfer MJ. A prospective evaluation of plasma prostate-specific antigen for detection of prostatic cancer. JAMA 1995;273:289–294.

19. Delongchamps NB, Singh A, Haas GP. The role of prevalence in the diagnosis of prostate cancer. Cancer Control 2006;13:158–168.

20. Carney PA, Miglioretti DL, Yankaskas BC, et al. Individual and combined effects of age, breast density, and hormone replacement therapy use on the accuracy of screening mammography. Ann Intern Med 2003;138:168–175.

21. Lansdorp-Vogelaar I, Knudsen AB, Brenner H. Cost-effectiveness of colorectal cancer screening. Epi Rev 2011;33:88–100.

22. Berrington de González A, Mahesh M, Kim K-P, et al. Radiation dose associated with common computed tomography examinations and the associated lifetime attributable risk of cancer. Arch Intern Med 2009;169:2071–2077.

23. D'Orsi CD, Shin-Ping Tu, Nakano C. Current realities of delivering mammography services in the community: do challenges with staffing and scheduling exist? Radiology 2005;235:391–395.

24. Buys SS, Partridge E, Black A, et al. Effect of screening on ovarian cancer mortality. The Prostate, Lung, Colorectal and Ovarian (PLCO) cancer screening randomized controlled trial. JAMA 2011;305:2295–2303.

25. Meador CK. The last well person. N Engl Med J 1994;330:440–441.

26. Croswell JM, Baker SG, Marcus PM, et al. Cumulative incidence of false-positive test results in lung cancer screening: a randomized trial. Ann Intern Med 2010;152:505–512.

27. Croswell JM, Kramer BS, Kreimer AR. Cumulative incidence of false-positive results in repeated multimodal cancer screening. Ann Fam Med 2009;7:212–222.

28. Fowler FJ, Barry MJ, Walker-Corkery BS. The impact of a suspicious prostate biopsy on patients' psychological, socio-behavioral, and medical care outcomes. J Gen Intern Med 2006; 21:715–721.

29. Schilling FH, Spix C, Berthold F, et al. Neuroblastoma screening at one year of age. N Engl J Med 2002;346:1047–1053.

30. Woods WG, Gao R, Shuster JJ, et al. Screening of infants and mortality due to neuroblastoma. N Engl J Med 2002;346:1041–1046.

31. Xiong T, Richardson M, Woodroffe R, et al. Incidental lesions found on CT colonography: their nature and frequency. Br J Radiol 2005;78:22–29.

32. Hubbard RA, Kerlikowske K, Flowers CI, et al. Cumulative probability of false-positive recall or biopsy recommendation after 10 years of screening mammography. Ann Intern Med 2011;155:481–492.

33. Mandelblatt JS, Cronin KA, Bailey S, et al. Effects of mammography screening under different screening schedules: model estimates of potential benefits and harms. Ann Intern Med 2009;151:738–747.

34. Gillman MW, Daniels SR. Is universal pediatric lipid screening justified? JAMA 2012;307:259–260.

35. Goldie SJ, Kohli M, Grima D. Projected clinical benefits and cost-effectiveness of a human papillomavirus 16/18 vaccine. J Natl Cancer Inst 2004;96:604–615.

Chapter 11

Chance

It is a common practice to judge a result significant, if it is of such a magnitude that it would have been produced by chance not more frequently than once in twenty trials. This is an arbitrary, but convenient, level of significance for the practical investigator, but it does not mean that he allows himself to be deceived once in every twenty experiments.
—Ronald Fisher
1929 (1)

KEY WORDS

Hypothesis testing
Estimation
Statistically
    significant
Type 1 (α) error
Type II (β) error
Inferential statistics
Statistical testing
P value
Statistical
    significance
Statistical tests
Null hypothesis

Non-parametric
    statistics
Two-tailed
One-tailed
Statistical power
Sample size
Point estimate
Statistical precision
Confidence interval
Multiple comparisons
Multivariable
    modeling
Bayesian reasoning

Learning from clinical experience, whether during formal research or in the course of patient care, is impeded by two processes: bias and chance. As discussed in Chapter 1, bias is systematic error, the result of any process that causes observations to differ systematically from the true values. Much of this book has been about where bias might lurk, how to avoid it when possible, and how to control for it and estimate its effects when bias is unavoidable.

On the other hand, random error, resulting from the play of chance, is inherent in all observations. It can be minimized but never avoided altogether. This source of error is called "random" because, on average, it is as likely to result in observed values being on one side of the true value as on the other.

Many of us tend to underestimate the importance of bias relative to chance when interpreting data, perhaps because statistics are quantitative and appear so definitive. We might say, in essence, "If the statistical conclusions are strong, a little bit of bias can't do much harm." However, when data are biased, no amount of statistical elegance can save the day. As one scholar put it, perhaps taking an extreme position, "A well designed, carefully executed study usually gives results that are obvious without a formal analysis and if there are substantial flaws in design or execution a formal analysis will not help" (2).

In this chapter, we discuss chance mainly in the context of controlled clinical trials because it is the simplest way of presenting the concepts. However, statistics are an element of all clinical research, whenever one makes inferences about populations based on information obtained from samples. There is always a possibility that the particular sample of patients in a study, even though selected in an unbiased way, might not be similar to the population of patients as a whole. Statistics help estimate how well observations on samples approximate the true situation.

TWO APPROACHES TO CHANCE

Two general approaches are used to assess the role of chance in clinical observations.

One approach, called hypothesis testing, asks whether an effect (difference) is present or is not by using statistical tests to examine the hypothesis

175

(called the "null hypothesis") that there is no difference. This traditional way of assessing the role of chance, associated with the familiar "P value," has been popular since statistical testing was introduced at the beginning of the 20th century. The hypothesis testing approach leads to dichotomous conclusions: Either an effect is present or there is insufficient evidence to conclude an effect is present.

The other approach, called estimation, uses statistical methods to estimate the range of values that is likely to include the true value—of a rate, measure of effect, or test performance. This approach has gained popularity recently and is now favored by most medical journals, at least for reporting main effects, for reasons described below.

HYPOTHESIS TESTING

In the usual situation, the principal conclusions of a trial are expressed in dichotomous terms, such as a new treatment is either better or not better than usual care, corresponding to the results being either statistically significant (unlikely to be purely by chance) or not. There are four ways in which the statistical conclusions might relate to reality (Fig. 11.1).

Two of the four possibilities lead to correct conclusions: (i) The new treatment really is better, and that is the conclusion of the study; and (ii) the treatments really have similar effects, and the study concludes that a difference is unlikely.

False-Positive and False-Negative Statistical Results

There are also two ways of being wrong. The new treatment and usual care may actually have similar effects, but it is concluded that the new treatment is more effective. Error of this kind, resulting in a "false-positive" conclusion that the treatment is effective, is referred to as a type I error or α error, the probability of saying that there is a difference in treatment effects when there is not. On the other hand, the new treatment might be more effective, but the study concludes that it is not. This "false-negative" conclusion is called a type II error or β error—the probability of saying that there is no difference in treatment effects when there is. "No difference" is a simplified way of saying that the true difference is unlikely to be larger than a certain size, which is considered too small to be of practical consequence. It is not possible to establish that there is no difference at all between two treatments.

Figure 11.1 is similar to 2 × 2 tables comparing the results of a diagnostic test to the true diagnosis (see Chapter 8). Here, the "test" is the conclusion of a clinical trial based on a statistical test of results from the trial's sample of patients. The "gold standard" for validity is the true difference in the treatments being compared—if it could be established, for example, by making observations on all patients with the illness or a large number of samples of these patients. Type I error is analogous to a false-positive test result, and type II error is analogous to a false-negative test result. In the absence of bias, random variation is responsible for the uncertainty of a statistical conclusion.

Because random variation plays a part in all observations, it is an oversimplification to ask whether chance is responsible for the results. Rather, it is a question of how likely random variation is to account for the findings under the particular conditions of the study. The probability of error due to random variation is estimated by means of inferential statistics, a quantitative science that, given certain assumptions about the mathematical properties of the data, is the basis for calculations of the probability that the results could have occurred by chance alone.

Statistics is a specialized field with its own jargon (e.g., null hypothesis, variance, regression, power, and modeling) that is unfamiliar to many clinicians. However, leaving aside the genuine complexity of statistical methods, inferential statistics should be regarded by the non-expert as a useful means to an end. Statistical testing is a means by which the effects of random variation are estimated.

The next two sections discuss type I and type II errors and place hypothesis testing, as it is used to estimate the probabilities of these errors, in context.

		TRUE DIFFERENCE	
		Present	Absent
CONCLUSION OF STATISTICAL TEST	Significant	Correct	Type I (α) error
	Not significant	Type II (β) error	Correct

Figure 11.1 ■ **The relationship between the results of a statistical test and the true difference between two treatment groups.** (*Absent* is a simplification. It really means that the true difference is not greater than a specified amount.)

Concluding That a Treatment Works

Most statistics encountered in the medical literature concern the likelihood of a type I error and are expressed by the familiar *P* value. The *P* value is a quantitative estimate of the probability that differences in treatment effects in the particular study at hand could have happened by chance alone, assuming that there is in fact no difference between the groups. Another way of expressing this is that *P* is an answer to the question, "If there were no difference between treatment effects and the trial was repeated many times, what proportion of the trials would conclude that the difference between the two treatments was at least as large as that found in the study?"

In this presentation, *P* values are called P_α, to distinguish them from estimates of the other kind of error resulting from random variation, type II errors, which are referred to as P_β. When a simple *P* is found in the scientific literature, it ordinarily refers to P_α.

The kind of error estimated by P_α applies whenever one concludes that one treatment is more effective than another. If it is concluded that the P_α exceeds some limit (see below) so there is no statistical difference between treatments, then the particular value of P_α is not as relevant; in that situation, P_β (probability of type II error) applies.

Dichotomous and Exact *P* Values

It has become customary to attach special significance to *P* values below 0.05 because it is generally agreed that a chance of <1 in 20 is a small enough risk of being wrong. A chance of 1 in 20 is so small, in fact, that it is reasonable to conclude that such an occurrence is unlikely to have arisen by chance alone. It could have arisen by chance, and 1 in 20 times it will, but it is unlikely.

Differences associated with $P_\alpha < 0.05$ are called statistically significant. However, setting a cutoff point at 0.05 is entirely arbitrary. Reasonable people might accept higher values or insist on lower ones, depending on the consequences of a false-positive conclusion in a given situation. For example, one might be willing to accept a higher chance of a false-positive statistical test if the disease is severe, there is currently no effective treatment, and the new treatment is safe. On the other hand, one might be reluctant to accept a false-positive test if usual care is effective and the new treatment is dangerous or much more expensive. This reasoning is similar to that applied to the importance of false-positive and false-negative diagnostic tests (Chapter 8).

To accommodate various opinions about what is and is not unlikely enough, some researchers report the exact probabilities of *P* (e.g., 0.03, 0.07, 0.11), rather than lumping them into just two categories (≤0.05 or >0.05). Users are then free to apply their own preferences for what is statistically significant. However, *P* values >1 in 5 are usually reported as simply *P* > 0.20, because nearly everyone can agree that a probability of a type I error >1 in 5 is unacceptably high. Similarly, below very low *P* values (e.g., *P* < 0.001) chance is a very unlikely explanation for an observed difference, and little further information is conveyed by describing this chance more precisely.

Another approach is to accept the primacy of *P* ≤ 0.05 and describe results that come close to that standard with terms such as "almost statistically significant," "did not achieve statistical significance," "marginally significant," or "a trend." These value-laden terms suggest that the finding should have been statistically significant but for some annoying reason was not. It is better to simply state the result and exact *P* value (or point estimate and confidence interval, see below) and let the reader decide for him or herself how much chance could have accounted for the result.

Statistical Significance and Clinical Importance

A statistically significant difference, no matter how small the *P*, does not mean that the difference is clinically important. A *P* value of <0.0001, if it emerges from a well-designed study, conveys a high degree of confidence that a difference really exists but says nothing about the magnitude of that difference or its clinical importance. In fact, trivial differences may be highly statistically significant if a large enough number of patients are studied.

Example

The drug donepezil, a cholinesterase inhibitor, was developed for the treatment of Alzheimer disease. In a randomized controlled trial to establish whether the drug produced worthwhile improvements, 565 patients with Alzheimer disease were randomly allocated to donepezil or placebo (3). The statistical significance of some trial end points was impressive: Both the mini-mental state examination and the Bristol Activities of Daily Living Scale were statistically different at *P* < 0.0001. However, the actual differences were small, 0.8 on a 30-point scale for the mini-mental state examination and 1 on a 60-point scale for the Bristol Activities of Daily Living Scale. Moreover, other outcomes, which more closely represented the burden of illness and care of these patients, were similar in the donepezil and placebo groups. These included entering institutional care and progression of disability (both primary end points) as well as behavioral and psychological symptoms, caregiver psychopathology, formal care costs, unpaid caregiver time, and adverse events or death. The authors concluded that the benefits of donepezil were "below minimally relevant thresholds."

On the other hand, very unimpressive P values can result from studies with strong treatment effects if there are few patients in the study.

Statistical Tests

Statistical tests are used to estimate the probability of a type I error. The test is applied to the data to obtain a numerical summary for those data called a test statistic. That number is then compared to a sampling distribution to come up with a probability of a type I error (Fig. 11.2). The distribution is under the null hypothesis, the proposition that there is no true difference in outcome between treatment groups. This device is for mathematical reasons, not because "no difference" is the working scientific hypothesis of the investigators conducting the study. One ends up rejecting the null hypothesis (concluding there is a difference) or failing to reject it (concluding that there is insufficient evidence in support of a difference). Note that not finding statistical significance is not the same as there being no difference. Statistical testing is not able to establish that there is no difference at all.

Some commonly used statistical tests are listed in Table 11.1. The validity of many tests depends on certain assumptions about the data; a typical assumption is that the data have a normal distribution. If the data do not satisfy these assumptions, the resulting P value may be misleading. Other statistical tests, called non-parametric tests, do not make assumptions about the underlying distribution of the data. A discussion of how these statistical tests are derived and calculated and of the assumptions on which they rest can be found in any biostatistics textbook.

Table 11.1

Some Statistical Tests Commonly Used in Clinical Research

Test	When Used
To Test the Statistical Significance of a Difference	
Chi square (χ^2)	Between two or more proportions (when there are a large number of observations)
Fisher's exact	Between two proportions (when there are a small number of observations)
Mann-Whitney U	Between two medians
Student t	Between two means
F test	Between two or more means
To Describe the Extent of Association	
Regression coefficient	Between an independent (predictor) variable and a dependent (outcome) variable
Pearson's r	Between two variables
To Model the Effects of Multiple Variables	
Logistic regression	With a dichotomous outcome
Cox proportional hazards	With a time-to-event outcome

The chi-square (χ^2) test for nominal data (counts) is more easily understood than most and can be used to illustrate how statistical testing works. The extent to which the observed values depart from what would have been expected if there were no treatment effect is used to calculate a P value.

Example

Cardiac arrest outside the hospital has a poor outcome. Animal studies suggested that hypothermia might improve neurologic outcomes. To test this hypothesis in humans, 77 patients who remained unconscious after resuscitation from out-of-hospital cardiac arrest were

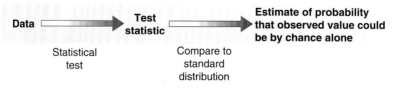

Figure 11.2 ■ **Statistical testing.**

randomized to cooling (hypothermia) or usual care (4). The primary outcome was survival to hospital discharge with relatively good neurologic function.

Observed Rates

	Survival with Good Neurological Function		
	Yes	No	Total
Hypothermia	21	22	43
Usual care	9	25	34
Total	30	47	77

Success rates were 49% in the patients treated with hypothermia and 26% in the patients on usual care. How likely would it be for a study of this size to observe a difference in rates as great as this or greater if there was in fact no difference in effectiveness? That depends on how far the observed results depart from what would have been expected if the treatments were of similar effectiveness and only random variation accounted for the different rates. If treatment had no effect on outcome, applying the success rate for the patients as a whole (30/77 = 39%) to the number of patients in each treatment group gives the expected number of successes in each group:

Expected Rates

	Success		
	Yes	No	Total
Hypothermia	16.75	26.25	43
Usual care	13.25	20.75	34
Total	30	47	77

The χ^2 statistic is the square of the differences between observed and expected divided by expected, summarized over all four cells:

$$\chi^2 = \sum \frac{(\text{Observed number} - \text{Expected number})^2}{\text{Expected number}}$$

The magnitude of the χ^2 statistic is determined by how different all of the observed numbers are from what would have been expected if there were no treatment effect. Because they are squared, it does not matter whether the observed rates exceed or fall short of the expected. By dividing the squared difference in each cell by the expected number, the difference is adjusted for the number of patients in that cell.

The χ^2 statistic for these data is:

$$\frac{(21 - 16.75)^2}{16.75} + \frac{(9 - 13.25)^2}{13.25} + \frac{(22 - 26.25)^2}{26.75}$$
$$+ \frac{(25 - 20.75)^2}{20.75} = 4.0$$

This χ^2 is then compared to a table (available in books and computer programs) relating χ^2 values to probabilities for that number of cells to obtain the probability of a χ^2 of 4.0. It is intuitively obvious that the larger the χ^2, the more likely chance is to account for the observed differences. The resulting P value for a chi-square test statistic of 4.0 and a 2 × 2 table was 0.046, which is the probability of a false-positive conclusion that the treatments had different effects. That is, the study results meet the conventional criterion for statistical significance, $P \leq 0.05$.

When using statistical tests, the usual approach is to test for the probability that an intervention is either more or less effective than another to a statistically important extent. In this situation, testing is called two-tailed, referring to both tails of a bell-shaped curve describing the random variation in differences between treatment groups of equal value, where the two tails of the curve include statistically unlikely outcomes favoring one or the other treatment. Sometimes there are compelling reasons to believe that one treatment could only be better or worse than the other, in which case one-tailed testing is used, where all of the type I error (5%) is in one of the tails, making it easier to reach statistical significance.

Concluding That a Treatment Does Not Work

Some trials are unable to conclude that one treatment is better than the other. The risk of a false-negative result is particularly large in studies with relatively few patients or outcome events. The question then arises: How likely is a false-negative result (type II or β error)? Could the "negative" findings in such trials have misrepresented the truth because these particular studies had the bad luck to turn out in a relatively unlikely way?

Example

One of the examples in Chapter 9 was a randomized controlled trial of the effects on cardiovascular outcomes of adding niacin versus placebo in patients with lipid abnormalities who were already taking statin drugs (5). It was a "negative" trial: Primary outcomes occurred in 16.4% of patients taking niacin and 16.2% in patients taking placebo, and the authors concluded that "there was no incremental clinical benefit from the addition of niacin to statin therapy." The statistical question associated with this assertion is: How likely was it that the study found no benefit when there really is one? After all, there were only a few hundred cardiovascular outcome events in the study so the play of chance might have obscured treatment effects. Figure 11.3 shows time-to-event curves for the primary outcome in the two treatment groups. Patients in the niacin and control groups had remarkably similar curves throughout follow-up, making a protective effect of niacin implausible.

Visual presentation of negative results can be convincing. Alternatively, one can examine confidence intervals (see Point Estimates and Confidence Intervals, below) and learn a lot about whether the study was large enough to rule out clinically important differences if they existed.

Of course, reasons for false-negative results other than chance also need to be considered: biologic reasons such as too short follow-up or too small dose of niacin, as well as study limitations such as noncompliance and missed outcome events.

Type II errors have received less attention than type I errors for several reasons. They are more difficult to calculate. Also, most professionals simply prefer things that work and consider negative results unwelcome. Authors are less likely to submit negative studies to journals and when negative studies are reported at all, the authors may prefer to emphasize subgroups of patients in which treatment differences were found. Authors may also emphasize reasons other than chance to explain why true differences might have been missed. Whatever the reason for not considering the probability of a type II error, it is the main question that should be asked when the results of a study are interpreted as "no difference."

HOW MANY STUDY PATIENTS ARE ENOUGH?

Suppose you are reading about a clinical trial that compares a promising new treatment to usual care

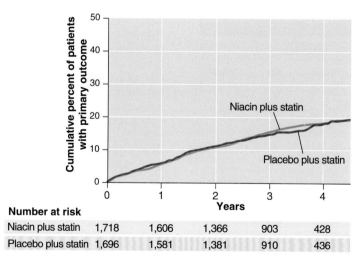

Figure 11.3 ■ **Example of a "negative" trial.** (Redrawn with permission from The AIM-HIGH Investigators. Niacin in patients with low HDL cholesterol levels receiving intensive statin therapy. N Engl J Med 2011;365:2255–2267.)

and finds no difference. You are aware that random variation can be the reason for whatever differences are or are not observed, and you wonder if the number of patients in this study is large enough to make chance an unlikely explanation for what was found. Alternatively, you may be planning to do such a study and have the same question. Either way, you need to understand how many patients would be needed to make a strong comparison of the effects of the two treatments?

Statistical Power

The probability that a study will find a statistically significant difference when a difference really exists is called the statistical power of the study. Power and P_β are complementary ways of expressing the same concept.

$$\text{Statistical power} = 1 - P_\beta$$

Power is analogous to the sensitivity of a diagnostic test. One speaks of a study being powerful when it has a high probability of detecting differences when treatments really do have different effects.

Estimating Sample Size Requirements

From the point of view of hypothesis testing of nominal data (counts), an adequate sample size depends on four characteristics of the study: the magnitude of the difference in outcome between treatment groups, P_α and P_β (the probability of the false-positive and false-negative conclusions you are willing to accept), and the underlying outcome rate.

These determinants of adequate sample size should be taken into account when investigators plan a study, to ensure that the study will have enough statistical power to produce meaningful results. To the extent that investigators have not done this well, or some of their assumptions were found to be inaccurate, readers need to consider the same issues when interpreting study results.

Effect Size

Sample size depends on the magnitude of the difference to be detected. One is free to look for differences of any magnitude and of course one hopes to be able to detect even very small differences, but more patients are needed to detect small differences, everything else being equal. Therefore, it is best to ask, "What is a sufficient number of patients

to detect the smallest degree of improvement that would be clinically meaningful?" On the other hand, if one is interested in detecting only very large differences between treated and control groups (i.e., strong treatment effects) then fewer patients need to be studied.

Type I Error

Sample size is also related to the risk of a type I error (concluding that treatment is effective when it is not). The acceptable probability for a risk of this kind is a value judgment. If one is prepared to accept the consequences of a large chance of falsely concluding that the treatment is effective, one can reach conclusions with fewer patients. On the other hand, if one wants to take only a small risk of being wrong in this way, a larger number of patients will be required. As discussed earlier, it is customary to set P_α at 0.05 (1 in 20) or sometimes 0.01 (1 in 100).

Type II Error

The chosen risk of a type II error is another determinant of sample size. An acceptable probability of this error is also a judgment that can be freely made and changed to suit individual tastes. Probability of P_β is often set at 0.20, a 20% chance of missing true differences in a particular study. Conventional type II errors are much larger than type I errors, reflecting a higher value placed on being sure an effect is really present when it is said to be.

Characteristics of the Data

The statistical power of a study is also determined by the nature of the data. When the outcome is expressed by counts or proportions of events or time-to-event, its statistical power depends on the rate of events: The larger the number of events, the greater the statistical power for a given number of people at risk. As Peto et al. (6) put it:

> In clinical trials of time to death (or of the time to some other particular "event"—relapse, metastasis, first thrombosis, stroke. recurrence, or time to death from a particular cause—the ability of the trial to distinguish between the merits of two treatments depends on how many patients *die* (or suffer a relevant event), rather than on the number of patients *entered.* A study of 100 patients, 50 of whom die, is about as sensitive as a study with 1,000 patients, 50 of whom die.

If the data are continuous, such as blood pressure or serum cholesterol, power is affected by the

Table 11.2

| Determinants of Sample Size | | | | |

		Determined by		
			Date Type	
	Investigator	**Means**		**Counts**
Sample size varies according to:	$\dfrac{1}{\text{Effect size, } P_\alpha, P_\beta}$	$\dfrac{1}{\text{Outcome rate}}$	OR	Variability

degree to which patients vary among themselves. The greater the variation from patient to patient with respect to the characteristic being measured, the more difficult it is to be confident that the observed differences (or lack of difference) between groups is not because of this variation, rather than a true treatment effect.

In designing a study, investigators choose the smallest treatment effect that is clinically important (larger treatment effects will be easier to detect) and the type I and type II errors they are willing to accept. They also obtain estimates of outcome event rates or variation among patients. It is possible to design studies that maximize power for a given sample size—such as by choosing patients with a high event rate or similar characteristics—as long as they match the research question.

Interrelationships

The relationships among the four variables that together determine an adequate sample size are summarized in Table 11.2. The variables can be traded off against one another. In general, for any given number of patients in the study, there is a trade-off between type 1 and type 2 errors. Everything else being equal, the more one is willing to accept one kind of error, the less it will be necessary to risk the other. Neither kind of error is inherently worse than the other. It is, of course, possible to reduce both type 1 and type 2 errors if the number of patients is increased, outcome events are more frequent, variability is decreased, or a larger treatment effect is sought.

For conventional levels of P_α and P_β, the relationship between the size of treatment effect and the number of patients needed for a trial is illustrated by the following examples. One represents a situation in which a relatively small number of patients was sufficient, and the other is one in which a very large number of patients was too small.

Example

A Small Sample Size That Was Adequate

For many centuries, scurvy, a vitamin C deficiency syndrome causing bleeding into gums and joints progressing to disability and death, was a huge problem for sailors. While aboard ship in 1747, James Lind studied the treatment of scurvy in one of the earliest controlled trials of treatment (7). He divided 12 badly affected sailors, who were confined to the ship's sick bay, into 6 treatment groups of 2 sailors each. Treatments were oranges and lemons, cider, elixir of vitriol, vinegar, seawater, or nutmeg. Except for the treatment, the sailors remained in the same place and ate the same food. Six days after treatment was begun, the two sailors given oranges and lemons, which contained ample amounts of vitamin C, were greatly improved: One was fit for duty and one was well enough to nurse the others. Sailors given other treatments were not improved. The *P* value (not calculated by Lind) for 2 of 2 successes versus 10 of 10 failures was 0.02 (assuming that Lind believed beforehand that oranges and lemons were the intervention of interest and that the other five interventions were inactive controls).

A Large Sample Size That Was Inadequate

Low serum vitamin D levels may be a risk factor for colorectal cancer, but results of studies of this question have been inconsistent with each other. In 1985, investigators established (originally, for another purpose) a cohort of 29,133 Finnish men aged 50 to 69 and measured their baseline serum vitamin D levels (8). Incident colon and rectal cancers were identified from the National Cancer Registry. After 12 years of follow-up, 239 colon cancers and 192 rectal cancers developed in the cohort. After adjustment for confounders, serum vitamin D levels were positively associated with colon cancer incidence and inversely associated to rectal cancer incidence, but neither of these findings was statistically significant.

For most of the therapeutic questions encountered today, a surprisingly large sample size is required. The value of dramatic, powerful treatments, such as antibiotics for pneumonia or thyroid replacement for hypothyroidism, was established by clinical experience or studying a small number of patients, but such treatments come along rarely and many of them are already well established. We are left with diseases, many of which are chronic and have multiple, interacting causes, for which the effects of new treatments are generally small. This makes it especially important to plan clinical studies that are large enough to distinguish real from chance effects.

Figure 11.4 shows the relationship between sample size and treatment difference for several baseline rates of outcome events. Studies involving fewer than 100 patients have a poor chance of detecting statistically significant differences for even large treatment effects. Looked at another way, it is difficult to detect effect sizes of <25%. In practice, statistical power can be estimated by means of readily available formulas, tables, nomograms, computer programs, or Web sites.

POINT ESTIMATES AND CONFIDENCE INTERVALS

The effect size that is observed in a particular study (such as treatment effect in a clinical trial or relative risk in a cohort study) is called the point estimate of the effect. It is the best estimate from the study of the true effect size and is the summary statistic usually given the most emphasis in reports of research.

However, the true effect size is unlikely to be exactly that observed in the study. Because of random variation, any one study is likely to find a result higher or lower than the true value. Therefore, a summary measure is needed for the statistical precision of the point estimate, the range of values likely to encompass the true effect size.

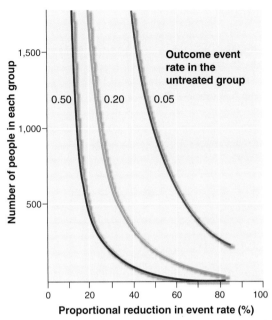

Figure 11.4 ■ The number of people required in each of two treatment groups (of equal size), for various rates of outcome events in the untreated group, to have an 80% chance of detecting a difference (P = 0.05) in reduction in outcome event rates in treated relative to untreated patients. (Calculated from formula in Weiss NS. Clinical epidemiology. The study of the outcome of illness. New York: Oxford University Press; 1986.)

Statistical precision is expressed as a confidence interval, usually the 95% confidence interval, around the point estimate. Confidence intervals are interpreted as follows: If the study is unbiased, there is a 95% chance that the interval includes the true effect size. The more narrow the confidence interval, the more certain one can be about the size of the true effect. The true value is most likely to be close to the point estimate, less likely to be near the outer limits of the interval, and could (5 times out of 100) fall outside these limits altogether. Statistical precision increases with the statistical power of the study.

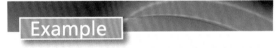

Example

The Women's Health Initiative included a randomized controlled trial of the effects of estrogen plus progestin on chronic disease outcomes in healthy postmenopausal women (9). Figure 11.5 shows relative risk and confidence

OUTCOME

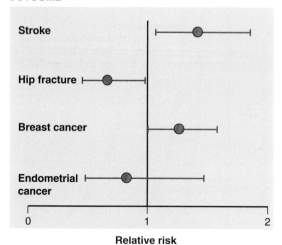

Figure 11.5 ■ **Example of confidence intervals.** The relative risk and confidence intervals for outcomes in the Women's Health Initiative: a randomized controlled trial of estrogen plus progestin in healthy postmenopausal women. (Data from Writing Group for the Women's Health Initiative Investigators. Risks and benefits of estrogen plus progestin in healthy postmenopausal women. JAMA 2002;288: 321–333.)

intervals for four of these outcomes: stroke, hip fracture, breast cancer, and endometrial cancer. The four illustrate various possibilities for how confidence intervals are interpreted. Estrogen plus progestin was a risk factor for stroke; the best estimate of this risk is the point estimate, a relative risk of 1.41, but the data are consistent with a relative risk as low as 1.07 or as high as 1.85. Estrogen plus progestin protected against hip fracture, preventing as much as 65% and as little as 2% of fractures. That is, the data are consistent with very little benefit, although substantial benefit is likely and even larger benefits are consistent with the results. Although risk of breast cancer is likely to be increased, the data are consistent with no effect (the lower end of the confidence interval includes a relative risk of 1.0). Finally, the study is not very informative for endometrial cancer. Confidence intervals are very wide, so not only was there no clear risk or benefit, but also the estimate of risk was so imprecise that substantial risk or benefit remained possible.

Statistical significance at the 0.05 level can be obtained from 95% confidence intervals. If the point corresponding to no effect (i.e., a relative risk of 1 or a treatment difference of 0) falls outside the 95% confidence intervals for the observed effect, the results are statistically significant at the 0.05 level. If the confidence intervals include this point, the results are not statistically significant.

Confidence intervals have advantages over P values. They put the emphasis where it belongs, on the size of the effect. Confidence intervals help the reader to see the range of plausible values and so to decide whether an effect size they regard as clinically meaningful is consistent with or ruled out by the data (10). They also provide information about statistical power. If the confidence interval is relatively wide and barely includes the value corresponding to no effect, readers can see that low power might have been the reason for the negative result. On the other hand, if the confidence interval is narrow and includes no effect, a large effect is ruled out.

Point estimates and confidence intervals are used to characterize the statistical precision of any rate (incidence and prevalence), diagnostic test performance, comparisons of rates (relative and attributable risks), and other summary statistics. For example, studies have shown that 7.0% (95% confidence interval, 5.2–9.4) of adults have a clinically important family history of prostate cancer (11); that the sensitivity of a high-sensitivity cardiac troponin assay (at the optimal cutoff point) for acute coronary syndrome was 84.8% (95% confidence interval 82.8–86.6) (12); and that return to usual activity after inguinal hernia repair was shorter for laparoscopic than open surgery (hazard ratio 0.56, 95% confidence interval 0.51–0.61) (13).

Confidence intervals have become the usual way of reporting the main results of clinical research because of their many advantages over the hypothesis testing (P value) approach. P values are still used because of tradition and as a convenience when many results are reported and it would not be feasible to include confidence intervals for all of them.

Statistical Power after a Study Is Completed

Earlier in the chapter, we discussed how calculation of statistical power based on the hypothesis testing approach is performed before a study is undertaken to ensure that enough patients will be entered to have a good chance of detecting a clinically meaningful effect if one is present. However, after the study is completed, this approach is less relevant (14). There

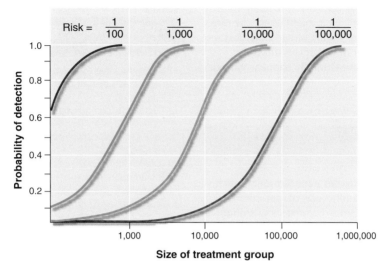

Figure 11.6 ■ **The probability of detecting one event according to the rate of the event and the number of people observed.** (Redrawn with permission from Guess HA, Rudnick SA. Use of cost effectiveness analysis in planning cancer chemoprophylaxis trials. Control Clin Trials 1983;4:89–100.)

is no longer a need to estimate effect size, outcome event rates, and variability among patients because they are all known. Rather, attention should be directed to point estimates and confidence intervals. With them, one can see the range of values that are consistent with the results and whether the effect sizes of interest are within this range or are ruled out by the data. In the niacin study, summarized earlier as an example of a negative trial, the hazard ratio was 1.02 and the 95% confidence interval was 0.87 to 1.21, meaning that the results were consistent with a small degree of benefit or harm. Whether this matters depends on the clinical importance attached to a difference in rates as large as represented by this confidence interval.

DETECTING RARE EVENTS

It is sometimes important to know how likely a study is to detect a relatively uncommon event (e.g., 1/1,000), particularly if that event is severe, such as bone marrow failure or life-threatening arrhythmia. A great many people must be observed in order to have a good chance of detecting even one such event, much less to establish a relatively stable estimate of its frequency. For most clinical research, sample size is planned to be sufficient to detect main effects, the answer sought for the primary research question. Sample size is likely to be well short of the number

needed to detect rare events such as uncommon side effects and complications. For that, a different approach, involving many more patients, is needed. An example is postmarketing surveillance of a drug, in which thousands of users are monitored for side effects.

Figure 11.6 shows the probability of detecting an event as a function of the number of people under observation. A rule of thumb is: To have a good chance of detecting a 1/x event, one must observe 3x people (15). For example, to detect at least one event if the underlying rate is 1/1,000, one would need to observe 3,000 people.

MULTIPLE COMPARISONS

The statistical conclusions of research have an aura of authority that defies challenge, particularly by non-experts. However, as many skeptics have suspected, it is possible to "lie with statistics" even if the research is well designed, the mathematics flawless, and the investigators' intentions beyond reproach.

Statistical conclusions can be misleading because the strength of statistical tests depends on the number of research questions considered in the study and when those questions were asked. If many comparisons are made among the variables in a large set of data, the P value associated with each individual comparison is an underestimate of how often the result of that comparison, among the others, is likely to arise by chance. As implausible as it might seem, the interpretation of the P value from a single statistical test depends on the context in which it is done.

To understand how this might happen, consider the following example.

Example

Suppose a large study has been done in which there are multiple subgroups of patients and many different outcomes. For instance, it might be a clinical trial of the value of a treatment for coronary artery disease for which patients are in 12 clinically meaningful subgroups (e.g., one-, two-, and three-vessel disease; good and bad ventricular function; the presence or absence of arrhythmias; and various combinations of these), and four outcomes are considered (e.g., death, myocardial infarction, heart failure, and angina). Suppose also that there are no true associations between treatment and outcome in any of the subgroups and for any of the outcomes. Finally, suppose that the effects of treatment are assessed separately for each subgroup and for each outcome—a process that involves a great many comparisons; in this case, 12 subgroups multiplied by 4 outcomes = 48 comparisons. With a $P_\alpha = .05$, 1 in 20 of these comparisons (in this case, 2 to 3) is likely to be statistically significant by chance alone. In the general case, if 20 comparisons are made, on average, 1 would be found to be statistically significant; if 100 comparisons are made, about 5 would be likely to be statistically significant, and so on. Thus, when a great many comparisons have been made, a few will be found that are strong enough, because of random variation, to appear statistical significant even if no true associations between variables exist in nature. As the saying goes, "If you torture the data long enough, they will confess!"

This phenomenon is referred to as the **multiple comparisons** problem. Because of this problem, the strength of evidence from clinical research depends on how focused its questions were at the outset.

Unfortunately, when the results of research are presented, it is not always possible to know how many

Table 11.3

How Multiple Comparisons Can Be Misleading

1. Make multiple comparisons within a study.
2. Apply tests of statistical significance to each comparison.
3. Find a few comparisons that are "interesting" (statistically significant).
4. Build an article around one of these interesting findings.
5. Do not mention the context of the individual comparison (how many questions were examined and which was considered primary before the data was examined).
6. Construct a *post hoc* argument for the plausibility of the isolated finding.

comparisons really were made. Sometimes, interesting findings have been selected from a larger number of uninteresting ones that are not mentioned. This process of deciding after the fact what is and is not important about a mass of data can introduce considerable distortion of reality. Table 11.3 summarizes how this misleading situation can arise.

How can the statistical effects of multiple comparisons be taken into account when interpreting research? Although ways of adjusting P values have been proposed, probably the best advice is to be aware of the problem and to be cautious about accepting positive conclusions of studies in which multiple comparisons were made. As put by Armitage (16):

> If you dredge the data sufficiently deeply and sufficiently often, you will find something odd. Many of these bizarre findings will be due to chance. I do not imply that data dredging is not an occupation for honorable persons, but rather that discoveries that were not initially postulated as among the major objectives of the trial should be treated with extreme caution.

A special case of multiple comparisons occurs when data in a clinical trial are examined repeatedly as they accrue, to assure that the trial is stopped as soon as there is an answer, regardless of how long the trial was planned to run. If this is done, as it often is for ethical reasons, the final P value is usually adjusted for the number of looks at the data. There is a statistical incentive to keep the number of looks to a minimum. In any case, if the accruing data are examined repeatedly, it will be more difficult to reach statistical significance after the multiple looks at the data are taken into account.

Another special case is genome-wide association studies, in which more than 500,000 single-nucleotide polymorphisms may be examined in cases and controls (17). A common way to manage multiple comparisons, to divide the usual P value of 0.05 by the number of comparisons, would require a genome-wide level of statistical significance of 0.0000001 (10^{-7}), which would be difficult to achieve because sample sizes in these studies are constrained and relative risks are typically small. Because of this, belief in results of genome-wide association studies relies on the consistency and strength of associations across many studies.

SUBGROUP ANALYSIS

It is tempting to go beyond the main results of a study to examine results within subgroups of patients with characteristics that might be related to treatment effect (i.e., to look for effect modification, as discussed in Chapter 5). Because characteristics present at the time of randomization are randomly allocated into treatment groups, the consequence of subgroup analysis is to break the trial as a whole into a set of smaller randomized controlled trials, each with a smaller sample size.

Example

Atrial fibrillation is treated with anticoagulants, vitamin K antagonists in high-risk patients, to prevent stroke. Investigators studied stroke prevention in patients with atrial fibrillation who could not take vitamin K antagonists. They randomly assigned these patients to a new anticoagulant, apixaban, or to aspirin (18). There were 164 outcome events and the hazard ratio was 0.45 (95% confidence interval 0.32–0.62) favoring apixaban. Figure 11.7 shows the hazard ratio for stroke in subgroups, with point estimates indicated by boxes (with their size proportional subgroup size) and confidence intervals. A total of 42 subgroups were reported, 21 for one outcome (stroke and systemic embolism, shown) and the same 21 for another outcome (major bleeding, not shown). The hazard ratios for most subgroups are around the hazard ratio for the study as a whole (shown by the vertical dashed line) and although some were higher or lower, none was statistically significant. This analysis suggests that effect modification was not present, but this conclusion was limited by low statistical precision in subgroups. Multiple comparisons, leading to a false-positive finding in subgroups, would have been an issue if there had been a statistically significant effect in one or more of the subgroups.

Subgroup analyses tell clinicians about effect modification so they can tailor their care of individual patients as closely as possible to study results in patients like them. However, subgroup analyses incur risks of misleading results because of the increased chance of finding effects in a particular subgroup that are not present, in the long run, in nature, that is, finding false-positive results because of multiple comparisons.

In practice, the effects of multiple comparisons may not be as extreme when treatment effects in the various subgroups are not independent of each other. To the extent that the variables are related to each other, rather than independent, the risk of false-positive findings is lessened. In the atrial fibrillation and anticoagulant example, age and prior stroke are components of the CHADS2 score (a metric for risk of stroke), but the three are treated as separate subgroups.

Another danger is coming to a false-negative conclusion. Within subgroups defined by certain kinds of patients or specific kinds of outcomes, there are fewer patients than for the study as a whole, often too few to rule out false-negative findings. Studies are, after all, designed to have enough patients to answer the main research question with sufficient statistical power. They are ordinarily not designed to have sufficient statistical power in subgroups, where the number of patients and outcome events is smaller. Guidelines for deciding whether a finding in a subgroup is real are summarized in Table 11.4.

Multiple Outcomes

Another version of multiple looks at the data is to report multiple outcomes—different manifestations of effectiveness, intermediate outcomes, and harms. Usually this is handled by naming one of the outcomes primary and the others secondary and then being more guarded about conclusions for the secondary outcomes. As with subgroups, outcomes

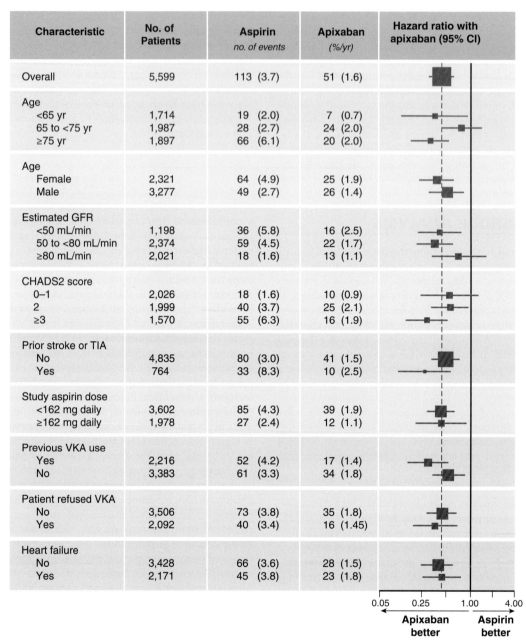

Characteristic	No. of Patients	Aspirin *no. of events*	Apixaban *(%/yr)*	Hazard ratio with apixaban (95% CI)
Overall	5,599	113 (3.7)	51 (1.6)	
Age				
<65 yr	1,714	19 (2.0)	7 (0.7)	
65 to <75 yr	1,987	28 (2.7)	24 (2.0)	
≥75 yr	1,897	66 (6.1)	20 (2.0)	
Age				
Female	2,321	64 (4.9)	25 (1.9)	
Male	3,277	49 (2.7)	26 (1.4)	
Estimated GFR				
<50 mL/min	1,198	36 (5.8)	16 (2.5)	
50 to <80 mL/min	2,374	59 (4.5)	22 (1.7)	
≥80 mL/min	2,021	18 (1.6)	13 (1.1)	
CHADS2 score				
0–1	2,026	18 (1.6)	10 (0.9)	
2	1,999	40 (3.7)	25 (2.1)	
≥3	1,570	55 (6.3)	16 (1.9)	
Prior stroke or TIA				
No	4,835	80 (3.0)	41 (1.5)	
Yes	764	33 (8.3)	10 (2.5)	
Study aspirin dose				
<162 mg daily	3,602	85 (4.3)	39 (1.9)	
≥162 mg daily	1,978	27 (2.4)	12 (1.1)	
Previous VKA use				
Yes	2,216	52 (4.2)	17 (1.4)	
No	3,383	61 (3.3)	34 (1.8)	
Patient refused VKA				
No	3,506	73 (3.8)	35 (1.8)	
Yes	2,092	40 (3.4)	16 (1.45)	
Heart failure				
No	3,428	66 (3.6)	28 (1.5)	
Yes	2,171	45 (3.8)	23 (1.8)	

0.05   0.25   1.00   4.00

← Apixaban better   Aspirin better →

Figure 11.7 ■ A subgroup analysis from a randomized controlled trial of the effectiveness of apixaban versus aspirin on stroke and systemic embolism in patients with atrial fibrillation. GFR (glomerular filtration rate) is a measure of kidney function. CHADS2 score is a prediction rule for the risk of embolism in patients with atrial fibrillation. (Redrawn with permission from Connolly SJ, Eikelboom J, Joyner C, et al. Apixaban in patients with atrial fibrillation. N Engl J Med 2011;364:806–817.)

Table 11.4

> **Guidelines for Deciding Whether Apparent Differences in Effects within Subgroups Are Real[a]**

From the study itself:

- Is the magnitude of the observed difference clinically important?
- How likely is the effect to have arisen by chance, taking into account:
  - the number of subgroups examined?
  - the magnitude of the *P* value?
- Was a hypothesis that the effect would be observed made before its discovery (or was justification for the effect argued for after it was found)?
- Was it one of a small number of hypotheses?

From other information:

- Was the difference suggested by comparisons within rather than between studies?
- Has the effect been observed in other studies?
- Is there direct evidence that supports the existence of the effect?

[a]Adapted from Oxman AD, Guyatt GH. A consumer's guide to subgroup analysis. Ann Intern Med 1992;116:78–84.

tend to be related to each other biologically (and as a consequence statistically), as is the case in the above example where stroke and systemic embolism are different manifestations of the same clinical phenomenon.

MULTIVARIABLE METHODS

Most clinical phenomena are the result of many variables acting together in complex ways. For example, coronary heart disease is the joint result of lipid abnormalities, hypertension, cigarette smoking, family history, diabetes, diet, exercise, inflammation, coagulation abnormalities, and perhaps personality. It is appropriate to try to understand these relationships by first examining relatively simple arrangements of the data, such as stratified analyses that show whether the effect of one variable is changed by the presence or absence of one or more of the other variables. It is relatively easy to understand the data when they are displayed in this way.

However, as mentioned in Chapter 7, it is usually not possible to account for more than a few variables using this method because there are not enough patients with each combination of characteristics to allow stable estimates of rates. For example, if 120 patients were studied, 60 in each treatment group, and just one additional dichotomous variable was

taken into account, there would only be, at most, about 15 patients in each subgroup; if patients were unevenly distributed among subgroups, there would be even fewer in some.

What is needed then, in addition to tables showing multiple subgroups, is a way of examining the effects of several variables together. This is accomplished by *multivariable modeling*—developing a mathematical expression of the effects of many variables taken together. It is "multivariable" because it examines the effects of multiple variables simultaneously. It is "modeling" because it is a mathematical construct, calculated from the data based on assumptions about characteristics of the data (e.g., that the variables are all normally distributed or all have the same variance).

Mathematical models are used in two general ways in clinical research. One way is to study the independent effect of one variable on outcome while taking into account the effects of other variables that might confound or modify this relationship (discussed under multivariable adjustment in Chapter 5). The second way is to predict a clinical event by calculating the combined effect of several variables acting together (introduced in concept under Clinical Prediction Rules in Chapter 7).

The basic structure of a multivariable model is:

$$\text{Outcome variable} = \text{constant} + (\beta_1 \times \text{variable}_1) + (\beta_2 \times \text{variable}_2) + \cdots,$$

where β_1, β_2, . . . are coefficients determined by the data, and variable$_1$, variable$_2$, . . . are the variables that might be related to outcome. The best estimates of the coefficients are determined mathematically and depend on the powerful calculating ability of modern computers.

Modeling is done in many different ways, but some elements of the process are basic.

1. Identify all the variables that might be related to the outcome of interest either as confounders or effect modifiers. As a practical matter, it may not be possible to actually measure all of them and the missing variables should be mentioned explicitly as a limitation.

2. If there are relatively few outcome events, the number of variables to be considered in the model might need to be reduced to a manageable size, usually no more than several. Often this is done by selecting variables that, when taken one at a time, are most strongly related to outcome. If a statistical criterion is used at this stage, it is usual to err on the side of including variables, for example, by choosing all variables showing an association

with the outcome of interest at a cutoff level of $P < 0.10$. Evidence for the biologic importance of the variable is also considered in making the selection.

3. Models, like other statistical tests, are based on assumptions about the structure of the data. Investigators need to check whether these assumptions are met in their particular data.

4. As for the actual models, there are many kinds and many strategies that can be followed within models. All variables—exposure, outcome, and covariates—are entered in the model, with the order determined by the research question. For example, if some are to be controlled for in a causal analysis, they are entered in the model first, followed by the variable of primary interest. The model will then identify the independent effect of the variable of primary interest. On the other hand, if the investigator wants to make a prediction based on several variables, the relative strength of their association to the outcome variable is determined by the model.

Example

Gastric cancer is the second leading cause of cancer death in the world. Investigators in Europe analyzed data from a cohort recruited from 10 European countries to see whether alcohol was an independent risk factor for stomach cancer (19). They identified nine variables that were known risk factors or potential confounders of the association between the main exposure (alcohol consumption) and disease (stomach cancer): age, study center, sex, physical activity, education, cigarette smoking, diet, body mass index, and physical activity, and in a subset of patients, serologic evidence of *Helicobacter pylori* infection. As a limitation, they mentioned that they would have included salt but did not have access to data on salt intake. Modeling was with the Cox proportional hazards model, so they checked that the underlying assumption, that risk does not vary with time, was met. After adjustment for the other variables, heavy but not light alcohol consumption was associated with stomach cancer (hazard ratio 1.65, 95% confidence interval 1.06–2.58); beer was associated, but not wine or liquor.

Some commonly used kinds of models are logistic regression (for dichotomous outcome variables such as those that occur in case-control studies) and Cox proportional hazards models (for time-to-event studies).

Multivariable modeling is an essential strategy for dealing with the joint effects of multiple variables. There is no other way to adjust for or to include many variables at the same time. However, this advantage comes at a price. Models tend to be black boxes, and it is difficult to "get inside" them and understand how they work. Their validity is based on assumptions about the data that may not be met. They are clumsy at recognizing effect modification. An exposure variable may be strongly related to outcome yet not appear in the model because it occurs rarely—and there is little direct information on the statistical power of the model for that variable. Finally, model results are easily affected by quirks in the data, the results of random variation in the characteristics of patients from sample to sample. It has been shown, for example, that a model frequently identified a different set of predictor variables and produced a different ordering of variables on different random samples of the same dataset (20).

For these reasons, the models themselves cannot be taken as a standard of validity and must be validated independently. Usually, this is done by observing whether or not the results of a model predicts what is found in another, independent sample of patients. The results of the first model are considered a hypothesis that is to be tested with new data. If random variation is mainly responsible for the results of the first model, it is unlikely that the same random effects will occur in the validating dataset, too. Other evidence for the validity of a model is its biologic plausibility and its consistency with simpler, more transparent analyses of the data, such as stratified analyses.

BAYESIAN REASONING

An altogether different approach to the information contributed by a study is based on Bayesian inference. We introduced this approach in Chapter 8 where we applied it to the specific case of diagnostic testing.

Bayesian inference begins with prior belief about the answer to a research question, analogous to pretest probability of a diagnostic test. Prior belief is based on everything known about the answer up to the point when new information is contributed by a study. Then, Bayesian inference asks how much the results of the new study change that belief.

Some aspects of Bayesian inference are compelling. Individual studies do not take place in an information vacuum; rather, they are in the context of all other information available at the time. Starting each study from the null hypothesis—that there is no effect—is unrealistic because something is already known about the answer to the question before the study is even begun. Moreover, results of individual studies change belief in relation to both their scientific strengths and the direction and magnitude of their results. For example, if all preceding studies were negative and the next one, which is of comparable strength, is found to be positive, then an effect is still unlikely. On the other hand, a weak prior belief might be reversed by a single strong study. Finally, with this approach it is not so important whether a small number of hypotheses are identified beforehand and multiple comparisons are not as worrisome. Rather, prior belief depends on the plausibility of the assertion rather than whether the assertion was established before or after the study was begun.

Although Bayesian inference is appealing, so far it has been difficult to apply because of poorly developed ways of assigning numbers to prior belief and to the information contributed by a study. Two exceptions are in cumulative summaries of research evidence (Chapter 13) and in diagnostic testing, in which "belief" is prior probability and the new information is expressed as a likelihood ratio. However, Bayesian inference is the conceptual basis for qualitative thinking about cause (see Chapter 12).

Review Questions

Read the following and select the best response.

11.1. A randomized controlled trial of thrombolytic therapy versus angioplasty for acute myocardial infarction finds no difference in the main outcome, survival to discharge from hospital. The investigators explored whether this was also true for subgroups of patients defined by age, number of vessels affected, ejection fraction, comorbidity, and other patient characteristics. Which of the following is *not* true about this subgroup analysis?

A. Examining subgroups increases the chance of a false-positive (misleading statistically significant) result in one of the comparisons.
B. Examining subgroups increases the chance of a false-negative finding in one of these subgroups, relative to the main result.
C. Subgroup analyses are bad scientific practice and should not be done.
D. Reporting results in subgroups helps clinicians tailor information in the study to individual patients.

11.2. A new drug for hyperlipidemia was compared with placebo in a randomized controlled trial of 10,000 patients. After 2 years, serum cholesterol (the primary outcome) was 238 mg/dL in the group receiving the new drug and 240 mg/dL in the group receiving the old drug ($P < 0.001$). Which of the following best describes the meaning of the P value in this study?

A. Bias is unlikely to account for the observed difference.
B. The difference is clinically important.
C. A difference as big or bigger than what was observed could have arisen by chance one time in 1,000.
D. The results are generalizable to other patients with hypertension.
E. The statistical power of this study was inadequate.

11.3. In a well-designed clinical trial of treatment for ovarian cancer, remission rate at 1 year is 30% in patients offered a new drug and 20% in those offered a placebo. The P value is 0.4. Which of the following best describes the interpretation of this result?

A. Both treatments are effective.
B. Neither treatment is effective.
C. The statistical power of this study is 60%.
D. The best estimate of treatment effect size is 0.4.
E. There is insufficient information to decide whether one treatment is better than the other.

11.4. In a cohort study, vitamin A intake was found to be a risk factor for hip fracture in women. The relative risk (highest quintile versus lowest quintile) was 1.48, and the 95% confidence interval was 1.05 to 2.07. Which of the following best describes the meaning of this confidence interval?

A. The association is not statistically significant at the $P < 0.05$ level.
B. A strong association between vitamin A intake and hip fracture was established.
C. The statistical power of this study is 95%.
D. There is a 95% chance that a range of relative risks as low as 1.05 and as high as 2.07 includes the true risk.
E. Bias is an unlikely explanation for this result.

11.5. Which of the following is the best reason for calling $P \leq 0.05$ "statistically significant?"

A. It definitively rules out a false-positive conclusion.
B. It is an arbitrarily chosen but useful rule of thumb.
C. It rules out a type II error.
D. It is a way of establishing a clinically important effect size.
E. Larger or smaller P values do not provide useful information.

11.6. Which of the following is the biggest advantage of multivariable modeling?

A. Models can control for many variables simultaneously.
B. Models do not depend on assumptions about the data.
C. There is a standardized and reproducible approach to modeling.
D. Models make stratified analyses unnecessary.
E. Models can control for confounding in large randomized controlled trials.

11.7. A trial randomizes 10,000 patients to two treatment groups of similar size, one offered chemoprevention and the other usual care. How frequently must a side effect of chemoprevention occur for the study to have a good chance of observing at least one such side effect?

A. 1/5,000
B. 1/10,000

C. 1/15,000
D. 1/20,000
E. 1/30,000

11.8. Which of the following is *least* related to the statistical power of a study with a dichotomous outcome?

A. Effect size
B. Type I error
C. Rate of outcome events in the control group
D. Type II error
E. The statistical test used

11.9. Which is the following best characterizes the application of Bayesian reasoning to a clinical trial?

A. Prior belief in the comparative effectiveness of treatment is guided by equipoise.
B. The results of each new study changes belief in treatment effect from what it was before the study.
C. Bayesian inference is an alternative way of calculating a P value.
D. Bayesian reasoning is based, like inferential statistics, on the null hypothesis.
E. Bayesian reasoning depends on a well-defined hypothesis before the study is begun.

11.10. In a randomized trial of intensive glucose lowering in type 2 diabetes, death rate was higher in the intensively treated patients: hazard ratio 1.22 (95% confidence interval 1.01–1.46). Which if the following is *not* true about this study?

A. The results are consistent with almost no effect.
B. The best estimate of treatment effect is a hazard ratio of 1.22.
C. If a P value were calculated, the results would be statistically significant at the 0.05 level.
D. A P value would provide as much information as the confidence interval.
E. The results are consistent with 46% higher death rates in the intensively treated patients.

Answers are in Appendix A.

REFERENCES

1. Fisher R in Proceedings of the Society for Psychical Research, 1929, quoted in Salsburg D. The Lady Tasting Tea. New York: Henry Holt and Co; 2001.

2. Johnson AF. Beneath the technological fix: outliers and probability statements. J Chronic Dis 1985;38:957–961.

3. Courtney C, Farrell D, Gray R, et al for the AD2000 Collaborative Group. Long-term donepezil treatment in 565 patients with Alzheimer's disease (AD2000): randomized double-blind trial. Lancet 2004:363:2105–2115.

4. Bernard SA, Gray TW, Buist MD, et al. Treatment of comatose survivors of out-of-hospital cardiac arrest with induced hypothermia. N Engl J Med 2002;346:557–563.

5. The AIM-HIGH Investigators. Niacin in patients with low HDL cholesterol levels receiving intensive statin therapy. N Engl J Med 2011;365:2255–2267.

6. Peto R, Pike MC, Armitage P, et al. Design and analysis of randomized clinical trials requiring prolonged observation of each patient. I. Introduction and design. Br J Cancer 1976;34: 585–612.

7. Lind J. A treatise on scurvy. Edinburgh; Sands, Murray and Cochran, 1753 quoted by Thomas DP. J Royal Society Med 1997;80:50–54.

8. Weinstein SJ, Yu K, Horst RL, et al. Serum 25-hydroxyvitamin D and risks of colon and rectal cancer in Finnish men. Am J Epidemiol 2011;173:499–508.

9. Rossouw JE, Anderson GL, Prentice RL, et al. for the Women's Health Initiative Investigators. Risks and benefits of estrogen plus progestin in healthy postmenopausal women: principle results from the Women's Health Initiative randomized controlled trial. JAMA 2002;288:321–333.

10. Braitman LE. Confidence intervals assess both clinical significance and statistical significance. Ann Intern Med 1991;114: 515–517.

11. Mai PL, Wideroff L, Greene MH, et al. Prevalence of family history of breast, colorectal, prostate, and lung cancer in a population-based study. Public Health Genomics 2010;13:495–503.

12. Venge P, Johnson N, Lindahl B, et al. Normal plasma levels of cardiac troponin I measured by the high-sensitivity cardiac troponin I access prototype assay and the impact on the diagnosis of myocardial ischemia. J Am Coll Cardiol 2009;54: 1165–1172.

13. McCormack K, Scott N, Go PMNYH, et al. Laparoscopic techniques versus open techniques for inguinal hernia repair. Cochrane Database Syst Rev 2003;(1):CD001785.

14. Goodman SN, Berlin JA. The use of predicted confidence intervals when planning experiments and the misuse of power when interpreting results. Ann Intern Med 1994;121: 200–206.

15. Sackett DL, Haynes RB, Gent M, et al. Compliance. In: Inman WHW, ed. Monitoring for Drug Safety. Lancaster, UK: MTP Press; 1980.

16. Armitage P. Importance of prognostic factors in the analysis of data from clinical trials. Control Clin Trials 1981;1:347–353.

17. Hunter DJ, Kraft P. Drinking from the fire hose—statistical issues in genomewide association studies. N Engl J Med 2007;357:436–439.

18. Connolly SJ, Eikelboom J, Joyner C, et al. Apixaban in patients with atrial fibrillation. N Engl J Med 2011;364: 806–817.

19. Duell EJ, Travier N, Lujan-Barroso L, et al. Alcohol consumption and gastric cancer risk in European Prospective Investigation into Cancer and Nutrition (EPIC) cohort. Am J Clin Nutr 2011;94:1266–1275.

20. Diamond GA. Future imperfect: the limitations of clinical prediction models and the limits of clinical prediction. J Am Coll Cardiol 1989;14:12A–22A.

Chapter 12

Cause

In what circumstances can we pass from observed association to a verdict of causation? Upon what basis should we proceed to do so?

—Sir Austin Bradford Hill
1965

KEY WORDS

Web of causation
Aggregate risk studies
Ecological studies
Ecological fallacy
Time-series studies
Multiple time-series studies

Decision analysis
Cost-effectiveness analysis
Cost–benefit analysis

This book has been about three kinds of clinically useful information. One is *description*, a simple statement of how often things occur, summarized by metrics such as incidence and prevalence, as well as (in the case of diagnostic test performance) sensitivity, specificity, predictive value, and likelihood ratio. Another is *prediction*, evidence that certain outcomes regularly follow exposures without regard to whether the exposures are independent risk factors, let alone causes. The third is either directly or implicitly about *cause and effect*. Is a risk factor an independent cause of disease? Does treatment cause patients to get better? Does a prognostic factor cause a different outcome, everything else being equal? This chapter considers cause in greater depth.

Another word for the study of the origination of disease is "etiology," now commonly used as a synonym for cause, as in "What is the *etiology* of this disease?" To the extent that the cause of disease is not known, the disease is said to be "idiopathic" or of "unknown etiology."

There is a longstanding tendency to judge the legitimacy of a causal assertion by whether it makes sense according to beliefs at the time, as the following historical example illustrates.

Example

In 1843, Oliver Wendell Holmes (then professor of anatomy and physiology and later dean of Harvard Medical School), published a study linking hand washing habits by obstetricians and childbed (puerperal) fever, an often-fatal disease following childbirth. (Puerperal fever is now known to be caused by a bacterial infection.) Holmes's observations led him to conclude that "the disease known as puerperal fever is so far contagious, as to be frequently carried from patient to patient by physicians and nurses (1)."

One response to Holmes's assertion was that the findings made no sense. "I prefer to attribute them [puerperal fever cases] to accident, or Providence, of which I can form a conception, rather than to contagion of which I cannot form any clear idea, at least as to this particular malady," wrote Charles Meigs, professor of midwifery and the diseases of women and children at Jefferson Medical College. Around that time, a Hungarian physician, Ignaz Semmelweis, showed that disinfecting physicians' hands reduced rates of childbed fever, and his studies were also dismissed because he had no generally accepted explanation for his findings. Holmes's and Semmelweis's assertions were made decades before pioneering work—by Louis Pasteur, Robert Koch, and Joseph Lister—established the germ theory of disease.

The importance attached to a cause-and-effect relationship "making sense," usually in terms of a biologic mechanism, is still imbedded in current thinking. For example, in the 1990s, studies showing that eradication of *Helicobacter pylori* infection prevented peptic ulcer disease were met with skepticism because everyone knew that ulcers of the stomach and duodenum were not an infectious disease. Now, *H. pylori* infection is recognized as a major cause of this disease.

In this chapter, we review concepts of cause in clinical medicine. We discuss the broader array of evidence, in addition to biologic plausibility, that strengthens or weakens the case that an association represents a cause-and-effect relationship. We also briefly deal with a kind of research design not yet considered in this book: studies in which exposure to a possible cause is known only for groups and not for the individuals in the groups.

BASIC PRINCIPLES

Single Causes

In 1882, 40 years after the Holmes-Meigs confrontation, Koch set forth postulates for determining that an infectious agent is the cause of a disease (Table 12.1). Basic to his approach was the assumption that a particular disease has one cause and that a particular cause results in one disease. This approach helped him to identify for the first time the bacteria causing tuberculosis, diphtheria, typhoid, and other common infectious diseases of his day.

Koch's postulates contributed greatly to the concept of cause in medicine. Before Koch, it was believed that many different bacteria caused any given disease. The application of his postulates helped bring order out of chaos. They are still useful today. That a unique infectious agent causes a particular infectious disease was the basis for the discovery in 1977 that Legionnaire disease is caused by a gram-negative bacterium; the discovery in the 1980s that a newly identified

Table 12.1

Koch's Postulates

1. The organism must be present in every case of the disease.
2. The organism must be isolated and grown in pure culture.
3. The organism must cause a specific disease when inoculated into an animal.
4. The organism must then be recovered from the animal and identified.

retrovirus causes AIDS; and the discovery in 2003 that a coronavirus caused an outbreak of severe acute respiratory syndrome (SARS) (2).

Multiple Causes

For some diseases, one cause appears to be so dominant that we speak of it as *the* cause. We say that *Mycobacterium tuberculosis* causes tuberculosis or that an abnormal gene coding for the metabolism of phenylalanine, an amino acid, causes phenylketonuria. We may skip past the fact that tuberculosis is also caused by host and environmental factors and that the disease phenylketonuria develops because there is phenylalanine in the diet.

More often, however, various causes make a more balanced contribution to the occurrence of disease such that no one stands out. The underlying assumption of Koch's postulates, one cause– one disease, is too simplified. Smoking causes lung cancer, coronary artery disease, chronic obstructive pulmonary disease, and skin wrinkles. Coronary artery disease has multiple causes, including cigarette smoking, hypertension, hypercholesterolemia, diabetes, inflammation, and heredity. Specific parasites cause malaria, but only if the mosquito vectors can breed, become infected, and bite people, and those people are not taking antimalarial drugs or are unable to control the infection on their own.

When many factors act together, it has been called the "web of causation" (3). A causal web is well understood in chronic degenerative diseases such as cardiovascular disease and cancer, but it is also the basis for infectious diseases, where the presence of a microbe is a necessary but not sufficient cause of disease. AIDS cannot occur without exposure to HIV, but exposure to the virus does not necessarily result in disease. For example, exposure to HIV rarely results in seroconversion after needlesticks (about 3/1,000) because the virus is not nearly as infectious as, say, the hepatitis B virus. Similarly, not everyone exposed to tuberculosis—in Koch's day or now—becomes infected.

When multiple causes act together, the resulting risk may be greater or less than would be expected by simply combining the effects of the separate causes. That is, they interact—there is effect modification. Figure 12.1 shows the 10-year risk of cardiovascular disease in a 60-year-old man with no prior history of cardiovascular disease according to the presence or absence of several common risk factors. The risk is greater than the sum of the effects of each individual risk factor. The effect of low HDL is more in the presence of elevated total cholesterol, the effect

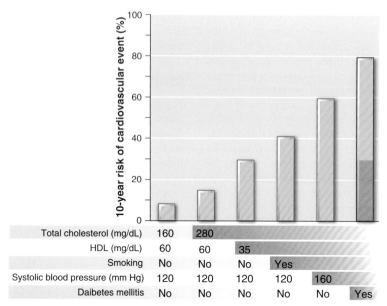

Figure 12.1 ■ **The interaction of multiple risk factors for cardiovascular disease.** Ten-year cardiovascular risk (%) for a 60-year-old man with no risk factors (left bar) and with the successive addition of five risk factors (bars to the right). Each risk factor alone adds relatively little (several percent) to risk whereas adding them to each other increases risk almost 10-fold, far more than the sum of the individual risk factors acting independently, which is shown by the shaded area of the right-hand bar. (Data from The Framingham Risk Calculator in UpToDate, Waltham, MA according to formulae in D'Agostino RB Sr, Vasan RS, Pencina MJ, et al. General cardiovascular risk profile for use in primary care. The Framingham Heart Study. Circulation 2008;117(6):743–753.)

of smoking is more in the presence of both elevated total cholesterol and low HDL, and so on. The consequence of exposure to each new risk factor is affected by exposure to the others, an example of effect modification. Age and sex are also risk factors and interact with the others (not shown).

When multiple causative factors are present and interact, it may be possible to make a substantial impact on a patient's health by changing just one or a few of them. In the previous example, treating hypertension and elevated serum cholesterol can substantially lower the risk of developing cardiovascular disease, even if the other risk factors are unchanged.

By and large, clinicians are more interested in treatable or reversible causes than immutable ones. For example, when it comes to cardiovascular disease, age and sex cannot be changed—they have to be taken as a given. On the other hand, smoking, blood pressure, and serum cholesterol can be changed. Therefore, even though risks related to age and sex are at least as big as for risk factors as the others and are taken into account when estimating cardiovascular risk, they do not offer a target for prevention or treatment.

Proximity of Cause to Effect

When biomedical scientists study cause, they usually search for the underlying pathogenetic mechanism or final common pathway of disease. Sickle cell anemia is an example. In simplified form, pathogenesis involves a gene coded for abnormal hemoglobin that polymerizes in low-oxygen environments (the capillaries of some tissues), resulting in deformed red cells, causing anemia as they are destroyed, and occluding vessels, causing attacks of ischemia with pain and tissue destruction.

Disease is also determined by less specific, more remote causes (risk factors) such as behavior and environments. These factors may have large effects on disease rates. For example, a large proportion of cardiovascular and cancer deaths in the United States can be traced to behavioral and environmental factors such as cigarette smoking, diet, and lack of exercise; AIDS is primarily spread through unsafe sexual behaviors and shared needles; and deaths from violence and unintended injuries are rooted in social conditions, access to guns, intoxication while driving, and seatbelt use.

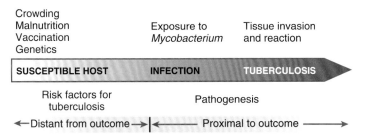

Figure 12.2 ■ Proximal and distal causes of tuberculosis.

Figure 12.2 shows how both risk factors and pathogenesis of tuberculosis—distant and proximal causes—lead on a continuum to the disease. Exposure to *M. tuberculosis* depends on the host's environment: close proximity to active cases. Infection depends on host susceptibility, which can be increased by malnutrition, decreased by vaccination, and altered by genetic endowment. Whether infection progresses to disease depends on these factors and others, such as immunocompetence, which can be compromised by HIV infection and age. Finally, active infection may be cured by antibiotic treatment.

Clinicians may be so intent on pathogenesis that they underestimate the importance of more remote causes of disease. In the case of tuberculosis, social and economic improvements influencing host susceptibility, such as less crowded living space and better nutrition, appear to have played a more prominent role in the decline in tuberculosis rates in developed countries than treatments. Figure 12.3 shows that the death rate from tuberculosis in England and Wales dropped dramatically before the tubercle bacillus was identified and a century before the first effective antibiotics were introduced in the 1950s.

The web of causation is continually changing, even for old diseases. Between 1985 and 1992, the number of tuberculosis cases in the United States, which had been falling for a century, began to increase (Fig. 12.4) (4). Why did this happen? There had been an influx of immigrants from countries with high rates of tuberculosis. The AIDS epidemic produced more people with a weakened immune system, making them more susceptible to infection with *M. tuberculosis*. When infected, their bodies allowed massive multiplication of the bacterium, making them more infectious. Rapid multiplication, especially in patients

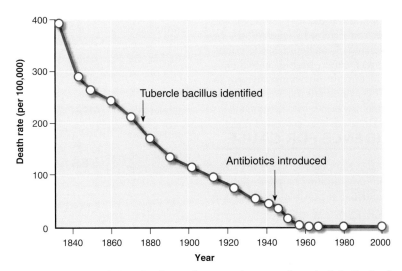

Figure 12.3 ■ Declining death rate from respiratory tuberculosis in England and Wales over the past 150 years. Most of the decrease occurred before antibiotic therapy was available. (Data from McKeown T. The Role of Medicine: Dream, Mirage, or Nemesis. London: Nuffield Provincial Hospital Trust; 1976 and from http://www. hpa.org.uk/Topics/InfectiousDiseases/InfectionsAZ/Tuberculosis/TBUKSurveillance Data/TuberculosisMortality)

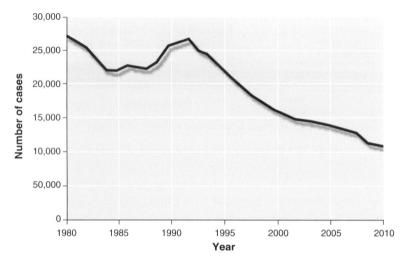

Figure 12.4 ■ **Tuberculosis cases in the United States, 1980 through 2010.** A longstanding decline was halted in 1985. The number of cases reached a peak in 1992 and then began to decline again. (Adapted from Centers for Disease Control and Prevention. Reported tuberculosis in the United States, 2010. Available at http://www.cdc.gov/Features/dsTB2010Data/. Accessed February 8, 2012.)

who did not follow prescribed drug regimens, favored the development of multidrug resistant strains. People who were more likely to have both AIDS and tuberculosis—the socially disadvantaged, intravenous drug users, and prisoners—were developing multidrug resistant disease and exposing others in the population to a difficult-to-treat strain. The interplay of environment, behavior, and molecular biology combined to reverse a declining trend in tuberculosis. To combat the new epidemic of tuberculosis, the public health infrastructure was rebuilt. Multidrug regimens (biologic efforts) and directly observing therapy to ensure compliance (behavioral efforts) were initiated and the rate of tuberculosis began to decline again.

INDIRECT EVIDENCE FOR CAUSE

In clinical medicine, it is not possible to prove causal relationships beyond any doubt, as one might a mathematic formula. What is possible is to increase one's conviction in a cause-and-effect relationship by means of empiric evidence to the point where, as a practical matter, cause has been established. Conversely, evidence against a cause can accumulate to the point where a cause-and-effect relationship becomes implausible.

A postulated cause-and-effect relationship should be examined in as many different ways as possible. In the remainder of this chapter, we discuss some commonly used approaches.

Examining Individual Studies

One approach to evidence for cause-and-effect has been discussed throughout this book: in-depth analysis of the studies themselves. When an association has been observed, a causal relationship is established to the extent that the association cannot be accounted for by bias and chance. Figure 12.5 summarizes a familiar approach. One first looks for bias and how much it might have changed the result, and then whether the association is unlikely to be by chance. For observational studies, confounding is always a

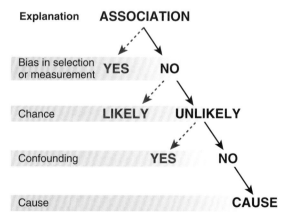

Figure 12.5 ■ **Association and cause.** Bias, chance, and confounding should be excluded before concluding that a causal association is likely.

possibility. Although confounding can be controlled in comprehensive, state-of-the science ways, it is almost never possible to rule it out entirely; therefore, confounding remains the enduring challenge to causal reasoning based on observational research.

Randomized trials can deal definitively with confounding, but they are not possible for studies of risk (i.e., causes) per se. For example, it is unethical (and would be unsuccessful) to randomize non-smokers to cigarette smoking to study whether smoking causes lung cancer. However, randomized controlled trials can contribute to causal inference in two situations. One is when the trial is to treat a possible cause, such as elevated cholesterol or blood pressure, and the outcome is prevented. Another is when a trial is done for another purpose and the intervention causes unanticipated harms. For example, the fact that there were an excess of cardiovascular events in randomized trials of the cyclooxygenase-2 inhibitor rofecoxib, which had been given for other reasons (e.g., pain relief), is evidence that this drug may be a cause of cardiovascular events.

Hierarchy of Research Designs

The various research designs can be placed in a hierarchy of scientific strength for the purpose of establishing cause (Table 12.2). At the top of the hierarchy are systematic reviews of randomized controlled trials because they can deal definitively with confounding. Randomized trials are followed by observational studies, with little distinction between cohort and case-control studies in an era when case-control analyses are nested in cohorts sampled from defined populations. Lower still are uncontrolled studies, biologic reasoning, and personal experience. Of course, this order is only a rough guide to strength of evidence. The manner in which an individual study is performed can go

a long way toward increasing or decreasing its validity, regardless of the type of design used. A bad randomized controlled trial contributes less to our understanding of cause than an exemplary cohort study.

With this hierarchy in mind, the strength of the evidence for cause and effect is sometimes judged according to the best studies of the question. Well-designed and well-executed randomized controlled trials trump observational studies, state-of-the-science observational studies trump case series, and so on. This is a highly simplified approach to evidence but is a useful shortcut.

THE BODY OF EVIDENCE FOR AND AGAINST CAUSE

What aspects of the research findings support cause and effect when only observational studies are available? In 1965, the British statistician Sir Austin Bradford Hill proposed a set of observations that taken together help to establish whether a relationship between an environmental factor and disease is causal or just an association (5) (Table 12.3). We review these "Bradford Hill criteria," mainly using smoking and lung cancer as an example. Smoking is generally believed to cause lung cancer even though there are not randomized controlled trials of smoking or an undisputed biologic mechanism.

Table 12.2

Hierarchy of Research Design Strength

Individual Risk Studies

Systematic reviews: consistent evidence from multiple randomized controlled trials

Randomized controlled trials

Observational studies
  Cohort studies
  Case-control, Case-cohort studies

Cross-sectional studies

Case series

Experience, expert opinion

Table 12.3

Evidence That an Association Is Cause and Effect	
Criteria	**Comments**
Temporality	Cause precedes effect
Strength	Large relative risk
Dose–response	Larger exposure to cause associated with higher rates of disease
Reversibility	Reduction in exposure is followed by lower rates of disease
Consistency	Repeatedly observed by different persons, in different places, circumstances, and times
Biologic plausibility	Makes sense according to biologic knowledge of the time
Specificity	One cause leads to one effect
Analogy	Cause-and-effect relationship already established for a similar exposure or disease

Adapted from Bradford Hill AB. The environment and disease: association and causation. Proc R Soc Med 1965;58:295–300.

Does Cause Precede Effect?

A cause should obviously occur before its effects. This seems self-evident, but the principle can be overlooked when interpreting cross-sectional and case-control studies, in which both the purported cause and the effect are measured at the same points in time. Smoking clearly precedes lung cancer by several decades, but there are other examples where the order of cause and effect can be confused.

Example

"Whiplash," is the occurrence of neck pain following a forceful flexion/extension injury, typically in an auto accident. Many people with whiplash recover quickly, but some go on to chronic symptoms, litigation, and requests for disability awards. Many patients with whiplash have anxiety and depression, and epidemiologic studies have linked the two. The injury and associated pain are generally thought to cause the psychological symptoms. Investigators in Norway tested the hypothesis that cause and effect was in the other direction (6). They analyzed a cohort with measurements of psychological symptoms before injuries and follow-up for 11 years. People with anxiety and depression before the injury were more likely to report whiplash.

Finding that what was thought to be a cause actually follows an effect is powerful evidence *against* cause, but temporal sequence alone is only minimal evidence *for* cause.

Strength of the Association

A strong association between a purported cause and an effect, as expressed by a large relative or absolute risk, is better evidence for a causal relationship than a weak association. The reason is that unrecognized bias could account for small relative risks but is unlikely to result in large ones.

Thus, the 20 times higher incidence of lung cancer among male smokers compared to non-smokers is much stronger evidence that smoking causes lung cancer than the finding that smoking is related to renal cancer, for which the relative risk is much smaller (about 1.5). Similarly, a 10- to 100-fold increase in risk of hepatocellular carcinoma in patients with hepatitis B infection is strong evidence that the virus is a cause of liver cancer.

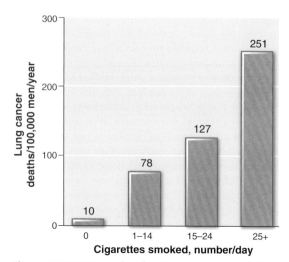

Figure 12.6 ■ Example of a dose–response relationship: lung cancer deaths in male physicians according to dose (number) of cigarettes smoked. (Data from data in Doll R, Peto R. Mortality in relation to smoking: 20 years' observations on male British doctors. Br Med J 1976;2:1525–1536.)

Dose–Response Relationships

A dose–response relationship is present if increasing exposure to the purported cause is followed by a larger and larger effect. In the case of cigarette smoking, "dose" might be the number of years of smoking, current packs per day, or "pack-years." Figure 12.6 shows a clear dose–response curve when lung cancer death rates (responses) are plotted against the number of cigarettes smoked (doses).

Demonstrating a dose–response relationship strengthens the argument for cause and effect, but its absence is relatively weak evidence against causation because not all causal associations exhibit a dose–response relationship within the range observed and because confounding remains possible.

Example

Both the strong association between smoking and lung cancer and the dose–response relationship could be examples of confounding. According to this argument, an unknown factor may exist that both causes people to smoke and increases their risk of developing lung cancer. The more the factor is present, the more smoking and lung cancer occur, hence the dose–response relationship. Such an argument is a theoretically possible explanation for the association between smoking and lung cancer, although just what the confounding factor might be has never been clarified. Short of a randomized controlled trial (which would, on average, allocate people with the confounding factor equally to smoking and non-smoking groups) the possibility of confounding is difficult to refute altogether.

Reversible Associations

A factor is more likely to be a cause of disease when its removal results in a decreased risk. Figure 12.7 shows that when people quit smoking, they decrease their likelihood of getting lung cancer in relation to the number of years since quitting.

Reversible associations are strong, but not infallible, evidence of a causal relationship because confounding could account for it. For example, Figure 12.7 is consistent with the (unlikely) explanation that people who are willing to quit smoking have smaller amounts of an unidentified confounding factor than those who continue to smoke.

Consistency

When several studies conducted at different times in different settings and with different kinds of patients all come to the same conclusion, evidence for a causal relationship is strengthened. Causation is particularly supported when studies using several different research designs, with complementary strengths and weaknesses, all produce the same result because studies using the same design might have all made the same mistake. For the association of smoking and lung cancer, many cohort, case-control, and time-series studies have shown that increased tobacco use is followed by increased lung cancer incidence, in both sexes, in various ethnic groups, and in different countries.

Different studies can produce different results. Lack of consistency does not necessarily mean that a causal relationship does not exist. Study results may differ because of differences in patients, interventions, follow-up, or outcome measures (i.e., they address somewhat different research questions). Also, the studies may vary in quality, and one good study may contribute more valid information than several poor ones.

Biologic Plausibility

As discussed at the beginning of this chapter, the belief that a possible cause is consistent with our knowledge of the mechanisms of disease, as it is currently understood, is often given considerable weight when assessing cause and effect. When one has absolutely no idea how an association might have arisen, one tends to be skeptical that the association is real. Such skepticism often serves us well.

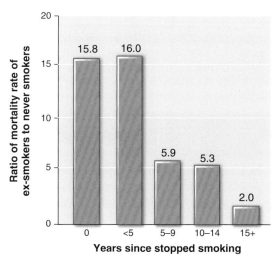

Figure 12.7 ■ Reversible association: declining mortality from lung cancer in ex-cigarette smokers. The data exclude people who stopped smoking after getting cancer. (Data from data in Doll R, Petro R. Mortality in relation to smoking: 20 years' observations on male British doctors. Br Med J 1976;2:1525–1536.)

Example

The substance Laetrile, extracted from apricot pits, was touted as a cure for cancer in the early 1980s. The scientific community was not convinced, mainly because it could think of no biologic reason why an extract of apricot pits that was not chemically related to compounds with known anticancer activity should be effective against cancer cells. Nevertheless, many cancer patients were taking Laetrile, which they obtained from unconventional sources, sometimes instead of mainstream chemotherapy. To resolve this controversy, researchers tested the effectiveness of Laetrile in a randomized controlled trial. The trial showed that Laetrile was, in fact, without activity against the cancers studied (7).

Biologic plausibility, when present, strengthens the case for causation, but the absence of biologic plausibility may just reflect the limitations of understanding of the biology of disease rather than the lack of a causal association.

Specificity

Specificity—one cause–one effect—is more often found for acute infectious diseases (e.g., poliomyelitis and tetanus) and for genetic diseases (e.g., familial adenomatous polyposis or ochronosis), although genetic effects are sometimes modified by gene–gene and gene–environment interactions. As mentioned earlier in this chapter, chronic, degenerative diseases often have many causes for the same effect and many effects from the same cause. Lung cancer is caused by cigarette smoking, asbestos, and radiation. Cigarette smoking not only causes lung cancer but also bronchitis, cardiovascular disease, periodontal disease, and wrinkled skin, to name a few. Thus, specificity is strong evidence for cause and effect, but the absence of specificity is weak evidence against it.

Analogy

The argument for a cause-and-effect relationship is strengthened when examples exist of well-established causes that are analogous to the one in question. Thus, the case that smoking causes lung cancer is strengthened by observations that other environmental toxins such as asbestos, arsenic, and uranium also cause lung cancer.

In a sense, applying the Bradford Hill criteria to cause is an example of Bayesian reasoning. For example, belief in causality based on strength of association and dose–response is modified (built up or diminished) by evidence concerning biologic plausibility or specificity, with each of the criteria contributing to a greater or lesser extent to the overall belief that an association is causal. The main difference from the Bayesian approach to diagnostic testing is that the various lines of evidence for cause (dose–response, reversibility, consistency, etc.) are being assembled concurrently in various scientific disciplines rather than in series by clinical research.

AGGREGATE RISK STUDIES

Until now, we have discussed studies in which exposure and disease are known for each individual in a study. To fill out the spectrum of research designs, we now consider a different kind of study, called aggregate risk studies, in which exposure to a risk factor is characterized by the average exposure of the group to which individuals belong. Another term is ecological studies, because people are classified by the general level of exposure in their environment, which may or may not correspond to their individual exposure. Examples are epidemiologic studies relating countries' wine consumption to rates of cardiovascular mortality and studies of regional cancer or birth defect rates in relation to regional exposures such as chemical spills.

The main problem with studies that simply correlate average exposure with average disease rates in groups is the potential for an ecological fallacy, in which affected individuals in a generally exposed group may not have been the ones actually exposed to the risk factor. Also, exposure may not be the only characteristic that distinguishes people in the exposed group from those in the non-exposed group; that is, there may be confounding factors. Thus, aggregate risk studies like these are most useful in raising hypotheses, which should then be tested by more rigorous research.

Evidence from aggregate risk studies can be strengthened when observations are made over a period of time bracketing the exposure and even further strengthened if observations are in more than one place and calendar time.

In a time-series study, disease rates are measured at several points in time, both before and after the purported cause has been introduced. It is then possible to see whether a trend in disease rate over time changes in relation to the time of exposure. If changes in the purported cause are directly followed by changes in the purported effect, and not at some other time, the association is less likely to be spurious. An advantage of time-series analyses is that they can distinguish between changes already occurring over time (secular trends) and the effects of the intervention itself.

Example

Health care–associated infections with methicillin-resistant *Staphylococcus aureus* (MRSA) are a major cause of morbidity, mortality, and cost in acute care hospitals. The U.S. Veterans Affairs (VA) initiated a national program to prevent these infections in VA hospitals (8). The VA introduced a "MRSA bundle" comprised a set of interventions including hand hygiene, universal nasal surveillance for MRSA, contact precautions for patients colonized or infected with MRSA, and changes in institutional

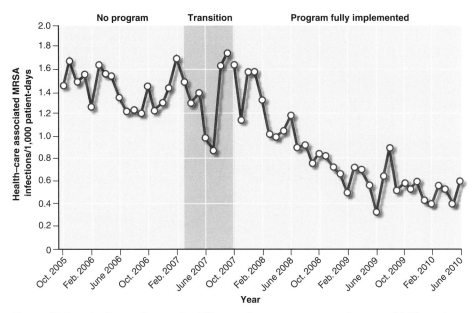

Figure 12.8 ■ A time-series study. Effects of a program to reduce methicillin-resistant *Staphylococcus aureus* **(MRSA) infections in Veterans Affairs facilities.** Results for intensive care units. (Redrawn with permission from Jain R, Kralovic SM, Evans ME, et al. Veterans Affairs initiative to prevent methicillin-resistant *Staphylococcus aureus* infections. N Engl J Med 2011;364:1419–1430.)

responsibilities for preventing infection. Data on MRSA infection rates were gathered from 2 years before the intervention thorough the time when the bundle was initiated to when it was fully implemented (Fig. 12.8). Rates in intensive care units were stable in the 2-year period before the bundle was introduced and fell progressively to 62% of the preintervention rate following the intervention, providing evidence that this particular intervention achieved its purposes.

Inference from time-series studies can be strengthened if it is possible to rule out other interventions occurring around the same time as the one under study that might have caused a change in rates. The case is also strengthened if intermediate outcomes (e.g., increased hand washing) follow the intervention (the MRSA package), as they did in the MRSA example.

In a multiple time-series studies, the suspected cause is introduced into several different groups at different times. Time-series measurements are then made in each group to determine whether the effect occurred in the same sequential manner in which the suspected cause was introduced. When an effect regularly follows

introduction of the suspected cause at various times and places, there is stronger evidence for cause than when this phenomenon is observed only once, as in the single time-series example, because it is even more improbable that the same extraneous factor(s) occurred at the same time in relation to the intervention in many different places and calendar times.

Example

Screening with Pap smears is done to prevent deaths from cervical cancer. This practice was initiated before there was strong evidence of effectiveness—indeed, before randomized controlled trials. The best available evidence of effectiveness comes from multiple time-series studies. An example is shown in Figure 12.9 (9). Organized Pap smear screening programs were implemented in Nordic countries at different times and with different intensities. Mortality rates from cervical cancer had been rising and then began to fall in the years just before screening began, illustrating the value of having information on time trends. Rates were roughly similar before screening programs

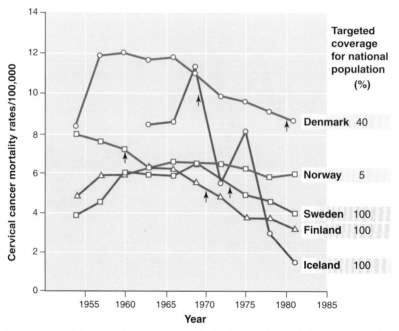

Figure 12.9 ■ A multiple time-series study. Change in cervical cancer mortality rates according to year organized Pap smear screening programs were implemented and targeted coverage. Arrows mark the year coverage was achieved for each country. (Redrawn with permission from Läärä E, Day NE, Hakama M. Trends in mortality from cervical cancer in Nordic countries: association with organized screening programmes. Lancet 1987;1(8544):1247–1249.

were started. Rates fell the most in countries (Iceland, Finland, and Sweden) with national programs with the broadest coverage and least in countries (Denmark and Norway) with the least coverage.

Multiple time series like this one are usually not planned experiments. Rather, the interventions were introduced in the different countries at different times and with different intensities for their own sociopolitical reasons. Researchers later took advantage of this "natural experiment," and data on cervical cancer death rates, to do a structured study.

The various ecological study designs are of vastly different scientific strength. Simply relating aggregate exposure to aggregate risk across regions may be useful for raising hypotheses to be tested by more rigorous studies. A single time series can provide convincing evidence of cause and effect if there is an unmistakable break in trend after the intervention and if concurrent interventions are ruled out. Multiple time series can provide strong evidence of cause, arguably on a par with randomized trials, because

it is so improbable that confounding would have produced the same effects following intervention at many different times and places.

MODELING

We have already discussed how mathematical models are used to control for confounding and to develop prediction rules. Another use of models is to describe the relative importance of various causes of disease and its prevention.

Example

The U.S. death rate from colorectal cancer fell by 26% from 1975 through 2000. What caused this change? Investigators modeled the respective contributions of changes in risk factors, screening, and treatment to the declining rate (10). Effects of primary prevention were entered into the model as the relative risk for both risk factors (smoking, obesity, red meat consumption) and protective factors (aspirin, multivitamin

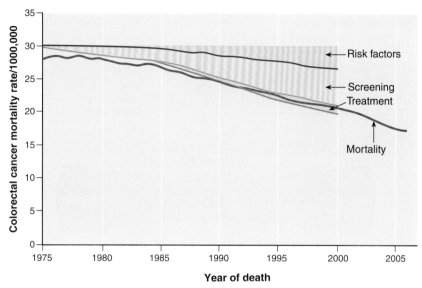

Figure 12.10 ■ Causes for the decline in colorectal cancer deaths, 1975–2000. (Redrawn with permission from Edwards BK, Ward E, Kohler BA, et al. Annual report to the Nation on the status of cancer, 1975–2006, featuring colorectal cancer trends and impact of interventions (risk factors, screening, and treatment) to reduce future rates. Cancer 2010; 116:544–573.)

use, and physical activity) along with the prevalence of each over time. Similarly, screening was entered as the rates of each type of screening test as they changed over time, and their sensitivity and specificity in detecting precancerous lesions. Treatment was modeled as the kinds of chemotherapy regimens available over time and their effectiveness in reducing mortality. The model included the many steps leading from adenomas (precursors of cancer) through cancer to treatment and survival. Figure 12.10 shows that the model predicted the actual fall in colorectal cancer death rates very closely. Changes in risk factors accounted for 35% of the decline in mortality, screening another 53% of the fall, and treatment only 12%.

Models take a group of people through the various possible steps in the natural history of the disease. In this case, it was the U.S. population from development of polyps through their transition to cancer, prevention by screening, and effects of treatment on cancer deaths. Data for the probabilities of transition from one to another state (e.g., from polyp to cancer or from cancer to cure) are from published research.

Other kinds of models are used for quantitative decision making, comparing the downstream consequences of alternative courses of action. Decision analysis identifies the decisions that lead to the best outcomes in human terms, such as survival or being disease-free. Cost-effectiveness analysis compares cost to outcomes (e.g., life saved or quality-adjusted lives saved) for alternative courses of action. In cost–benefit analysis, both cost and benefits are expressed in money terms. Whenever cost is taken into account in these models, it is adjusted for the change in the value of money over time, because the money is spent or saved at various points in time over the course of disease. In all these models, if some of the inputted data are weak, sensitivity analysis can be used to see the effects of various values for these data.

Modeling can provide answers to questions that are so broad in scope that they are not available from individual research studies—and perhaps never will be. They are increasingly relied on to complement other forms of research when trying to understand the consequences of clinical decisions.

WEIGHING THE EVIDENCE

When determining cause, one must consider the evidence from all available studies. After examining the research design, the quality of studies, and whether their results are for and against cause, the case for causality can be strengthened or eroded.

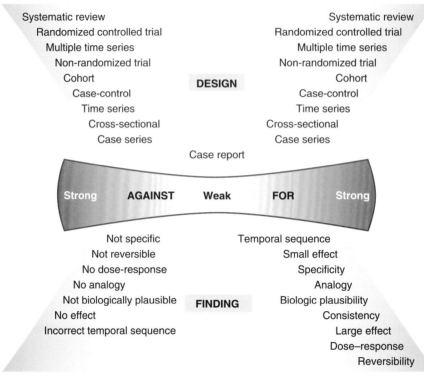

Figure 12.11 ■ Relative strength of evidence for and against a causal effect. Note that with study designs, the strength of evidence *for* a causal relationship is a mirror image of that *against*. With findings, evidence *for* a causal effect does not mirror evidence *against* an effect.

Figure 12.11 summarizes the different types of evidence for and against cause, depending on the research design, and results that strengthen or weaken the evidence for cause. The figure roughly indicates relative strengths in helping to establish or discard a causal hypothesis. Thus, a carefully done cohort study showing a strong association and a dose–response relationship that is reversible is strong evidence for cause, whereas a cross-sectional study finding no effect is weak evidence against cause.

Belief in a cause-and-effect relationship is a judgment based on both the scientific strength and results of all research bearing on the question. As a practical matter, at issue is whether the weight of the evidence is convincing enough for us to behave as if something were a cause, not whether it is established beyond all reasonable doubt.

Review Questions

Read the following statements and select the best response.

12.1. One of your patients read that cell phones cause brain cancer, and she wants to know your opinion. You discover that the incidence of malignant brain tumors is increasing in the United States. Results of several observational studies of cell phone use and brain cancer have not agreed with each other. A randomized controlled trial might resolve the question. What is the main reason why a randomized controlled trial (RCT) would be unlikely for this question?

A. It would cost too much.
B. People would not agree to be randomized to cell phone use.

C. It would take too long.

D. Even if done well, a randomized trial could not answer the question.

12.2. Which of the following would be least consistent with the belief that cell phone use is a cause of brain cancer?

A. A dose–response relationship

B. A large effect size (such as relative risk)

C. Separate analyses of patients with right- and left-sided tumors in relation to the side they usually listened to their cell phone

D. A biologic explanation for why cell phones might cause cancer

E. Cell phone use is associated with many different kinds of cancers

12.3. Which of the following is the most accurate description of a causal relationship?

A. Tuberculosis has a single cause, the tubercle bacillus.

B. Most genetic diseases are caused only by an abnormal gene.

C. Coronary heart disease has multiple interacting causes.

D. Effective treatment has been the main cause of decline in tuberculosis rates.

12.4. Which of the following is *not* one of the Bradford Hill criteria for causation?

A. Dose–response

B. Statistical significance

C. Reversibility

D. Biologic plausibility

E. Analogy

12.5. A study of the colorectal cancer screening comparing fecal occult blood testing to no screening finds that screening costs $20,000 per year of life saved. This study is an example of which of the following?

A. Cost–benefit analysis

B. Decision analysis

C. Cost-effectiveness analysis

D. A clinical decision rule

12.6. Which of the following is true about aggregate risk studies?

A. Aggregate risk studies are not susceptible to confounding.

B. Multiple time-series studies cannot provide strong evidence of cause and effect.

C. Studies relating average exposure to average risk can provide a strong test of a causal hypothesis.

D. An ecological fallacy might affect their validity.

12.7. Which of the following would weaken belief that the "MRSA package" (Fig. 12.6) caused the observed decline in MRSA infections in VA acute care hospitals?

A. Hand washing, a part of the MRSA package, increased after the program was introduced.

B. Better antibiotics became available around the time of the program

C. The rate of MRSA infections was stable for the years before the program was introduced.

D. Decline in rates began just after the program was introduced.

12.8. Randomized controlled trials are the strongest research designs for establishing cause and effect. Which of the following is the main limitation of trials for this purpose?

A. Randomized trials cannot control for unmeasured confounders.

B. Clinical trials may not be ethical or feasible for some questions.

C. Type of study design is only a crude measure of the scientific strength.

D. Results of poorly designed and conducted trials are no better than for observational studies.

12.9. Which of the following provides the *strongest* evidence for a cause-and-effect relationship?

A. Observational studies that have controlled for bias and minimized the role of chance.

B. A biologic mechanism can explain the relationship.

C. The purported cause clearly precedes the effect.

D. There is a dose–response relationship.

E. The evidence as a whole is consistent with the Bradford Hill criteria.

12.10. You discover that case-control studies have been done to determine whether cell phone use is associated with the development of brain cancer. In one study, patients with brain cancer and matched controls without brain cancer were asked about cell phone use. The estimated relative risk for at least 100 hours of use compared to no use was 1.0 for all types of brain cancers combined (95% confidence interval 0.6–1.5). This finding is consistent with all of the following *except:*

A. Use of cell phones increases the incidence of brain cancers by 50%.
B. Use of cell phones protects against brain cancers.
C. Specific types of cancers might be associated with cell phone use.
D. The study has adequate statistical power to answer the research question.

Answers are in Appendix A.

REFERENCES

1. Holmes OW. On the contagiousness of puerperal fever. Med Classics 1936;1:207–268. [Originally published, 1843.]
2. Fouchier RA, Kuiken T, Schutten M, et al. Aetiology: Koch's postulates fulfilled for SARS virus. Nature 2003;423:240.
3. MacMahon B, Pugh TF. Epidemiology: Principles and Methods. Boston: Little, Brown & Co.; 1970.
4. Burzynski J, Schluger NW. The epidemiology of tuberculosis in the United States. Sem Respir Crit Care Med 2008;29:492–498.
5. Bradford Hill A. The environment and disease: association or causation? Proc R Soc Med 1965;58:295–300.
6. Mykletun A, Glozier N, Wenzel HG, et al. Reverse causality in the association between whiplash and symptoms of anxiety and depression. The HUNT Study. Spine 2011;36:1380–1386.
7. Moertel CC, Fleming TR, Rubin J, et al. A clinical trial of amygdalin (Laetrile) in the treatment of human cancer. N Engl J Med 1982;306:201–206.
8. Jain R, Kralovic SM, Evans ME, et al. Veterans Affairs initiative to prevent methicillin-resistant *Staphylococcus aureus* infections. N Engl J Med 2011;364:1419–1430.
9. Läärä E, Day NE, Hakama M. Trends in mortality from cervical cancer in the Nordic countries: association with organized screening programmes. Lancet 1987;1(8544):1247–1249.
10. Edwards BK, Ward E, Kohler BA, et al. Annual report to the nation on the status of cancer, 1975-2006, featuring colorectal cancer trends and impact of interventions (risk factors, screening, and treatment) to reduce future rates. Cancer 2010;116:544–573.

Summarizing the Evidence

When the research community synthesizes existing evidence thoroughly, it is certain that a substantial proportion of current notions about the effects of health care will be changed. Forms of care currently believed to be ineffective will be shown to be effective; forms of care thought to be useful will be exposed as either useless or harmful; and the justification for uncertainty about the effects of many other forms of health care will be made explicit.

—*Ian Chalmers and Brian Haynes*
1994

KEY WORDS

Narrative review
Systematic review
PICO
Publication bias
Funnel plot
Forest plot
Meta-analysis
Heterogeneity

Patient-level meta-
analysis
Fixed effect model
Random effects model
Meta-regression
Network meta-analysis
Cumulative meta-
analysis

Clinical decisions are based on the weight of evidence bearing on a question. Sometimes the results of large, strong studies are so compelling that they eclipse all other studies of the same question. More often, however, clinicians depend on the accumulation of evidence from many less definitive studies. When considering these individual studies, clinicians need to establish the context for that one piece of evidence by asking, "Have there been other good studies of the same question, what have they shown, and do their results establish a pattern when the studies' scientific strengths and statistical precision are taken into account?" Reviews are intended to answer these kinds of questions.

Reviews are made available to users in many different forms. They may be articles in journals, chapters in textbooks, summaries prepared by the Cochrane Collaboration, or monographs published by professional or governmental organizations. If the authors of individual research articles are doing their job properly, they will provide information about results of previous studies in the Introduction or Discussion sections of the article.

However a review is made available, the important issue is how well it is done. There are many different ways, each with strengths and weaknesses. In this chapter, we briefly describe traditional reviews and then address in more detail a powerful and more explicitly scientific approach called "systematic reviews."

TRADITIONAL REVIEWS

In traditional reviews, called narrative reviews, an expert in the field summarizes evidence and makes recommendations. An advantage of these reviews is that they can address broad-gauged topics, such as "management of the diabetic patient," and consider a range of issues, such as diagnostic criteria, blood glucose control and monitoring, cardiovascular risk factor modification, and micro- and macrovascular complications. Compliance and cost-effectiveness may also be included. Clinicians need guidance on such a broad range of questions and experts are in a good position to provide it. Authors usually have experience with the disease, know the pertinent evidence base, and have been applying their knowledge in the care of patients.

A disadvantage of narrative reviews is that evidence and recommendations in them may be colored by value judgments that are not made explicit. The lack of structure of traditional reviews may hide important threats to validity. Original research might be cited without a clear account of how articles were found, raising the danger that they were selectively cited to support a point of view. Personal experience and conventional wisdom are often included and may be difficult to distinguish from bedrock research evidence. The strength of the original research may not be carefully critiqued, but instead suggested by shorthand indicators of quality—such as the prestige of the journal, eminence of the author, how recently the study was published, the number of articles for and against a given conclusion, and perhaps general research design (e.g., as randomized trial)—without regard for how well studies were actually designed and executed. Also, there may be no explicit rationale for why one research finding was valued over another.

Of course, a traditional review may *not* have these limitations, especially if it has been peer reviewed by other experts with complementary expertise and if the author has included evidence from more structured reviews. However, concern about the limitations of traditional reviews, especially lack of structure and transparency, has prompted a new approach.

SYSTEMATIC REVIEWS

Systematic reviews are rigorous reviews of the evidence bearing on specific clinical questions. They are "systematic" because they summarize original research following a scientifically based plan that has been decided on in advance and made explicit at every step. As a result, readers can see the strength of the evidence for whatever conclusions are reached and, in principle, check the validity for themselves. Sometimes it is possible to combine studies, giving a more precise estimate of effect size than is available in individual studies.

Systematic reviews are especially useful for addressing a single, focused question such as whether angiotensin-converting enzyme inhibitors reduce the death rate in patients with congestive heart failure

Table 13.1

Elements of a Systemic Review

1. Define a specific question.
2. Find all relevant studies (published and unpublished).
3. Select the strongest studies.
4. Describe the scientific strength of the selected studies.
5. Determine if quality is associated with results.
6. Summarize the studies in figures (forest plots) and tables.
7. Determine if pooling of studies (meta-analysis) is justified.
8. If so, calculate a summary effect size and confidence interval.
9. Identify reasons for heterogeneity if present.

or whether skin adhesives are better than sutures for closing superficial lacerations. For a systematic review to be useful, strong studies of the question should be available. There should not be so few studies of the question that one could just as well critique the individual studies directly. The study results should disagree or at least leave the question open; if all the studies agree with one another, there is nothing to reconcile in a review. Systematic reviews are also useful when there is reason to believe that politics, intellectual passion, or self-interest are accounting for how research results are being interpreted.

Systematic reviews can provide a credible answer to targeted (but not broad-gauged) questions and offers a set of possibilities for how traditional reviews can be done better. They complement, but cannot replace, traditional reviews. Systematic reviews are most often used to summarize randomized controlled trials; therefore, we will base our comments on trials. However, the same methods are used to summarize observational studies of risk and studies of diagnostic test performance.

The elements of a systematic review are summarized in Table 13.1 and will be addressed one at a time throughout the remainder of this chapter.

Defining a Specific Question

Systematic reviews are of specific questions. For effects of interventions, the elements of specificity have been defined under the acronym PICO (1):

P = Patients
I = Intervention
C = Comparison
O = Outcomes

To these, some have added T for time (e.g., follow-up in a cohort study or randomized trial) and S for study design (e.g., randomized trial or cohort) to make PICOTS. Elements of targeted questions for other kinds of studies (e.g., studies of diagnostic test accuracy or observational studies of risk or prognostic factors) are less well defined but include many of the same features.

Finding All Relevant Studies

The first step in a systematic review is to find all the studies that bear on the question at hand. The review should include a complete sample of the best studies of the question, not just a biased sample of studies that happen to have come to attention. Clinicians who review topics less formally—for colleagues in rounds, morning report, and journal clubs—face a similar challenge and should use similar methods, although the process cannot be as exhaustive.

How can a reviewer be reasonably sure that he or she has found all the best studies, considering that the medical literature is vast and widely dispersed? No one method of searching is sufficient for this task, so multiple complementary approaches are used (Table 13.2).

Most reviews start by searching online databases of published research, among them MEDLINE, (the National Library of Medicine's electronic database of published articles) EMBASE, and the Cochrane Database of Systematic Reviews. There are many others that can be identified with a librarian's help. Some, such as MEDLINE, can be searched both for a content area (such as treatment of atrial fibrillation) and for a quality marker (e.g., randomized controlled trial). However, even in the best hands the sensitivity of MEDLINE searches (even for articles that are in MEDLINE) is far from perfect. Also, the contents of the various databases tend to complement each other. Therefore, database searching is useful but not sufficient.

Other ways of finding the right articles make up for what database searches might have missed. Recent reviews and textbooks (particularly electronic

textbooks that are continually updated) are a source. Experts in the content area (e.g., rheumatic heart disease or *Salmonella* infection) may recommend studies that were not turned up by the other approaches. References cited in articles already found are another possibility. There are a growing number of registries of clinical trials and funded research that can be used to find unpublished results.

The goal of consulting all these sources is to avoid missing any important article, even at the expense of inefficiency. In diagnostic test terms, the reviewer uses multiple parallel tests to increase the sensitivity of the search, even at the expense of many false-positive results (i.e., unwanted or redundant citations), which need to be weeded out by examining the studies themselves.

In addition to exercising due diligence in finding articles, authors of systematic reviews explicitly describe the search strategy for their review, including search terms. This allows readers to see the extent to which the reviewer took into account all the studies that were available at the time.

Limit Reviews to Scientifically Strong, Clinically Relevant Studies

To be included in a systematic review, studies must meet a threshold for scientific strength. The assumption is that only the relatively strong studies should count. How is that threshold established? Various expert groups have proposed criteria for adequate scientific strength, and their advantages and limitations are discussed later in this chapter.

Usually only a small proportion of studies are selected from a vast number of potential articles on the topic. Many articles describe the biology of disease and are not ready for clinical application. Others communicate opinions or summaries of existing evidence, not original clinical research. Many studies are not scientifically strong, and the information they contain is eclipsed by stronger studies. Relatively few articles report evidence bearing directly on the clinical question and are both scientifically strong and clinically relevant. Table 13.3 shows how articles were selected for a systematic review of statin drugs for the prevention of infections; only 11 of 632 publications identified were included in the review.

Are Published Studies a Biased Sample of All Completed Research?

The articles cited in systematic reviews should include all scientifically strong studies of the question, regardless of whether have been published. **Publication bias** is the tendency for published studies to be

Table 13.2

Approaches to Finding All the Studies Bearing on a Question

- Search online database such as MEDLINE, EMBASE, and the Cochrane Database of Systemic Reviews.
- Read recent reviews and textbooks.
- Seek the advice of experts in the content area.
- Consider articles cited in the articles already found by other approaches.
- Review registries of clinical trials and funded research (to identify unpublished studies).

Table 13.3

Systematic Reviews Include Only a Small Proportion of All Articles on a Question. Articles Considerer and Included in a Systematic Review of Statins and Prevention of Infections

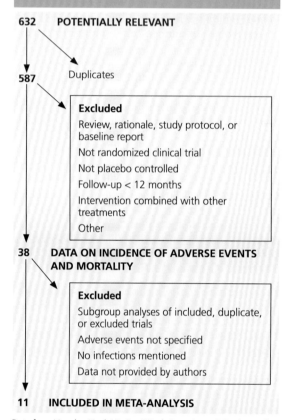

632   POTENTIALLY RELEVANT

587   Duplicates

Excluded

Review, rationale, study protocol, or baseline report

Not randomized clinical trial

Not placebo controlled

Follow-up < 12 months

Intervention combined with other treatments

Other

38   DATA ON INCIDENCE OF ADVERSE EVENTS AND MORTALITY

Excluded

Subgroup analyses of included, duplicate, or excluded trials

Adverse events not specified

No infections mentioned

Data not provided by authors

11   INCLUDED IN META-ANALYSIS

Data from Van den Hoek HL, Bos WJ, de Boer A, et al. Statins and the prevention of infections: systematic review and meta-analysis of data from large randomized placebo controlled trials. BJM 2011; 343:d7281.

systematically different from all completed studies of a question. In general, published studies are more likely to be "positive" (i.e., to find an effect) for several reasons, related to a general preference for positive results. Investigators are less likely to complete studies that seem likely to end up negative and less likely to submit negative studies to journals. Journal peer reviewers are less likely to find negative studies interesting news, and editors are less likely to publish them.

Other selective pressures may favor positive studies. Authors may report outcomes that were not identified or made primary before data were collected and were selected for emphasis in publications after the results were available.

To get around these problems, some authors of systematic reviews make a concerted effort to find unpublished studies, including those that were funded and begun but not completed. They are aided in this effort by public registries of all studies that have been started.

Funnel plots are a graphical way of detecting bias in the selection of studies for systematic reviews. For each study, the effect size is plotted against some measure of the study's size or precision, such as sample size, number of outcome events, or confidence interval (Fig. 13.1).

In the absence of publication bias (Fig. 13.1A), large trials (plotted at the top of the figure) are likely to be published no matter what they find and yield estimates of comparative effectiveness that are closely grouped around the true effect size. Small studies (plotted in the lower part of the figure) are more likely to vary in reported effect size because of statistical imprecision, and so to be spread out at the bottom of the figure, surrounding the true effect size. In the absence of publication bias, they would be as often in the lower right as the lower left of the figure. The result, in the absence of bias, is a symmetrical, peaked distribution—an inverted funnel. Publication bias, particularly the tendency for small studies to be published only if they are positive, shows up as asymmetry in the funnel plot (Fig. 13.1B). There are disproportionately fewer small studies that favor the control group, seen as a paucity of studies in the lower right corner of the figure.

Other factors, not directly related to distaste for negative studies, can cause publication bias. Funding of research by agencies with a financial interest in the results can also lead to distortions in the scientific record. Outcomes of studies sponsored by industry (usually drug and device companies) are more likely to favor the sponsor's product than those with other funding sources. One possible reason is that industry sponsors sometimes require, as a condition of funding research, that they approve the resulting articles before they are submitted to journals. Industry sponsors have blocked publication of research they have funded that has not, in their opinion, found the "right" result.

How Good Are the Best Studies?

Clinicians need to know just how good the best studies of a question are so that they will know how seriously to take the conclusions of the systematic review. Are the studies so strong that it would be irresponsible to discount them? Or are they weak, suggesting that it is reasonable to not follow their lead?

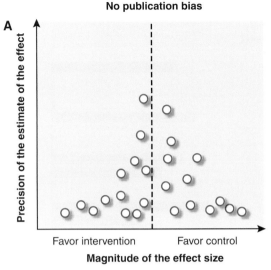

No publication bias

A

Precision of the estimate of the effect

Favor intervention   Favor control

Magnitude of the effect size

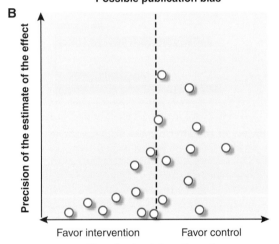

Possible publication bias

B

Precision of the estimate of the effect

Favor intervention   Favor control

Magnitude of the effect size

Figure 13.1 ■ Funnel plots to detect publication bias. Each trial is indicated by a circle. **A.** Trials are symmetrical in the shape of an inverted funnel, suggesting no publication bias. **B.** There are no trials in the lower right corner, suggesting that small trials not favoring the intervention were not published. (Redrawn with permission from Guyatt GH, Oxman AD, Montori V, et al. GRADE guidelines: 5. Rating the quality of evidence = publication bias. J Clin Epidemiol 2011;64:1277–1282.)

Many studies have shown that the individual elements of quality discussed throughout this book, such as concealment of treatment assignment, blinding, follow-up, and sample size, are systematically related to study results. The quality of the evidence identified by the systematic review can be summarized by a table showing the extent to which markers of quality are present in the studies included in the review.

Example

A systematic review summarized published reports of the effectiveness of the supplement chondroitin on pain intensity in patients with osteoarthritis of the hip or knee (2). The investigators found 20 published trials comparing glucosamine to placebo. Figure 13.2 shows the proportion of trials meeting several criteria for quality. (Ignore, for the moment, effect sizes, shown on the right.) A substantial proportion of trials did not meet basic standards for scientific quality such as concealment of allocation, intention-to-treat analysis, and sample size, so the evidence base for this question was not particularly strong.

Individual measures of quality can also be combined into summary measures. A simple, commonly used scale for studies of treatment effectiveness, the Jadad Scale, includes whether the study was described as randomized and double-blinded and whether there was a description of withdrawals and dropouts (3). However, there is not a clear relationship between summary scores for study quality and results (4). Why might this be? The component studies in systematic reviews are already highly selected and, therefore, might not differ much from one another in quality. Also, summary measures of quality typically add up scores for the presence or absence of each element of quality, and there is no reason to believe that each makes an equal contribution to the overall validity of the study. It is not difficult to imagine, for example, that weakness in one aspect of a study might be so damaging as to render the entire study invalid, even though all the other aspects of quality are exemplary.

Example

In a randomized, placebo-controlled trial, women with unexplained fatigue but no anemia had less fatigue after taking an iron supplement (5). The effect was small, only about 1 point on a 10-point scale for fatigue, but statistically significant. Most aspects of the study, such as

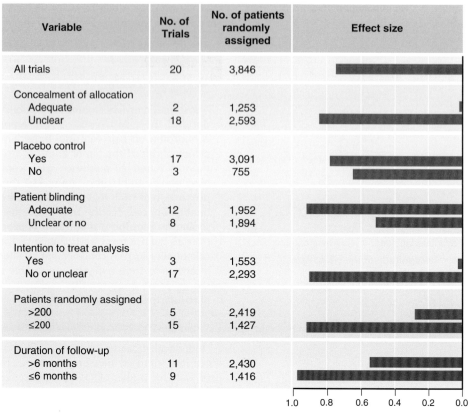

Figure 13.2 ■ **Quality of 20 trials in a systematic review of the effectiveness of glucosamine on pain in patients with osteoarthritis of the knee or hip.** (Data from Reichenbach S, Sterchi R, Scherer M, et al. Meta-analysis: chondroitin for osteoarthritis of the knee and hip. Ann Intern Med 2007; 146:580–590.)

randomization, allocation concealment, sample size, and follow-up, were strong. Also, the iron and placebo pills were visually identical. However, iron causes characteristic side effects (e.g., dark stools and constipation) that could have prompted women to recognize whether they were taking iron or the placebo. Also, fatigue is a relatively "soft" outcome that might be influenced by belief in the effectiveness of iron supplements. Even if all other aspects of the study were beyond reproach (and the overall quality score was excellent), this one aspect of quality—patients being aware of which treatment they were taking coupled with an outcome easily influenced by this knowledge—could have accounted for the small observed difference, rather than a true treatment effect.

Therefore, while quality checklists and scores have their place, they are no substitute for critically examining the individual studies in a systematic review with an eye toward how much any imperfections in the studies might have influenced their results.

Is Scientific Quality Related to Research Results?

Studies meeting higher standards for methods should come closer to the truth than weak ones. Therefore, it may be informative for reviewers to show if there is a relationship between study quality and study conclusion. This is often done by examining the relationship between individual quality measures and outcomes because of the limitations of summary scores.

Example

Figure 13.2 shows the relationship between several markers of quality and effect size with confidence intervals for trials of chondroitin versus placebo or no intervention for relief of pain of osteoarthritis of the knee or hip (2). In general, effect sizes were larger in trials in which the quality measure was absent; this effect was statistically significant for concealment of allocation, intention-to-treat analysis, and larger studies. An analysis restricted to the three largest studies with intention-to-treat analyses found an effect size of –0.03 (95% confidence interval –0.13 to 0.07), where an effect size of –0.30 was considered minimally clinically relevant. That is, there was no clinically important effect.

Summarizing Results

The results of a systematic review are typically displayed as a forest plot showing the point estimate of effectiveness and confidence interval for each study in the review. Figure 13.3 illustrates a summary of studies comparing quinine to placebo for muscle cramps (6). The measure of effectiveness in this example is change in the number of leg cramps in a 2-week period. In other systematic reviews, it might be relative risk, attributable risk, or any other measure of effect. Point estimates are represented by boxes with their size proportional to the size of the study. A vertical line marks where neither quinine nor placebo was more effective.

The origin of the name "forest plot" is uncertain, but it is variously attributed to a researcher's name or the appearance resembling a "forest of lines" (7). We believe they help readers "see the forest and the trees."

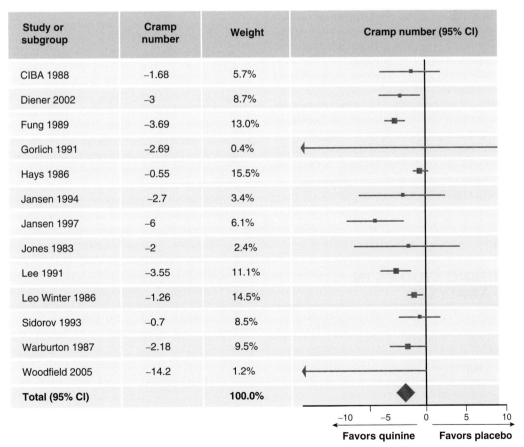

Figure 13.3 ■ **Example of a forest plot.** Summary of 13 randomized trials of the effectiveness of quinine versus placebo on number of cramps in 2 weeks. (Redrawn with permission from El-Tawil S, Al Musa T, Valli H, et al. Quinine for muscle cramps. Cochrane Database Syst Rev 2010;(12):CD005044.)

Forest plots summarize a tremendous amount of information that would otherwise require a great deal of effort to find.

1. *Number of studies.* The rows show the number of studies meeting stringent criteria for quality, in this case, 13.
2. *What studies and when.* The first column identifies names and year of publication for the component studies so that readers can see how old the studies are and where they can be found. (Full references to studies are not shown in the figure but are included in the article).
3. *Pattern of effect sizes.* The 13 point estimates, taken as a whole, show what the various studies reported for effect sizes. In the example, all of the 13 studies favored quinine, but the size of the effects varies.
4. *Precision of estimates.* Many studies (6 of 13) were "negative" (their confidence intervals included no effect). This would give the impression, in a simple accounting of the number of "positive" and "negative" studies, that treatment is not effective or at least that effectiveness is questionable. The forest plot gives a different impression: All point estimates favor quinine, and the negative studies tend to be imprecise yet consistent with effectiveness.
5. *The effects for the big studies.* The large, statistically precise studies (seen by both narrow confidence intervals and large boxes representing point estimates) deserve more weight than small ones. In the example, the confidence intervals for the two largest studies do not include "no change in muscle cramp rate" (although one touches it).

In these ways, a single picture conveys in a glance a lot of basic information about the very best studies of a question.

COMBINING STUDIES IN META-ANALYSES

Meta-analysis is the practice of combining ("pooling") the results of individual studies, if they are similar enough to justify a quantitative summary effect size. When appropriate, meta-analyses provide more precise estimates of effect sizes than are available in any of the individual studies.

Are the Studies Similar Enough to Justify Combining?

It makes no sense to pool the results of very different studies—studies of altogether different kinds of patients, interventions, doses, follow-ups, and outcomes. Treating "apples and oranges" as if they are all just fruits disregards useful information.

Investigators use two general approaches to decide whether it is appropriate to pool study results. One is to make an informed judgment about whether the research questions addressed by the trials are similar enough to constitute studies of the same question (or a set of reasonably similar questions).

Example

Do antioxidant supplements prevent gastrointestinal cancers? Investigators sought the answer to this question is a systematic review (8). The antioxidants were vitamins A, C, E, and B_6, beta-carotene (which has vitamin A activity), and the minerals zinc and selenium, singly and in combination at various doses. Cancers were of the esophagus, stomach, colon, rectum, pancreas, and liver. The investigators calculated a pooled estimate of relative risk for the 14 randomized trials they found. The point estimate was close to 1 (no effect) and the confidence interval was narrow, indicating no overall effect. But should they have pooled these studies? On the face of it, the study questions were very different from each other. Although the various vitamins and minerals do have in common that they are antioxidants (as are countless other compounds in the diet), they have altogether different chemical structures, roles in metabolism, and deficiency syndromes. Similarly, the gastrointestinal cancers have very different genetics, risk factors, and pathogenesis. For example, stomach cancer follows infection with the bacterium *Helicobacter pylori*, whereas liver cancer is often a complication of viral hepatitis. It seems improbable that these supplements and these cancers have enough in common to justify treating them as simply "antioxidant supplements" and "gastrointestinal cancers" and finding a meaningful result. That the investigators found no effect may be because of the differences among the studies and does not rule out effects of specific supplements on specific cancers.

Reasonable people might disagree on how similar studies must be to justify combining them. We have been critical of pooling in this study, but other capable people thought that pooling was justified and that the study was worth publishing in a leading journal.

Another approach is to use a statistical test for heterogeneity, the extent to which the trial results are different from each other beyond what might be expected by chance. Here the null hypothesis is that there is no difference among study results and the statistical test is used to see if there is a statistically significant difference among them. Failing to reject the null hypothesis of no difference among the studies may seem reassuring, but there is a problem. Most meta-analyses are of relatively few studies, so the tests have limited statistical power. The risk of a false-negative result, a conclusion that the studies are not heterogeneous when they are, is often high. Power is also affected by the number of patients in these studies and how evenly they are distributed among the studies. If one of the component studies is much larger than the others, it contributes most of the information bearing on the question. It may be more informative to examine the large study carefully and then contrast it with the others. In the antioxidant and gastrointestinal cancers example, the statistical test did show heterogeneity.

What Is Combined—Studies or Patients?

Until now, we have been discussing how *studies* are combined, which is the usual way meta-analyses are done, An even more powerful approach is to obtain data on each individual *patient* in each of the component studies and to pool these data to produce, in effect, a single large study called a patient-level meta-analysis. Relatively few meta-analyses are done this way because of the difficulties in obtaining all these data from many different investigators and reconciling how variables were coded. However, when patient-level meta-analyses can be done, it becomes possible to look for effects in clinically important subgroups of patients. The numbers of patients in these subgroups may be too small in the individual studies to produce stable estimates of effects but large enough when patients in several studies are pooled.

Example

Inhaled nitric oxide is effective in full-term infants with pulmonary hypertension and hypoxic respiratory failure. However, it was uncertain whether nitric oxide is effective in preterm infants. Investigators did a patient-level meta-analysis of trials of nitric oxide in preterm infants (9). They pooled data on 3,298 preterm infants in 12 trials and found no effect on death or chronic lung disease (59% versus 61% favoring nitric oxide, relative risk 0.96, 95% confidence interval 0.92–1.01). Because there were data for each patient, it was possible to look for effectiveness in clinically relevant subgroups of preterm infants just as one might in a single large trial. Effectiveness did not differ according to gestational age, birth weight, multiple births, race, antenatal steroids, and seven other infant characteristics.

How Are the Results Pooled?

When study results are pooled, each individual study contributes to the summary effect in relation to its size (strictly speaking, the inverse of its variance). Those that contribute large amounts of information are weighted more heavily than those that make small contributions. This is made explicit in the quinine example (Fig. 13.3), where the weight of each study is reported in the third column, with the total adding up to 100%. Four of the largest studies contribute more to the summary effect than the other nine smaller studies.

Two kinds of mathematical models are used to summarize studies in meta-analyses. These models differ in what is being summarized and in how conservative they are in estimating overall confidence intervals.

With the fixed effect model (Fig. 13.4A), it is assumed that each of the studies is of exactly the same question so that the results of the studies differ only by chance. This model is called "fixed effect" because it is assumed that there is only one underlying effect size for all the studies, although the results of the individual studies do differ from one another because of the play of chance.

The main problem with this approach is that, on the face of it, the studies rarely resemble one another so closely (in terms of patients, interventions, follow-up, and outcomes) that they can be considered simple replications of one another. Should vitamins A, C, and E and selenium really be considered simply examples of "antioxidant supplements," even though they have different biochemical structures and mechanisms of action? Or are they different enough from one another that they might have different effects? To the extent that the study questions differ somewhat,

A Fixed effects model

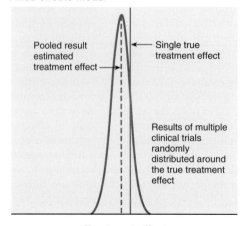

Treatment effects

B   Random effects model

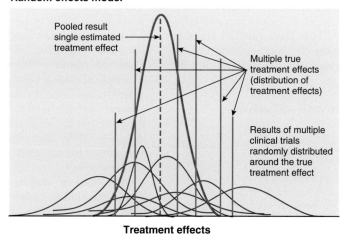

Treatment effects

Figure 13.4 ■ Models for combining studies in a meta-analysis. A. Fixed effect model. **B.** Random effects model. (Redrawn with permission from UpToDate, Waltham, MA.)

the width of the summary confidence intervals calculated by the fixed effect model tends to imply a greater degree of precision than is actually the case. Also, by combining dissimilar studies, one loses useful information that might have resulted from contrasting them. The fixed effect model is used when the studies in a systematic review are clearly quite similar to each other.

The random effects model (Fig. 13.4B) assumes that the studies address somewhat different questions but that they form a closely related family of studies of a similar question. The studies are considered a random sample of all studies bearing on that question. Even if clinical judgment and a statistical tests both suggest heterogeneity, it may still be reasonable to combine studies using a random effects model, as long as the studies are similar enough to one another (which is obviously a value judgment). Random effects models produce wider confidence intervals than fixed effect models and for this reason are thought to be more realistic. However, it is uncertain how the family of similar studies is defined and whether the studies are really a random sample of all such studies of a question. Nevertheless, because random effects models at least take heterogeneity into account and are, therefore, less likely to overestimate precision, they are the model used when (as if often the case) heterogeneity is present.

When an overall effect size is calculated, it is usually displayed at the bottom of the forest plot of component studies as a diamond representing the summary point estimate and confidence interval (see Fig. 13.3). The summary effect is a more precise and formalized presentation of what might have been concluded from the pattern of results available in the forest plot.

Identifying Reasons for Heterogeneity

Random effects models are a way of taking heterogeneity into account when calculating a summary effect size, but a separate need is to identify characteristics of patients or treatments that are responsible for the variation in effects.

The most straightforward way to identify reasons for heterogeneity is to do subgroup analyses. This is possible in patient-level meta-analyses, as described in the example about nitric oxide treatment of preterm infants. However, if trials, not patients, are pooled, one must rely on less direct methods.

Another approach to understanding the reasons for heterogeneity is to do a sensitivity analysis, as discussed in Chapter 7. Summary effects are examined with and without trials that seem, either for clinical or statistical reasons, to be different from the others. For example, investigators might look at summary effects (or statistical tests for heterogeneity) after removing relatively weak trials or those in which the dose of drug was relatively small to see if study strength or drug dose account for differences in results across studies.

A modeling approach called meta-regression, similar to multivariable analysis (discussed in Chapter 11) can be used to explore reasons for heterogeneity when trials, not patients, are pooled. The independent variables are those reported in aggregate in each individual trial (e.g., the average age or proportion of men and women in those trials) and the outcomes are the reported treatment effect for each of those trials. The number of observations is the number of trials in the meta-analysis. This approach is limited by the availability of data on the covariates of interest in the individual trials, the compatibility of the data across trials, and the stability of models based on just a few observations (the number of trials in the meta-analysis). Another limitation, as with any aggregate-risk study, is the possibility of an "ecological fallacy," as discussed in Chapter 12.

The various studies in a systematic review sometimes address the effectiveness of a set of interrelated interventions, not just a single comparison between an intervention and control group. For example, there are several techniques for bariatric surgery such as jejunoileal bypass, sleeve gastrectomy, adjustable gastric banding, among others. Randomized trials have compared various combinations of these to each other and to usual care, but no study has compared each technique to all the others. Network meta-analysis is a mathematical way of estimating the comparative effectiveness of interventions that are not directly compared in actual studies but can be indirectly compared by use of modeling. Using a network meta-analysis, investigators were able to estimate the respective effects of each bariatric surgery method compared to usual care, showing that each was effective and identifying the hierarchy of effectiveness (10).

CUMULATIVE META-ANALYSES

Usually the studies in a forest plot are represented separately in alphabetical order by first author or in chronological order. Another way to look at the same information is to present a cumulative meta-analysis. Component studies are put in chronological order, from oldest to most recent, and a new summary effect size and confidence interval is calculated for each time the results of a new study became available. In this way, the figure represents a running summary of all the studies up to the time of each new trial. This is a Bayesian approach, as described in Chapter 11, where each new trial modifies prior belief in comparative effectiveness, established by the trials that went before.

The following example illustrates the kind of insights a cumulative meta-analyses can provide and also shows how meta-analyses in general and cumulative meta-analyses in particular are useful for establishing harmful effects. Individual trials, which are powered to detect effectiveness, are usually underpowered to detect harms because harms occur at a substantially lower rate. Pooling data may accumulate enough events to detect harmful effects.

Example

Rofecoxib is a non-steroidal anti-inflammatory drug (NSAID) that is less likely to cause gastrointestinal complications than older NSAIDs. Studies of patients taking this drug reported an increased rate of cardiovascular events, but this was not attributed to the drug because confidence intervals were wide, including no effect, and also because the risk in the largest study was explained as a protective effect of the comparator, naproxen. Investigators did a meta-analysis of 16 randomized trials of rofecoxib versus control (a placebo or another NSAID) (11). All but one of the studies was small, with only 1 to 6 cardiovascular events per trial, but there were 24 cardiovascular events in the one large trial. The summary relative risk of rofecoxib for myocardial infarction, including data from the large trial, was 2.24 (95% confidence interval 1.24–4.02). When was risk first apparent? A cumulative meta-analysis (Fig. 13.5) shows that a statistically significant effect was apparent in 2000, mainly because of

the information contributed by the one large study. Subsequent studies tended to consolidate this finding and increase statistical precision. Rofecoxib was taken off the market in 2004, 4 years after a cumulative meta-analysis would have shown cardiovascular risk was present at conventional levels of statistical significance.

Cumulative meta-analyses have been used to show when the research community *could have known* about effectiveness or harm if it had available a meta-analysis of the evidence, but now it

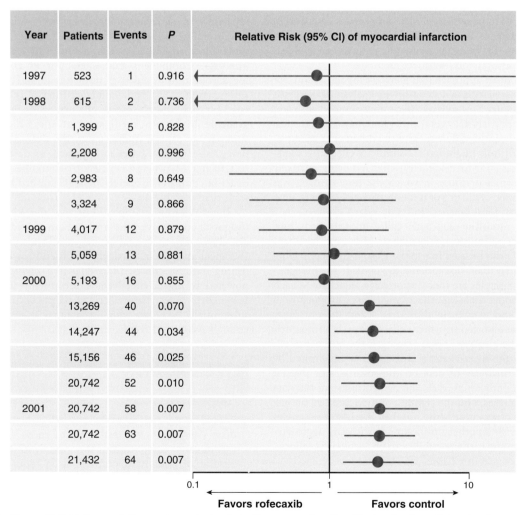

Figure 13.5 ■ **A cumulative meta-analysis of studies comparing the effects of rofecoxib to placebo on rates of myocardial infarction.** (Redrawn with permission from Juni P, Nartey L, Reichenbach S, et al. Risk of cardiovascular events and rofecoxib: cumulative meta-analysis. Lancet 2004;364:2021–2029.)

is possible to have the results of meta-analyses in real time. In the Cochrane Collaboration, meta-analyses are updated every time a new trial becomes available. For each new meta-analysis, the summary effect size represents the accumulation of evidence up to the time of the update, though without explicitly showing what summary effect sizes had been in the past.

SYSTEMATIC REVIEWS OF OBSERVATIONAL AND DIAGNOSTIC STUDIES

We have discussed systematic reviews and meta-analyses, using randomized controlled trials as examples. However, systematic reviews are also useful for other kinds of studies, as illustrated by the following summary of observational studies.

Example

Patients with venous thromboembolism may have recurrences after anticoagulation is stopped. Investigators obtained patient-level data from 2,554 patients in seven cohort studies that followed up patients after anticoagulation was stopped (12). Because there were data for each patient, incidence was estimated by time-to-event analysis. Men had a higher risk of thromboembolism than women (HR=2.2). After adjusting for hormone-associated initial thromboembolism in women, the excess risk in men persisted. Recurrence rate did not differ between men and women among patients whose initial event occurred after exposure to a major risk factor. Examination of both main question (whether recurrence rates differed in men and women) and secondary questions (whether effects were different according to whether women took menopausal hormone or the initial event followed exposure to a major risk factor) were made possible because of the larger sample size afforded by pooled results and by the availability of patient-level data.

The performance of a diagnostic test, being a relatively targeted question, is also well suited for systematic reviews, as the following example illustrates.

Example

Patients with low back and leg pain may have a herniated intervertebral disc pressing on a spinal nerve root. Primary care physicians rely on information from history and physical examination to select patients who might benefit from imaging and surgery. Pain on straight leg raising is one of the core diagnostic tests for a herniated disc. How well does this test perform? Investigators in the Cochrane Collaboration did a systematic review of studies describing the sensitivity and specificity of straight leg raising (13). They found 10 studies that used surgical findings as the gold standard (Fig. 13.6). Sensitivity was consistently high, but the corresponding specificities were low, imprecisely estimated, and quite variable. Because of heterogeneity, especially for specificity, results were not pooled. The investigators reported that there was no single explanation for heterogeneity, but there was variation in both how the test was interpreted as positive and how the reference standard was interpreted as abnormal. An ROC curve suggested a trade-off between sensitivity and specificity at different cut-points for an abnormal test. Most of the studies were too small to support a more complete evaluation of the reasons for heterogeneity.

STRENGTHS AND WEAKNESSES OF META-ANALYSES

Meta-analyses, when justified by relatively homogeneous results of component studies, can make many contributions to systematic reviews. They can establish that an effect is present or absent with more authority than individual trials or less formal ways of summing up effects. Pooling makes it possible to estimate effects sizes more precisely so that clinicians can have a better understanding of how big or small the true effect might be. Meta-analyses can detect treatment complications or differences in effects among subgroups, questions that individual trials usually do not have the statistical power to address. They make it possible to recognize the point in time when effectiveness or harm has been established whereas this is much more difficult with less formal reviews.

Disadvantages of meta-analyses include the temptation to pool quite dissimilar studies, providing a

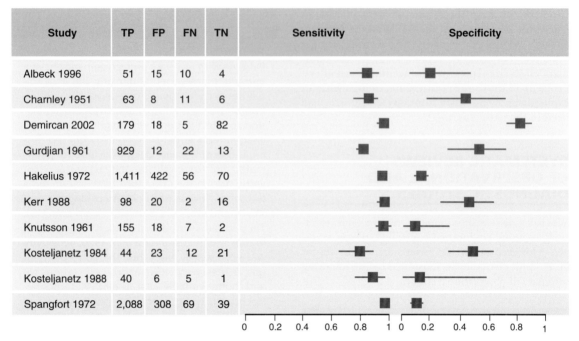

Study	TP	FP	FN	TN	Sensitivity	Specificity
Albeck 1996	51	15	10	4		
Charnley 1951	63	8	11	6		
Demircan 2002	179	18	5	82		
Gurdjian 1961	929	12	22	13		
Hakelius 1972	1,411	422	56	70		
Kerr 1988	98	20	2	16		
Knutsson 1961	155	18	7	2		
Kosteljanetz 1984	44	23	12	21		
Kosteljanetz 1988	40	6	5	1		
Spangfort 1972	2,088	308	69	39		

Figure 13.6 ■ **A systematic review of diagnostic test performance.** The sensitivity and specificity of straight leg raising as a test for lumbar disc herniation in patients with low back pain and leg pain. (Redrawn with permission from van der Windt DA, Simons E, Riphagen II, et al. Physical examination for lumbar radiculopathy due to disc herniation in patients with low-back pain. Cochrane Database Syst Rev 2010;(2):CD007431.)

misleading estimate of effects and directing attention away from why differences in effects exist. Meta-analyses do not include information based on the biology of disease, clinical experience, and the practical application of best evidence to patient care—other dimensions of care that may have as large influence on patient-centered outcomes as do choice of drugs or procedures.

Which comes closer to the truth, the best individual research or meta-analyses? It is a false choice. Meta-analyses cannot be better than the scientific strength of the individual studies that they summarize. Sometimes most of the weight in a meta-analysis is vested in a single trial, so there is relatively little difference between the information in that trial and in a summary of all studies of the same question. For the most part, the two—large strong studies and meta-analyses of all related studies—complement each other rather than compete. When they disagree, the main issue is why they disagree, which should be sought by examination of the studies themselves, not the methods in general.

Review Questions

Read the following and select the best response.

13.1. A systematic review of observational studies of antioxidant vitamins to prevent cardiovascular disease combined the results of 12 studies to obtain a summary effect size and confidence interval. Which of the following would be the strongest rationale for combining study results?

A. You wish to obtain a more generalizable conclusion.
B. A statistical test shows that the studies are heterogeneous.
C. Most of the component studies are statistically significant.
D. The component studies have different, and to some extent complementary, biases.
E. You can obtain a more precise estimate of effect size.

13.2. You are asked to critique a review of the literature on whether alcohol is a risk factor for breast cancer. The reviewer has searched MEDLINE and found several observational studies of this question but has not searched elsewhere. All of the following are limitations of this search strategy *except*:

A. Studies with negative results tend to not be published.
B. MEDLINE searches typically miss some articles, even those included in the database.
C. MEDLINE does not include all of the world's journals.
D. MEDLINE can be simultaneously searched for both content area and methods.

13.3. A systematic review of antiplatelet drugs for cardiovascular disease prevention combined individual patients, not trials. Which of the following is an advantage of this approach?

A. It is more efficient for the investigator.
B. Subgroup analyses are possible.
C. It is not necessary to choose between fixed and random effects models when combining data.
D. Publication bias is less likely.

13.4. Which of the following is *not* generally used to define a specific clinical question studied by randomized controlled trials?

A. Covariates that were taken into account
B. Interventions (e.g., exposure or experimental treatment)
C. Comparison group (e.g., patients taking placebo in a randomized trial)
D. Outcomes
E. Patients in the trials

13.5. Which of the following best describes ways of measuring study quality?

A. The validity of summary measures of study quality is well established.
B. A description of study quality is a useful part of systematic reviews.
C. In a summary measure of quality, strengths of the study can make up for weaknesses.

D. Individual measures of quality such as randomization and blinding are not associated with study results.

13.6. Which of the following kinds of studies is least likely to be published?

A. Small positive studies
B. Large negative studies
C. Large positive studies
D. Small negative studies

13.7. Which of the following is a comparative advantage of traditional ("narrative") reviews over systematic reviews?

A. Readers can confirm that evidence cited is selected without bias.
B. Narrative reviews can review a broad range of questions bearing on the care of a condition.
C. They rely on the experience and judgment of an expert in the field.
D. They provide a quantitative summary of effects.
E. The scientific strength of the studies cited is explicitly evaluated.

13.8. Which of the following is not always part of a typical forest plot?

A. The number of studies that meet high standards for quality
B. A summary or pooled effect size with confidence interval
C. Point estimates of effect size for each study
D. Confidence intervals for each study
E. The size or weight contributed by each study

13.9. Which of the following cannot be used for identifying severity of illness as a reason for heterogeneity in a systematic review with meta-analysis?

A. Controlling for severity of illness in a study-level meta-analysis
B. A mathematical model relating average severity of illness to outcome across the component studies
C. A comparison of summary effect sizes in studies stratified by mean severity of illness
D. Subgroup analyses of patient-level data

13.10. Which of the following is the best justification for combining the results of five studies into a single summary effect?

    A. The patients, interventions, and outcomes are relatively similar.

    B. All studies are of high quality.

    C. A statistical test does not detect heterogeneity.

    D. Publication bias has been ruled out by a funnel plot.

    E. The random effects model will be used to calculate the summary effect size.

13.11. Which of the following is an advantage of the random effects model over the fixed effect model?

    A. It can be used for studies with time-to-event analyses.

    B. It describes the summary effect size for a single, narrowly defined question.

    C. It is better suited for meta-analyses of diagnostic test performance.

    D. It gives more realistic results when there is heterogeneity among studies.

    E. Confidence intervals tend to be narrower.

Answers are in Appendix A.

REFERENCES

1. Sackett DL, Richardson WS, Rosenberg W, et al. Evidence-based medicine. How to practice and teach EBM. New York; Churchill Livingstone; 1997.

2. Reichenbach S, Sterchi R, Scherer M, et al. Meta-analysis: chondroitin for osteoarthritis of the knee and hip. Ann Intern Med 2007;146:580–590.

3. Jadad AR, Moore RA, Carroll D, et al. Assessing the quality of reports of randomized clinical trials: Is blinding necessary? Controlled Clinical Trials 1996;17:1–12.

4. Balk EM, Bonis PAL, Moskowitz H, et al. Correlation of quality measures with estimates of treatment effect in meta-analyses of randomized controlled trials. JAMA 2002;287:2973–2982.

5. Verdon F, Burnand B, Stubi CL, et al. Iron supplementation for unexplained fatigue in nonanemic women: double-blind, randomized placebo controlled trial. BMJ 2003;326:1124–1228.

6. El-Tawil S, Al Musa T, Valli H, et al. Quinine for muscle cramps. Cochrane Database Syst Rev 2010;(12):CD005044.

7. Lewis S, Clarke M. Forest plots: trying to see the wood and the trees. BMJ 2001;322:1479–1480.

8. Bjelakovic G, Nikolova D, Simonetti RG, et al. Antioxidant supplements for prevention of gastrointestinal cancers: a systematic review and meta-analysis. Lancet 2004;364:1219–1228.

9. Askie LM, Ballard RA, Cutter GR, et al. Inhaled nitric oxide in preterm infants: an individual-level data meta-analysis of randomized trials. Pediatrics 2011;128:729–739.

10. Padwal R, Klarenbach S, Wiebe N, et al. Bariatric surgery: a systematic review and network meta-analysis of randomized trials. Obes Rev 2011;12:602–621.

11. Juni P, Nartey L, Reichenbach S, et al. Risk of cardiovascular events and rofecoxib: cumulative meta-analysis. Lancet 2004;364:2021–2029.

12. Douketis J, Tosetto A, Marcucci M, et al. Risk of recurrence after venous thromboembolism in men and women: patient level meta-analysis. BMJ 2011;342:d813.

13. van der Windt DA, Simons E, Riphagen II, et al. Physical examination for lumbar radiculopathy due to disc herniation in patients with low-back pain. Cochrane Database Syst Rev 2010;(2):CD007431.

Chapter 14

Knowledge Management

Where is the wisdom we have lost in knowledge?
Where is the knowledge we have lost in information?
—T.S. Eliot
1934

KEY WORDS

Knowledge
    management
Conflict of interest
Scientific misconduct
Point of care
Just-in-time
    learning

Clinical practice
    guidelines
MEDLINE
EMBASE
PubMed
Peer review
Structured abstract

Finding the best available answer to a specific clinical question is like finding a needle in a haystack. Essential information is mixed with a vast amount of less credible "factoids" and opinions, and it is a daunting task to sort the wheat from the chaff. Yet, that is what clinicians need to do. Critical reading is only as good as the information found.

Knowledge management is the effective and efficient organization and use of knowledge. This was a difficult task in the days of print media only. Fortunately, knowledge management has become a great deal easier in the era of electronic information. There are more and better studies on a broad range of clinical questions, widely available access to research results, and efficient ways to rapidly sort articles by topic and scientific strength. These opportunities followed the widespread availability of computers, the World Wide Web, and electronic information for clinical purposes.

Finding information may seem to be a low priority for clinicians still in training. They are surrounded by information, far more than they can

handle comfortably, and they have countless experts to help them decide what they should take seriously and what they should disregard. However, developing one's own plan for managing knowledge becomes crucial later on, whether in practice or academe.

Even with recent developments, effective and efficient knowledge management is a challenging task. In this chapter, we review modern approaches to clinical knowledge management. We will discuss four basic tasks: looking up information, keeping up with new developments in your field, remaining connected to medicine as a profession, and helping patients find good health information themselves.

BASIC PRINCIPLES

Several aspects of knowledge management cut across all activities.

Do It Yourself or Delegate?

Clinicians must first ask themselves, "Will I find and judge clinical research results for myself or delegate this task to someone else?" The answer is both. Clinicians should be capable of finding and critiquing information on their own; it is a basic skill in clinical medicine. But as a practical matter, it is not possible to go it alone for all of one's information needs. There are just too many questions in a day and too little time to answer them on one's own. Therefore, clinicians must find trustworthy agents to help them manage knowledge.

Which Medium?

One can obtain information via a rich array of media. They range from printed books and journals to digital information on the Web accessed through stationary and handheld platforms. There are audiotapes, videotapes, and more. The information is neither more nor less sound because of how it happens to come to you. Validity depends on authors, reviewers, and editors, not the medium. However, the availability of various media, with complementary advantages and disadvantages, makes it easier to find ones that match every user's preferences.

A modern knowledge management plan should be based on electronic information on the Internet. The information base for clinical medicine is changing too fast for print media alone to be sufficient. For example, clinically important discoveries in antiviral therapy for HIV, innovative scanning technologies, and state-of-the-science cancer chemotherapy emerge from year to year, even month to month. The Internet can keep pace with such rapid change and also complement, but not replace, traditional sources.

Grading Information

Grading makes it possible for clinicians to grasp the basic value of information in seconds. Usually, the quality of the evidence (confidence in estimates of effects) and strength of recommendations are graded separately. Table 14.1 shows an example of one widely used grading scheme called GRADE, similar in principle to other approaches in general use. This grading is for interventions; grading of other kinds of information is less well developed. Notice that recommendations are based on the strength of the research evidence, depend on the balance of benefits and harms, and vary in how forcefully and widely the intervention should be offered to patients. Although criteria for grading are explicit, assigning grades still depends partly on judgment.

Misleading Reports of Research Findings

Until now, we have acted as if the only threats to the validity of published clinical research stem from the difficulties of applying good scientific principles to the study of human illness. That is, validity is about the management of bias and chance. Unfortunately, there are other threats to the validity of research results, related to the investigators themselves and the social, political, and economic environment in which they work. We are referring to the all-too-human tendency to report the results of research according to one's own stake in the results.

Conflict of interest exists when investigators' private interests compete with their responsibilities to be unbiased investigators. There are many possible competing interests:

- Financial conflict of interest: When personal or family income is related to research results (this conflict is usually considered the most powerful and most difficult to detect)
- Personal relationships: Supporting friends and putting down rivals
- Intellectual passion: Being for one's own ideas and against competing ones
- Institutional loyalties: Putting the interests of one's own school, company, or organization above others
- Career advancement: Investigators get more academic credit for publishing interesting results in elite journals.

Conflict of interest exists in relation to a specific topic, not in general, and regardless of whether it has actually changed behavior.

How is conflict of interest expressed? Scientific misconduct—fraud, fabrication, and plagiarism—are extreme examples. Less extreme is selective reporting of research results, either by not reporting unwelcome results (publication bias) or reporting results according to whether they seem to be the "right" ones. Industry sponsors of research can sometimes block publication or alter how results are reported. To create a public record of whether this has occurred, randomized controlled trials are now registered on publically available Web sites before data collection, making to possible to follow-up on whether the results were published when expected and whether the reported endpoints were the same as when the trial began (1).

More subtle and more difficult to detect are efforts to "spin" results by the way they are described, for example, by implying that a very low P value means the results are clinically important or by describing effects as "large" when most of us would think they were not (2). All of us depend on peer reviewers and editors to limit the worst of this kind of editorializing in scientific articles.

We mention these somewhat sordid influences on the information clinicians (and their patients) depend on because they are, in some situations, every bit as real and important as the well-informed application of confidence intervals and control of confounding, the usual domain of clinical epidemiology. Research and its interpretation are human endeavors and will, therefore, always be tinged, to some extent, with

Table 14.1

Grading Recommendations for Treatment According to the Quality of Evidence (Confidence in Estimate of Effect, A–C) and Strength of Recommendation (1–2) with Implications. Based on GRADE Guidelines

Grade of Recommendation	Clarity of Risk/Benefit	Quality of Supporting Evidence	Implications
1A. Strong recommendation, high-quality evidence	Benefits clearly outweigh risks and burdens, or vice versa	Consistent evidence from well-performed randomized controlled trials, or overwhelming evidence in some other form. Further research is unlikely to change confidence in the estimates of benefits and risks	Strong recommendations apply to most patients in most circumstances without reservation. Clinicians should follow a strong recommendation unless there is a clear and compelling rationale for an alternative approach.
1B. Strong recommendation, moderate-quality evidence	Benefits clearly outweigh risks and burdens, or vice versa	Evidence from randomized controlled trials with important limitations (inconsistent results, methodologic flaws, or imprecision), or very strong evidence of some other research design. Further research (if performed) is likely to change our confidence in the estimates of benefits and risk	Strong recommendation that applies to most patients. Clinicians should follow a strong recommendation unless there is a clear and compelling rationale for an alternative approach.
1C. Strong recommendation, low-quality evidence	Benefits appear to outweigh risk and burdens, or vice versa	Evidence from observational studies, unsystematic clinical experience, or randomized controlled trials with serious flaws. Any estimate of effect is uncertain.	Strong recommendation that applies to most patients. Some of the evidence base supporting the recommendation is of low quality.
2A. Weak recommendation, high-quality evidence	Benefits closely balanced with risks and burdens	Consistent evidence from well-performed randomized controlled trials or overwhelming evidence of some other form. Further research is unlikely to change our confidence in the estimates of benefits and risks.	Weak recommendation. Best action may differ depending on circumstances or patient or societal values
2B. Weak recommendation, moderate-quality evidence	Benefits closely balanced with risks and burdens, with some uncertainty in the estimates of benefits, risks, and burdens	Evidence from randomized controlled trials with important limitations (inconsistent results, methodologic flaws or imprecision), or very strong evidence from some other research design. Further research (if performed) is likely to change confidence in estimates of benefits and risks.	Weak recommendation. Alternative approaches likely to be better for some patients under some circumstances.
2C. Weak recommendation, low-quality evidence	Uncertainty in the estimates of benefits, risks, and burdens; benefits may be closely balanced with risks and burdens	Evidence from observational studies, unsystematic clinical experience, or randomized controlled trials with serious flaws. Any estimate of effect is uncertain.	Very weak recommendation. Other alternatives may be equally reasonable.

Adapted from Guyatt GH, Oxman AD, Vist GE, et al. for the GRADE Working Group. GRADE: an emerging consensus on rating quality of evidence and strength of recommendations. BMJ 2008;336:924–926.

self-serving results. There are ongoing efforts to limit bias related to conflicts of interest, mainly by insisting on full disclosure but also by excluding people with obvious conflicts of interest from peer review of manuscripts and grants, authorship of review articles and editorials, and from guidelines panels.

LOOKING UP ANSWERS TO CLINICAL QUESTIONS

Clinicians need to be able to look up answers to questions that arise during the care of their patients. They need this for things they do not know but also to check facts they think they know but might not, because the information base for patient care is always changing.

It is best to get answers to questions just at the time and place where they arise during the care of patients. This has been called the point of care and the associated learning just-in-time-learning. Answers can then be used to guide clinical decision making for the patient at hand. Also, what is learned is more likely to be retained than information encountered out of context in a classroom, lecture hall, book, or journal, apart from the need to know for a specific patient. In any case, postponing the answering of questions to a later time too often means they do not get answered at all.

For just-in-time learning to happen, several conditions must be in place (Table 14.2). Most patient care settings are time-pressured, so the answer must come quickly. As an office pediatrician pointed out, "If I added just 1 to 2 extra minutes to each patient visit, I would get home an hour later at the end of the day!" What clinicians need is not *an* answer but the best available answer, given the state of knowledge at the time. They need information that corresponds as closely as possible to the specific clinical situation their patient is in; if the patient is elderly and has several diseases, the research information should be about elderly patients with comorbidities. Clinicians need information sources that move with them as they travel from their office to home (where they take night and weekend call) and to hospitals and nursing homes.

When all this happens, and it certainly can, the results are extraordinarily powerful.

Table 14.2

Conditions in Which Information Is Available at the Point of Care

Condition	Rationale
Rapid access	The information must be available within minutes for it to fit into the busy workflow of most patient care settings.
Current	Because the best information base for clinical decisions is continually changing, the information usually needs to be electronic (as a practical matter, on the Internet).
Tailored to the specific question	Clinicians need information that matches as closely as possible the actual situation of their individual patient.
Sorted by scientific strength	There is a vast amount of information for almost any clinical question but only a small proportion of it is scientifically strong and clinical relevant.
Available in clinical situations	Clinicians cannot leave their place of work to look up answers; they must find it right where they work.

susceptibility to antimalarial drugs varies across the globe and that it is continually changing. The Centers for Disease Control and Prevention have a Web site (http://www.cdc.gov) with current information for travelers to all parts of the world. Using the computer in your clinic, you quickly find out which prophylactic drug this patient should take and for how long before, during, and after the trip. You are also reminded that he should have a booster dose of polio vaccine and be vaccinated for hepatitis A and B, typhoid, and yellow fever. The site lists clinics where these vaccines are available. The site also shows that northern Ghana, where your patient will be visiting, is in the "meningitis belt," so he should also be vaccinated against meningococcal disease. The information you are relying on is an up-to-date synthesis of the world's best advice and is available to you within seconds.

Example

A patient sees you because he will be traveling to Ghana and wants advice on malaria prophylaxis. You are aware that the malaria parasite's

Solutions

Clinical Colleagues

A network of colleagues with various and complementary expertise is a time-honored way of getting point of care information. Many clinicians have identified local opinion leaders for this purpose. Of course, those opinion leaders must have their own sources of information, presumably more than just other colleagues.

Electronic Textbooks

Textbooks, even libraries, are on the Internet and made available to clinicians by their medical schools, health systems, and professional societies. For example, UpToDate (http://www.uptodate.com) is an electronic information resource for clinicians, the product of thousands of physician–authors and editors covering 9,000 topics in the equivalent of 90,000 printed pages (if it were ever printed).[†] Information is continually updated, peer reviewed, searchable and linked to abstracts of the original research, and recommendations are graded. UpToDate is available at the point of care throughout the world wherever the Internet can be accessed by computers or mobile platforms.

Example

One author was seeing patients in Boston during the anthrax scare in 2001. Around that time, biologic terrorists spread anthrax spores through the U.S. postal system, resulting in dozens of cases and five deaths. A young woman came to urgent care because she was worried that a recent skin lesion was caused by anthrax. When told it was not, she responded (somewhat impolitely), "How do you know, you've never seen it?" To which her doctor responded, "Of course not, none of us has, but we know what it looks like. Come with me and I'll show you." Using UpToDate on an office computer, he was able to show the patient several pictures of anthrax skin lesions, which looked quite different from hers, and she gained confidence that she was not, in fact, the next anthrax victim.

Other textbooks, such as ACP Medicine, Harrison's Online, and many subspecialty textbooks, are also available in electronic form.

Clinical Practice Guidelines

Clinical practice guidelines are advice to clinicians about the care of patients with specific conditions. In addition to giving recommendations, good guidelines also make explicit the evidence base and rationale for those recommendations. Like evidence-based medicine, guidelines are meant to be a starting place for decision making about individual patients, to be modified by clinical judgment; that is, they are guidelines, not rules. High-quality guidelines represent the wise application of research evidence to the realities of clinical care, but guidelines vary in quality. Table 14.3

Table 14.3

Standards for Trustworthy Clinical Practice Guidelines

Standard	Explanation
Transparency	How the guideline was developed and funded has been made explicit and is publically accessible.
Conflict of Interest	Group members' conflicts of interest related to financial, intellectual, institutional, and patient/public activities bearing on the guideline are disclosed.
Group Composition	Group membership was multidisciplinary and balanced, comprising a variety of methodological experts and clinicians, and populations expected to be affected by the guideline.
Systematic Review	Recommendations are based on systematic reviews that met high standards for quality.
Evidence and Strength of Recommendation	Each recommendation is accompanied by an explanation for its underlying reasoning, the level of confidence in the evidence, and the strength of the recommendation.
Description of Recommendations	The guideline states precisely what the recommended action is and under what circumstances it should be performed.
External Review	The guideline has been reviewed by the full spectrum of relevant stakeholders (e.g., scientific and clinical experts, organizations, and patients).
Updating	The guideline reports the date of publication and evidence review and plans for updating when there is new evidence that would substantially change the guideline.

Modified from Institute of Medicine. Clinical Practice Guidelines We Can Trust. Washington, DC: National Academies Press; 2011. The standards were for developing guidelines and have been modified to guide users in recognize guidelines they can trust.

[†]Robert and Suzanne Fletcher are among hundreds the editors of UpToDate.

summarizes criteria for credible guidelines developed by the U.S. Institute of Medicine. A relatively comprehensive listing of guidelines can be found at the National Guideline Clearinghouse, which is available online at http://www.guidelines.gov.

The Cochrane Library

Clinical scientists throughout the world have volunteered to review the world's literature on specific clinical questions, to synthesize this information, store it in a central site, and to keep it up to date. The collection of reviews is available at http://www.cochrane.org. Although the Cochrane Library is incomplete, given the vast number of questions it might address, it is an excellent source of systematic reviews, with meta-analyses when justified, on the effects of interventions and, more recently, of diagnostic test performance.

Citation Databases (PubMed and Others)

MEDLINE is a bibliographic database, compiled by the U.S. National Library of Medicine, covering approximately 5,000 journals in biomedicine and health, mostly published in English. It is available free of charge using a search engine, usually PubMed (http://www.ncbi.nlm.nih.gov/pubmed). MEDLINE can be searched by topic, journal, author, year, and research design. In addition to citations, some abstracts are available. EMBASE (http://www.embase.com) is also used and complements what is found in MEDLINE; beyond these two are many other bibliographic databases for more specialized purposes.

PubMed searches are limited by two kinds of misclassification. First, they produce false-negative results; that is, they miss articles that really are wanted. Second, searches produce many false-positive results; that is, they find more citations than are actually wanted on the basis of scientific strength and clinical relevance. For example, when Canadian nephrologists were asked to use PubMed to answer unique clinical questions in their field, they were able to retrieve 46% of relevant articles and the ratio of relevant to non-relevant articles was 1/16 (3). Both problems can be reduced, but not totally overcome, by better searching techniques.

PubMed searches are a mainstay for investigators and educators who have the time to construct careful searches and sort through the resulting articles, but PubMed searches are too inefficient to be of much practical value in helping clinicians, especially in answering day-to-day questions quickly. However, PubMed is particularly useful for looking up whether rare events have been reported.

Example

You are seeing a patient who you thought had cat scratch disease and who now has abdominal pain. After ruling out other causes, you wonder whether the abdominal pain might be from lymphadenopathy. To find out if this has ever been reported, you do a PubMed search and find a case report of cat scratch fever and abdominal lymphadenopathy (4). Armed with this information, even though it is just a report of one case, you are somewhat more confident in your diagnosis and management.

Other Sources on the Internet

A vast amount of health information is posted on the Internet, some of which is quite helpful for health professionals. It can be found by a search engine such as Google or Google Scholar and by sites sponsored by the U.S. government such as MedlinePlus (http://www.nlm.nih.gov/medlineplus) and HealthFinder (http://healthfinder.gov) for health information and Health Hotlines (http://healthhotlines.nlm.nih.gov) for contact information of health related organizations. Other countries have their own Internet resources.

SURVEILLANCE ON NEW DEVELOPMENTS

Keeping up with new developments in any clinical field is a daunting task. It is not that the pace of practice-changing discoveries is unmanageable. Rather, the relevant information is widely dispersed across many journals and mixed with a vast number of less important articles.

Example

How widely are the best articles in a field dispersed among journals? The editors of *ACP Journal Club* regularly review more than 100 journals and select scientifically strong, clinically relevant articles in internal medicine for publication every month. This process provides an opportunity to describe, at least for internal medicine, the degree to which key articles are dispersed among journals. Figure 14.1 shows the proportion of key articles a reader would

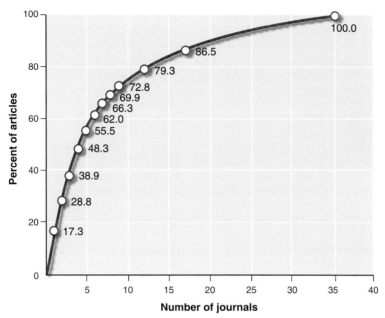

Figure 14.1 ■ How many journals would you have to read to keep up with the literature in your field? The proportion of scientifically strong, clinically relevant articles in internal medicine according to the number of journals, in descending order of yield. (Data from ACP Journal Club, 2011).

encounter according to the number of journals read, starting with the highest yield journal and adding journals in order of descending yield. One would need to regularly review 4 journals to find 50% of these articles, 8 journals to find 75%, and 20 journals to find 90% of the key articles in internal medicine.

Therefore, it is not possible for individual readers, even with great effort, to find all of the essential articles in a field on their own. They need to delegate the task to a trusted intermediary, one who will review many journals and select articles according to criteria they agree with.

Fortunately, help is available. Most clinical specialties sponsor publications that summarize major articles in their field. These publications vary in how explicit and rigorous their selection process is. At one extreme, *ACP Journal Club* publishes its criteria for each kind of article (e.g., studies of prevention, treatment, diagnosis, prognosis) and provides a critique of each article it selects. At the other extreme, many newsletters include summaries of articles without making explicit either how they were selected or what their strengths and limitations are.

There are now various ways to have new information—published research articles, guidelines, white papers, and news articles—in your specific areas of interest sent to you. One way is to identify specific topics and have new information about them automatically sent to you as it arises by means of RSS feeds and other services. Another is to participate in one of a growing number of social media, such as Facebook and blogs, where other people discover and select information you might want to know about and send it to you, just as you send new information to them. Less structured examples are research teams who share articles and news stories related to their work and ward teams in teaching hospitals where residents, students, and attending physicians share articles about their patients' medical problems. Social media can be effective and efficient if you choose the right colleagues to participate with.

JOURNALS

Journals have a central role in the health professions. Everything we have said about clinical epidemiology and knowledge management is based on a foundation of original research published in peer-reviewed journals.

Research reports are selected and improved before publication by a rigorous process involving critical review by editors guided by peer review, comments by experts in the article's content area and methods who provide advice on whether to publish and how a manuscript (the term for the article before it is published) could be improved. The reviewers are advisors to the editor (or editorial team), not the ones who directly decide the fate of the manuscript. Peer-review and editing practices, along with the evidence base and rationale for them, are summarized on the official Web site of the World Association of Medical Editors (http://www.wame.org) and the International Committee of Medical Journal Editors (http://www.icmje.org). Peer review and editing improve manuscripts, but published articles are far from perfect (5); therefore, readers should be grateful for the journals' efforts to make articles better but also maintain a healthy skepticism about the quality of the end result.

Working groups have defined the information that should be in a complete research article according to the type of study (randomized controlled trial, diagnostic test evaluation, systematic review, etc.) (Table 14.4). Readers can use these checklists to see if all the necessary information is included in an article, just as investigators use them to assure that their articles are complete.

Journals themselves are not particularly helpful for some elements of knowledge management. Reading individual journals is not a reliable way of keeping up with new scientific developments in a field or for looking up the answers to clinical questions.

But journals do add another dimension: exposing readers to the full breadth of their profession. Opinions, stories, untested hypotheses, commentary on published articles, expressions of professional values, as well as descriptions of the historical, social, and political context of current-day medicine and much more, reflect the full nature of the profession (Table 14.5). The richness of this information completes the clinical picture for many readers. For example, when *Annals of Internal Medicine* began publishing stories about being a doctor (6), many readers remarked that while reports

Table 14.4

Guidelines for Reporting Research Studies		
Study Type	**Name of Statement**	**Citation**
Randomized Controlled Trials	Consolidated Standards of Reporting Trials (CONSORT)	http://www.consort-statement.org
Diagnostic Tests	Standards for Reporting of Diagnostic Test Accuracy (STARD)	http://www.stard.org
Observational Studies	Strengthening the Reporting of Observational Studies in Epidemiology (STROBE)	http://www.strobe-statement.org
Non-Randomized Studies of Educational, Behavioral, and Public Health Interventions	Transparent Reporting of Evaluations with Nonrandomized Design (TREND)	http://www.cdc.gov/trendstatement
Meta-analyses of Randomized Controlled Trials	Quality of Reporting of Meta-analyses (QUOROM)	Moher D, Cook DJ, Eastwood S, et al. Improving the quality of reports of meta-analyses of randomized controlled trials: the QUOROM statement. Lancet 1999;354:1896–900.
Meta-analyses of Observational Studies	Meta-analyses of Observational Studies in Epidemiology (MOOSE)	Stroup DF, Berlin JA, Morton SC, et al. Meta-analysis of observational studies in epidemiology: a proposal for reporting. Meta-analysis Of Observational Studies in Epidemiology (MOOSE) group. JAMA 2000;283:2008–2012.
Systematic Reviews of Diagnostic Accuracy Studies	Quality Assessment of Diagnostic Accuracy Studies (QUADAS)	Whiting PF, Rutjes AWS, Westwood ME, et al. QUADAS-2: a revised tool for the quality assessment of diagnostic accuracy studies. Ann Intern Med 2011;155:529–536.
Genetic Risk Prediction Studies	Genetic Risk Prediction Studies (GRIPS)	Janssens AC, Ioannidis JP, van Duijn CM, et al. Strengthening the reporting of genetic risk prediction studies: the GRIPS statement. Ann Intern Med 2011;154:421–425.

Table 14.5

The Diverse Contents of a General Medical Journal

Science	The Profession
Original research	Medical education
Preliminary studies	History
Review articles	Public policy
Editorials (for synthesis and opinion)	Book reviews
Letters to the editor	News
Hypotheses	Stories and poems

of research and reviews were essential, the experience of being a doctor was what they cared about the most.

"Reading" Journals

The ability to critique research on one's own is a core skill for clinicians. But this skill is used selectively

and to different degrees, just as the completeness of the history and physical examination, which is part of a clinician's repertoire, is used to a varying extent from one patient encounter to another. It is not necessary to read journals from cover to cover, any more than one would read a newspaper from front to back. Rather, one browses—reads in layers—according to the time available and the strength and relevance of each individual article.

Approaches to streamlined reading vary. It is a good idea to at least survey the titles (analogous to newspaper headlines) of all articles in an issue to decide which articles matter most to you. For those that do, you might read more deeply, adjusting the depth as you go (Fig. 14.2). The abstract is the best place to start, and many responsible readers stop there. If the conclusions are interesting, the methods section might come next; there, one finds basic information bearing on whether the conclusions are credible. One might want to look at the results section to see a more detailed description of what was found. Key figures (e.g., a survival curve for the main results of a randomized trial)

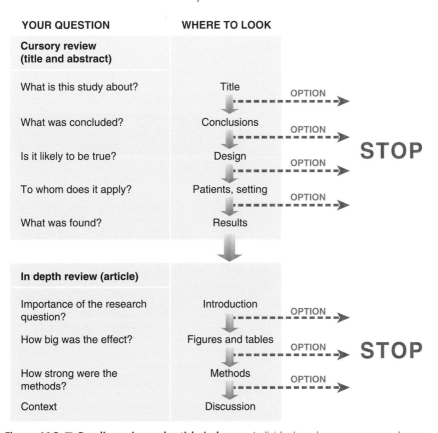

Figure 14.2 ■ Reading a journal article in layers. Individual readers can progress deeper into an article or stop and go on to another, according to its scientific strength and clinical importance to them.

Table 14.6

The Organization of a Structured Abstract

Heading	Value to Reader
Context	Burden of suffering from the disease/illness. Why is the research question important? What is already known?
Objective	What the investigators set out to learn
Setting	The setting to which results can be generalized, such as community, primary care practices, referral centers, and the like
Participants	What kinds of patients (regarding generalizability)? How many (regarding statistical power/precision)?
Design	How strong is the study? How well is it matched to the research question?
Intervention (if any)	Is the intervention state-of-the-art? Is it feasible in your setting?"
Main outcome measures	Are the outcomes clinically important?
Results	What was found?
Limitations	What aspects of the study threaten the validity of the conclusions?
Conclusion	Do the authors believe that the result answers their question? How convincingly?

may communicate the "bottom line" efficiently. A few articles are so important, in relation to one's particular needs, that they are worth reading word for word, perhaps for participation in a journal club.

Structured abstracts are organized according to the kinds of information that critical readers depend on when deciding whether to believe a study's results. Table 14.6 shows headings of abstracts in structured form, along with the kind of information associated with them. (Traditional abstracts, with headings for Introduction, Methods, Results, and Discussion, are a shortened version.) These headings make it easier for readers to find the information they need and also force authors to include this information, some of which might otherwise have been left out if the abstract were less structured.

Unfortunately, many clinicians set goals for journal reading that are higher than they can achieve. They believe they must look at each article in detail, which requires a lot of time with each journal issue. Too often, this results in postponing reading and perhaps never getting to it at all, and it can generate a lot

of anxiety, self-reproach, and cluttered workspaces. If such negative feelings are associated with reading medical journals, something is wrong.

GUIDING PATIENTS' QUEST FOR HEALTH INFORMATION

Patients now look up health information on the Internet. As a result, clinicians have different responsibilities for teaching their patients.

One responsibility is to guide patients to the most credible Web sites. Simple searches, such as for migraine headaches or weight loss, find a rich array of sites, some among the best in the world, others zealous and misguided, and still others commercial and self-serving. Clinicians should be able to suggest especially good Web sites for the patient's particular questions. There are many that are sponsored by governments, medical schools, professional organizations, and patient advocacy groups. Clinicians can also help patients recognize the best health information on the Web, guided by criteria formulated by the Medical Library Association (Table 14.7).

Another responsibility is to help patients weigh the value of information they do find. Here, clinicians have a great deal to offer based on their understanding of clinical epidemiology, the biology of

Table 14.7

Criteria Patients Can Use to Evaluate Health Information on the Web

1. Sponsorship
   - Can you easily identify the site sponsor? Are advisory board members and consultants listed?
   - What is the Web address (gov = government, edu = educational institution, org = professional organization, com = commercial)?
2. Currency
   - The site should have been updated recently, and the date of the latest revision posted.
3. Factual Information
   - The information should be about facts, not opinions, and can be verified from primary sources such as professional articles.
   - When opinions are stated, the source (a qualified professional or organization) should be identified.
4. Audience
   - The Web site should clearly state whether the information is for consumers or health professionals. (Some sites have separate areas for consumers and health professionals).

Modified from Medical Library Association. A User's Guide to Finding and Evaluating Health Information on the Web. Available at http://mlanet.org/resources/userguide.html. Accessed August 1, 2012.

disease, the clinical presentations of illness, the difference between isolated observations and consistent patterns of evidence, and much more. All of this is a valuable complement to what patients bring to the encounter—intense interest in a specific clinical question and the willingness to spend lots of time searching for answers.

PUTTING KNOWLEDGE MANAGEMENT INTO PRACTICE

Clinical epidemiology, as described in this book, is intended to make clinicians' professional lives easier and more satisfying. Armed with a sound grounding in the principles by which the validity and generalizability of clinical information are judged, clinicians can more quickly and accurately detect whether the scientific basis for assertions is sound. For example, they can see when confidence intervals are consistent with clinically important benefit or harm or that a study of the effects of an intervention includes neither randomization nor other efforts to deal with confounding. They are better prepared to participate in discussions with colleagues outside their specialty about patient care decisions. They have a better basis for deciding how to delegate some aspects of their information needs. They can gain more confidence and experience greater satisfaction with the intellectual aspects of their work.

Beyond that, every clinician should have a plan for knowledge management, one that fits his or her particular needs and resources. The Internet must be an important part of the plan because no other medium is so comprehensive, up-to-date, and flexible. Much of the information needed to guide patient care decisions should be available at the point of care so that it can be brought to bear on the patient at hand. There is no reason why the information you use cannot be the best available in the world at the time, as long as you have access to the Internet.

A workable approach to knowledge management must be active. Clinicians should set aside time periodically to revisit their plan, to learn about new opportunities as they arise, and to acquire new skills as they are needed. There has never been a time when the evidence base for clinical medicine was so strong and accessible. Why not make the most of it?

Review Questions

Read the following statements and select the best answer.

14.1. You are finishing residency and will begin practice. You want to establish a plan for keeping up with new developments in your field even though there are few professional colleagues in your community. All of the following might be useful, but which will be *most* useful to you?

   A. Subscribe to a few good journals.
   B. Buy new editions of printed textbooks.
   C. Subscribe to a service that reviews the literature in your field.
   D. Search MEDLINE at regular intervals.
   E. Keep up contacts with colleagues in your training program by e-mail and telephone.

14.2. You can rely on the best general medical journals in your field to:

   A. Provide answers to clinical questions.
   B. Assure that you have kept up with the medical literature.

   C. Guarantee that the information they contain is beyond reproach.
   D. Expose you to the many dimensions of your profession.

14.3. Many children in your practice have attacks of otitis media. You want to base your management on the best available evidence. Which of the following is the *least* credible source of information on this question?

   A. A clinical practice guideline by a major medical society
   B. A systematic review published in a major journal
   C. The Cochrane Database of Systematic Reviews
   D. The most recent research article on this question

14.4. A search of MEDLINE is especially useful for which of the following?

   A. Finding all of the best articles bearing on a clinical question
   B. An efficient strategy for finding the good articles

C. Looking for reports of rare events
D. Keeping up with the medical literature
E. Being familiar with the medical profession as a whole

14.5. Which of the following is accomplished by peer review of research manuscripts before they are published?

A. Exclude articles by authors with a conflict of interest.
B. Make the published article accurate and trustworthy.
C. Relieve readers of the need to be skeptical about the study.
D. Decide for the editors about whether they should publish the manuscript.

14.6. An author of an article showing that screening colonoscopy is more effective in preventing colorectal cancer than other forms of screening would have conflicts of interest if he or she had any of the following *except:*

A. Clinical income from performing colonoscopies
B. Investment in a company that makes colonoscopies
C. Investment in medical products in general
D. Publications of articles that have consistently advocated colonoscopy as the best screening test
E. Rivalry with other scholars who advocate another screening test

14.7. Which of the following is the least useful way of looking up answers to clinical questions at the point of care?

A. Subscribing to several journals and keeping them available where you see patients
B. Guidelines on http://www.guidelines.gov
C. The Cochrane Library on the Internet
D. A continually updated electronic textbook

14.8. Which of the following should be *least* reassuring to a patient about the quality of a Web site providing information about HIV?

A. The site is sponsored by a governmental agency and names its advisory board members.
B. The site provides facts, not opinions.
C. The primary source of information is stated.
D. The author is a well-known expert in the field.
E. The date of the last revision is posted and recent.

14.9. Which of the following is *not* part of grading clinical recommendations using the GRADE system?

A. Deciding whether to use a diagnostic test
B. Takes into account the balance of benefits and harms
C. Rates the quality of scientific evidence separately
D. Suggests how commonly and how forcefully a treatment should be recommended
E. Rates the strength of the evidence and of recommendations separately

14.10. A comprehensive approach to managing knowledge in your field would include which of the following?

A. Subscribing to some journals and browsing them
B. Establishing a plan for looking up information at the point of care
C. Finding a publication that helps you keep up with new developments in your field
D. Identifying Web sites you can recommend to your patients
E. All of the above

Answers are in Appendix A.

REFERENCES

1. Laine C, Horton, R, DeAngelis CD, et al. Clinical trial registration: looking back and moving ahead. Lancet 2007;369:1909–1911.
2. Fletcher RH, Black B. "Spin" in scientific writing: scientific mischief and legal jeopardy. Med Law 2007;26(3):511–525.
3. Shariff SZ, Sontrop JM, Haynes RB, et al. Impact of PubMed search filters on the retrieval of evidence for physicians. CMAJ 2012;184:303.
4. Losanoff JE, Sauter ER, Rider KD. Cat scratch disease presenting with abdominal pain and retroperitoneal lymphadenopathy. J Clin Gastroenterol 2004;38:300–301.
5. Goodman SN, Berlin J, Fletcher SW, et al. Manuscript quality before and after peer review and editing at Annals of Internal Medicine. Ann Intern Med 1994;121:11–21.
6. Lacombe MA, ed. On Being a Doctor. Philadelphia: American College of Physicians; 1995.

Answers to Review Questions

CHAPTER 1   INTRODUCTION

1.1 **D.** Samples can give a misleading impression of the situation in the parent population, especially if the sample is small.

1.2 **E.** Generalizing the results of a study of men to the care of a woman assumes that the effectiveness of surgery for low back pain is the same for men and women.

1.3 **B.** The two treatment groups did not have an equal chance of having pain measured.

1.4 **A.** The difference in recovery between patients who received surgery versus medical care may be the result of some other factor, such as age, that is different between the two treated groups and not the result of surgery itself.

1.5 **B.** These are biases related to measurement of the outcome (recovery from pain).

1.6 **C.** The other medical conditions confound the relationship between treatment and outcome; that is, they are related to both treatment and recovery and might be the reason for the observed differences.

1.7 **C.** The observation that histamines mediate inflammation in hay fever leads to a promising hypothesis that blocking histamines will relieve symptoms, but the hypothesis needs to be tested in people with hay fever. The other answers all assume more about the causes of symptoms than is actually stated. For example, histamine is only one of many mediators of inflammation in hay fever.

1.8 **C.** Samples may misrepresent populations by chance, especially when the samples are small.

1.9 **A.** Generalizing from younger to older patients is a matter of personal judgment based on whatever facts there are that bear on whether older patients respond to treatment the same as younger patients. Internal validity is about whether the results are correct for the patients in the study, not about whether they are correct for other kinds of patients. Both bias and chance affect internal validity.

1.10 **B.** If volunteers had the same amount of exercise as the non-volunteers, a difference in the rate of CHD could not be explained by this variable. Differences in the groups (selection bias) or in the methods used to determine CHD (measurement bias) could account for the finding.

1.11 **C.** The drug's effect on mortality is the most important thing to determine. It is possible that some arrythmia-suppressing drugs can increase the rate of sudden death (in fact, this has happened). In such situations, the intermediate biologic outcome of decreased arrhythmias is an unreliable marker of the clinical outcome—sudden death.

1.12 **B.** Measurement bias is frequently an issue when patients are asked to recall something that may be related to the illness, because those with illness may have heightened recall for preceding events that they think might be related to their illness.

1.13 **B.** The questioning (measurement) about contraceptive use was not the same in the two groups.

1.14 **D.** Small study numbers increase the possibility that chance accounts for differences between groups.

1.15 **A.** Different neighborhoods often are surrogates for socioeconomic variables that are related to numerous health outcomes, which may mean the two groups are different in terms of important covariates.

CHAPTER 2   FREQUENCY

2.1 C. The population at risk is dynamic—people are entering and leaving it continually, so the rates from cancer registries should be reported as person-years.

2.2 A. This is point prevalence because cases are described for a point in time in the course of their life.

2.3 A. There is no follow-up (no time dimension) in a prevalence study.

2.4 D. A random or probability sample is representative of the population sampled in the long run, if enough people in the population are sampled.

2.5 B. In a steady state, duration of disease = prevalence/incidence. In this case, it is 1/100 divided by 40/10,000/year = 25 years.

2.6 D. A study beginning with existing patients with a disease and looking back at their previous experience with the disease would not be a cohort study, which begins with patients with something in common (e.g., new onset of disease) and follows them forward in time for subsequent health events.

2.7 C. Even though sampling every 10th patient might produce a representative sample, it would not be random and could misrepresent the population sampled.

2.8 C. Children with another seizure were all part of the original cohort of children with a first seizure.

2.9 E. A larger sample would produce an estimate of incidence that is closer to the true one by reducing random error. It would not introduce a systematic difference in incidence as A–D would.

2.10 A. It is endemic because it is confined to a geographic area.

2.11 E. The cases existed any time in a 3-month period.

2.12 C. Dynamic populations, such as residents of the State of North Carolina, are continually turning over because of births and deaths as well as out-migration and in-migration.

2.13 A. Children in the cohort have in common being born in North Carolina in 2012 and are followed up for scoliosis as it develops over time.

2.14 D. Prevalence studies are not useful for diseases of short duration because there will be few cases at a point in time. They do not measure incidence and cannot provide much evidence bearing on cause.

2.15 E. A number like 800,000 without an associated denominator is not a rate and is, therefore, not any of the incidence and prevalence rates given in A–D.

CHAPTER 3   ABNORMALITY

3.1 D. Ordinal

3.2 B. Dichotomous

3.3 A. Interval—continuous

3.4 E. Interval—discrete

3.5 C. Nominal

3.6 C. This approach, called construct validity, is one of the ways of establishing the validity of a measurement. Note that answers B and D relate to reliability, not validity.

3.7 D. All except D are reasons for variation in measurements on a single patient, whereas D is about variation among patients.

3.8 D. Because clinical distributions do not necessarily follow a normal distribution, abnormality should not be defined by whether or not they do.

3.9 A. Naturally occurring distributions may or may not resemble the normal curve.

3.10 C. Although ultimately you and the patient may decide on a trial of statin therapy, this is not an emergency situation. The cholesterol test should be repeated; elevated values are often lower on repeat testing. A trial of exercise and weight loss can also lower cholesterol. Patients who are otherwise healthy and with a <10% 10-year risk of cardiovascular diseases are usually not immediately prescribed medication to lower cholesterol.

3.11 B. The figure shows one mode (hump). The median and mean are similar to each other, and are both below 4,000 g.

3.12 C. Two standard deviations encompass 95% of the values. The distribution is not skewed. Range is sensitive to extreme values.

3.13 B. One standard deviation encompasses about 2/3 of values around the mean. Looking at the figure, 2/3 of the values around the mean would be approximately 3,000 to 4,000 g.

3.14 D. Panel A of Figure 3.13 shows approximately even dispersion of measurements above and below the true value, suggesting chance variation. The effect of different observers making the measurements (interobserver variability) could also be at play.

3.15 G. Panel B shows skewed measurements to the right of the true value. In other words, the hospital staff tended to overestimate the electronic monitor results and record normal fetal heart rates when they were abnormal on electronic monitoring, thus demonstrating biased measurements. Chance and interobserver variability may also be involved because not all the measurements are the same.

3.16 G. Panel C shows similar results to Panel B except that the bias is in the other direction, that is, the hospital staff tended to underestimate the electronic monitor results. In both Panels B and C, the hospital staff measurements tended to "normalize" what were abnormal electronic monitor measurements.

CHAPTER 4   RISK: BASIC PRINCIPLES

4.1 A. When a risk factor is common in a population, it is important to compare its prevalence in people with and without disease. There is no comparison in the example. Lung cancer is a common cancer, and smoking is a strong, not weak, risk factor for cancer. The fact that there are other risk factors for lung cancer is not relevant.

4.2 B. Risk factors are sought when a new disease appears, as was the case with HIV.

4.3 D. Risk prediction models are used in all situations.

4.4 C. Because so many more women were assigned to the low-risk stratum, the largest number of cases will likely come from that group. Risk prediction models give probabilities but do not predict which persons in a group will develop disease. The figure does not give information about incorrect assignments to the strata.

4.5 C. The patient is unlikely to develop colorectal cancer in the next 5 years because he is a member of the group with a low probability, but he could be one of the 2% who develops disease. Even for a common cancer, there are subgroups of people with a low probability of developing it. For example, few young people develop colorectal cancer.

4.6 B. Well-constructed risk models are more likely to be highly calibrated (able to predict the percentage of a group that develops disease) than have good discrimination (able to predict which individuals in the group will develop disease).

4.7 A. Markers help identify groups with increased risk of disease, but because they are not causes of disease, removing the marker does not prevent disease. Markers are usually confounded with cause of disease (see Chapters 1 and 5).

4.8 B. Symptoms, physical examination findings, and laboratory tests are generally more important than risk factors when diagnosing disease.

4.9 D. The overlap of the two groups demonstrates that the risk model does not discriminate well between women who did and did not develop breast cancer over 5 years. The figure gives no direct information about calibration and stratification. Few women who developed breast cancer were at high risk.

4.10 C. Good calibration does not impair discrimination. However, risk models can discriminate poorly even if they are highly calibrated, as the example in the text shows.

CHAPTER 5   RISK: EXPOSURE TO DISEASE

5.1 C. Retrospective cohort studies do not allow investigators the luxury of deciding what data to collect. They can only choose from the available data collected at a time before the study originated. Also, these data, which are often collected for clinical purposes, may not have been collected systematically and in the same way. Answers A, B, and D are correct for both prospective and retrospective cohort studies.

5.2 B. Relative risk is the ratio of incidence of an outcome (disease) in exposed ÷ non-exposed. Therefore, the relative risk of stroke in smokers compared to non-smokers in their 40s is 29.7 ÷ 7.4 = 4.0

5.3 D. Attributable risk (AR) is the risk of disease attributable to the risk factor and is calculated as the difference in absolute risk (incidence) of exposed persons minus that in non-exposed persons. Therefore, the attributable risk of stroke in smokers compared to non-smokers in their 60s is 110.4 – 80.2 = 30.2.

5.4 C. Relative risk gives no information about incidence, whereas attributable risk does, so the statement in C is incorrect. The other answers are all correct. To calculate population attributable risk, one must know the prevalence of a risk factor in the population, which is not given in the question. The incidence of stroke among smokers was higher in the 60s than in the 40s. The RR of stroke among smokers in the 40s was 4.0, compared to 1.4 in the 60s. Stronger relative risks are better evidence for a causal relationship than weaker ones. In the analysis of this study, age could be treated as either a confounding variable and controlled for or, as in the information presented, as an effect modifier showing that the effect of smoking varies by age.

5.5 A. Absolute risk is another term for incidence. DVT is a rare event in most women, and the incidence in this study was 0.8/10,000/yr among women who neither had the mutation nor took OCs.

5.6 C. A good way to organize your thinking for questions 5.6–5.10 is to create a 2 × 2 table of the incidence of DVT according to OC use (present/absent) and factor V Leiden (present/absent).

Incidence (per 10,000/yr) of DVT According to OC Use and Mutation for Factor V Leiden

		OC Use	
		Present	**Absent**
Factor V Leiden	*Present*	28.5	5.7
	Absent	3.0	0.8

The table shows that among women who do not carry the factor V Leiden mutation the attributable risk of DVT for taking OC compared to those who do not take OC is 3.0/10,000 – 0.8/10,000 = 2.2/10,000.

5.7 E. The attributable risk of DVT among OC users who also carry factor V Leiden is substantial when compared to most women using OC, 28.5/10,000 – 3.0/10,000 = 25.5/10,000.

5.8 B. Population attributable risk = attributable risk (25.5/10,000 women/yr) × prevalence of factor V Leiden (0.05) = 1.3/10,000 women/yr

5.9 C. Relative risk is calculated by dividing the incidence of DVT among women carrying the factor V Leiden mutation and using OCs by the incidence of DVT in women who take OCs but do not carry the mutation (28.5/10,000/yr ÷ 3.0/10,000 = 9.5)

5.10 A. Among women without the mutation, the relative risk for DVT and using OCs is calculated by dividing the incidence among those taking OCs by the incidence among those not using OCs (3.0/10,000/yr ÷ 0.8/10,000/yr = 3.8).

5.11 C. Using OCs in a woman heterozygous for factor V Leiden is an example of a risk factor with a substantial relative risk (prescribing OCs to such a woman increases her chance of developing DVT with a relative risk of 5.0) but a relatively small absolute risk—28.5 women out of 10,000 who have the mutation and use OCs would develop DVT in the next year. Even more relevant for this patient is that her absolute risk would rise from about 6 to about 28 per 10,000 over the next year. It is important for a known carrier who wants to take OCs to understand that her risk is increased and to know how much that increased risk is in absolute terms. A prudent clinician would also want to be sure that the patient does not have other indications of increased risk of thrombosis such as age, smoking, or a family or personal history of clotting problems. This kind of decision requires careful judgment from both patient and clinician. However, using absolute or attributable risk will clarify the risk for the patient better than using relative risk when discussing clinical consequences.

5.12 B. The degree of illness may have confounded the results in this study so that sicker patients are more likely to take aspirin. One way to examine this possibility and adjust for confounding if it is present is to stratify the users and non-users into groups with similar indications for using aspirin and compare death rates in the subgroups.

CHAPTER 6   RISK: FROM DISEASE TO EXPOSURE

6.1 B. If exposure to oral contraceptives was recorded just after the myocardial infarction, it could not have been a cause of it. All of the other choices could have artificially increased exposure in cases, resulting in a falsely elevated odds ratio.

6.2 E. Even an exemplary cases-control study such as this one should not claim that it has identified a cause because unmeasured confounding is always possible.

6.3 E. Case-control studies produce only odds ratios, which can be used to estimate relative risk.

6.4 C. Epidemic curves describe the rise and fall in the number of cases over the time of the outbreak.

6.5 A. One can always obtain a crude relative risk from a cohort study. However, if the cohort data do not contain all of the variables that should be controlled for, a case-control analysis of the cohort study is a more efficient approach to including the additional data because the data needs to be collected only for cases and controls, not for the entire cohort.

6.6 D. It would be better to sample cases and controls from a cohort rather than a dynamic population, especially if exposure or disease is changing rapidly over time and if controls are not matched to the date of onset of disease for cases.

6.7 E. Multiple control groups (not to be confused with multiple controls per case) are a way of examining whether the results are "sensitive" to the types of controls chosen, that is, whether the results using the different control groups are substantially different, calling the results into question.

6.8 C. Case-control studies do not provide information on incidence (although if they are nested in a cohort, a cohort analysis of the same data can).

6.9 B. Matching is used to control for variables that might be strongly related to exposure or disease, to be sure that at least the cases and controls do not differ on those variables.

6.10 C. The crude odds ratio is obtained by creating a 2×2 table relating the number of cases versus controls to the number of exposed versus non-exposed people and dividing the cross products. In this case, the odds ratio is 60×60 divided by $40 \times 40 = 2.25$.

6.11 E. Case-control studies cannot study multiple outcomes because they begin with the presence or absence of only one disease, cannot report incidence, and cases should be incident (new onset), not prevalent.

6.12 D. Odds ratios based on prevalent cases can provide a rough measure of association but not a comparison of risk, which is about incident (new-onset) cases.

6.13 D. During the early phases of an outbreak, the offending microbe or toxin is usually known, but even if it is not, the most pressing question is how the disease is being spread. This information can then be used to stop the outbreak and identify the source.

6.14 C. If a case-control study is based on all or a random sample of cases and a random sample of controls from a population or cohort, the cases and controls should be similar to each other on characteristics other than exposure.

6.15 D. Case-controls studies do not provide information on incidence.

6.16 E. The odds ratio approximates the relative risk when the disease is rare; a rule of thumb is $<1/100$.

CHAPTER 7 PROGNOSIS

7.1 A. Zero time is at the onset of disease (in this case, Barrett's esophagus), not the time of outcome events (in this case, esophageal cancer).

7.2 C. Different rates of dropping out would bias results only if those who dropped out had a systematically different prognosis from those who remained.

7.3 E. Responses A–D are all possible reasons for measurement bias, whereas a true difference in incontinence rates between patients treated with surgery versus medical care would not be a systematic error.

7.4 E. Responses A–D are all features of clinical prediction rules.

7.5 C. Case series are a hybrid research strategy, not describing clinical course in a cohort nor relative risk with a case-control approach nor studying a representative sample of prevalent cases.

7.6 C. Patients would be censored for any reason that removes them from the study or causes them not to be in the study for as long as 3 years. If the outcome is survival, having another potentially fatal disease would not matter if they had not yet died of it.

7.7 A. Prognosis is about disease outcomes over time, and prevalence studies do not measure events over time.

7.8 B. Survival curves estimate survival in a cohort, after taking into account censored patients, and do not directly describe the proportion of the original cohort who survived.

7.9 E. All of the responses might be correct depending on the research question. For example, it would be useful to know prognosis both among patient in primary care and also among those referred to specialists.

7.10 B. Because patients had to meet stringent criteria to be included in the trial, the clinical course of those assigned to usual care would not be representative of patients with the disease, as they occur in the general population or in a defined clinical setting. Therefore, the results would not be generalizable to any naturally occurring group of patients with multiple sclerosis.

7.11 B. Even if clinical prediction rules are constructed using the best available methods, the strongest test of their ability to predict is that they have been shown to do so in patients other that the ones used to develop the rule.

7.12 D. A hazard ratio is calculated from information in a survival curve and is similar but not identical to relative risk.

7.13 C. Outcome events in time-to-event analyses are either/or events that occur only once.

CHAPTER 8 DIAGNOSIS

First, determine the numbers for each of the four cells in Figure 8.2: a = 49; b = 79; c = 95 – 49 (or 46); d = 152 – 79 (or 73). Add the numbers to determine the column and row totals.

8.1 C. 52% Sensitivity = 49/95 = 52%

8.2 B. 48% Specificity = 73/152 = 48%

8.3 A. 38% Positive predictive value = 49/128 = 38%

8.4 D. 61% Negative predictive value = 73/119 = 61%

8.5 A. 38% Prevalence of sinusitis in this practice = 95/247 = 38%

8.6 A. 38%

1. Calculate LR of a positive test (patient has facial pain)

$$LR+ = \frac{49/(49+46)}{79/(79+73)} = 1.0$$

2. Convert pretest probability to pretest odds

$$\text{Pretest odds} = \text{prevalence}/(1 - \text{prevalence}) = 0.38/(1 - 0.38) = 0.61$$

3. Calculate posttest odds by multiplying pretest odds by LR+

$$\text{Posttest odds} = 0.61 \times 1.0 = 0.61$$

4. Convert posttest odds to posttest probability

Posttest
probability = posttest odds/(1 + posttest odds)
= 0.61/(1 + 0.61)
= 0.38 or 38%

(Another, simpler, approach is that posttest probability = positive predictive value)

+ PV = 49/128
= 38%

8.7 D. ~75% The LR for "high probability" of sinusitis was 4.7 and the pretest probability (prevalence) was 38%. You can use one of three methods to determine the posttest probability of sinusitis among patients with "high probability" of sinusitis: (1) the mathematical approach outlined in Figure 8.8 (or on Web sites), (2) using a nomogram, or (3) using the bedside "rule of thumb" approach outlined in Table 8.3.

1. Mathematical approach:
   Pretest odds = 0.38/(1.38) = 0.61
   LR+ × pretest odds = 4.7 × 0.61 = 2.9
   Posttest probability = 2.9/(1 + 2.9)
   = 0.74 or 74%

2. Nomogram:
   Put ruler on 38% for prevalence and 4.7 for LR; it crosses the posttest number at approximately 75%.

3. Bedside "rule of thumb":
   An LR of 4.7 (close to 5) increases the probability of sinusitis approximately 30 percentage points, from 38% to 68%.

8.8 C. ~45%

8.9 B. ~20%

8.10 C. As prevalence becomes smaller, the predictive value of a test decreases (see Fig. 8.7). Clinicians are more likely to treat a patient with a 75% probability of sinusitis than to forego treatment for one with 20% probability. (For the latter, further testing, such as sinus x-rays, may be warranted.) The posttest probability of "intermediate probability" of sinusitis is 45%, close to a coin toss.

8.11 D. Requiring two independent tests to be abnormal, that is, using them in series, increases specificity and positive predictive value. (See example on page 126–7 and Table 8.4). However, this approach lowers sensitivity; therefore, B is incorrect. Using tests in parallel increases sensitivity (making A incorrect) but usually decreases positive predictive value (making C incorrect). Work with Figure 8.2 and 8.3 to convince yourself.

8.12 A. The most important requirement when using multiple tests is that each contributes independent information not already evident from a previous test. When using tests in series, performing the test with the highest specificity first is most efficient and requires fewer patients to undergo both tests. In parallel testing, performing the test with the highest sensitivity is most efficient.

CHAPTER 9   TREATMENT

9.1 A. Every effort was made to make this trial as true to life as possible by comparing drugs in common use, having broad eligibility criteria, not blinding participants, allowing care to proceed as usual, and relying on a patient-centered outcome rather than a laboratory measurement. Although the trial is for efficacy, it is better described as practical and it is certainly not large.

9.2 D. Intention-to-treat analysis, counting outcomes according to the treatment group that patients `were randomized to, tests the effects of offering treatment, regardless of whether patients actually take it. It is, therefore, about effectiveness in ordinary circumstances and the measure of effect, like usual care, is affected by drop-outs, reducing the observed treatment effect over what it would have been if everyone took the treatment they were assigned to.

9.3 A. All characteristics at the time of randomization, such as severity of disease, are randomly allocated. Characteristics arising after randomization, such as retention, response to treatment, and compliance, are not.

9.4 D. The greatest advantage of randomized trials over observational studies is prevention of confounding. Randomization creates comparison groups that would have the same outcome rates, on average, were it not for intervention effects.

9.5 E. The study had extensive inclusion and exclusion criteria. This would increase the extent to which patients in the trial were similar to each other, making it easier to detect treatment differences if they exist, but at the expense of generalizability, the ability to extrapolate from study results to ordinary patient care.

9.6 A. Intention-to-treat analyses describe the effects of being offered treatments, not necessarily taking them. To describe the effects of actually receiving the intervention, one would have to treat the data as if they were from a cohort study and use a variety of methods to control for confounding.

9.7 B. Stratified randomization is one approach to control of confounding, especially useful when a characteristic is strongly related to outcome—and also when the study is small enough that one worries that randomization might not create groups with similar prognosis.

9.8 C. In explanatory analyses, outcomes are attributed to the treatment patients actually receive, not the treatment group they were randomized to, which is an intention-to-treat analysis.

9.9 B. Side effects of the drug, both symptoms and signs, would alert patients and doctors to who is taking the active drug but could not affect random allocation, which was done before drug was begun.

9.10 C. For a randomized controlled trial to be ethical, there should not be conclusive evidence that one of the experimental treatments is better or worse than the other—that is, the scientific community should be in a state of "equipoise" on that issue. There may be opinions as to which is better, but no consensus. There may

be some evidence bearing on the comparison, but the evidence should not be conclusive.

9.11 D. Because the new drug has advantages over the old one, but comparative effectiveness is unknown, the appropriate randomized trial comparing the two would be a non-inferiority trial to establish whether the new drug is no less efficacious.

9.12 A. Making the primary outcome of a trial a composite of clinically important and related outcomes increases the number of outcome events and, therefore, the ability of the trial to detect an effect if it is present. The disadvantage is that the intervention may affect the component outcomes differently, and reliance on the composite outcome alone might mask this effect.

9.13 C. Both bad luck in randomization and breakdown in allocation concealment (by bad methods or cheating) would show up as differences in baseline characteristics of patients in a trial. Small differences are expected and the challenge is to decide how large the differences must be for them to raise concern.

9.14 C. The usual drug trials reported in the clinical literature are "Phase III" trials, intended to establish efficacy or effectiveness. Further study, with postmarketing surveillance, is needed to detect uncommon side effects. Responses A and D are about what Phase I and Phase II trials are meant to establish.

9.15 B. Prevention of confounding is the main advantage of randomized controlled trials, which is why they are valued despite being ethically complicated, slower, and more expensive. Whether they resemble usual care depends on how the trial is designed.

CHAPTER 10   PREVENTION

10.1 A. 33%. The relative risk reduction of colorectal cancer mortality is the absolute risk reduction divided by the cancer mortality rate in the control group. (See Chapter 9.)

The colorectal cancer mortality rate in the screened group = 82/15,570 = 0.0053

The colorectal cancer mortality rate in the control group = 121/15,394 = 0.0079

Absolute risk reduction = 0.0079 − 0.0053 = 0.0026

Relative risk reduction of colorectal cancer mortality due to screening = 0.0026/0.0079 =

0.33 or 33% reduction. An alternative approach calculates the complement of relative risk. In the example, the relative risk of colorectal mortality in the screened compared to the control group was 0.0053/0.0079 = 0.67. The complement of 0.67 = 1.00 − 0.67 = 0.33 or 33%.

10.2 C. 385. The number needed to screen is the reciprocal of absolute risk reduction, 1/0.0026, or 385.

10.3 **C.** If 30% of the screened group were found to have polyps, at least 4,671 (0.3 × 15,570) had a false-positive test for colon cancer. If the sensitivity of the test was 90% and the number of cancers was 82, about 74 people (0.9 × 82) had a true-positive result. The positive predictive value of the test, therefore, would be about 74/(74 + 4,671), or 1.6%. (Using exact numbers, the authors calculated a positive predictive value of 2.2%). Negative predictive value was not calculated, but it would be high because the incidence of cancer over 13 years was low (323/15,570 or 21 per thousand) and about 90% of tests were negative.

10.4 **B.** Lead time (the period time between the detection of a disease on screening and when it would ordinarily be diagnosed because the patient seeks medical care due to symptoms) can be associated with what appears to be an improvement in survival. The fact that mortality did not improve after screening in this randomized trial raises the possibility that lead-time bias is responsible for the result. Another possible cause of the finding is overdiagnosis.

10.5 **A.** See answer for **10.4.**

10.6 **C.** Overdiagnosis, the detection of lesions that would not have caused clinical symptoms or morbidity, is likely because, even after 20 years, the number of cancers in the control group remained fewer than that in the screened group. Increased numbers of cancers in the screened group could occur if there were more smokers in the screened group, but randomization should have made that possibility unlikely.

10.7 **D.** Several important questions are to be considered when assessing a new vaccine, including: (i) Has the vaccine been shown to be efficacious (did it work under ideal circumstances when everyone in the intervention group received the vaccine and no one in a comparable control group did) and was it effective (under every day circumstances, in which some people in the intervention group did not receive the vaccine)? (ii) Is the vaccine safe? (iii) Is the burden of suffering of the condition the vaccine protects against important enough to consider a preventive measure? and (iv) Is it cost-effective? Cost of the vaccine is only one component of an analysis of cost-effectiveness.

10.8 **C.** Disease prevalence is lower in presumably well people (screening) than in symptomatic patients (diagnosis). As a result, positive predictive value will be lower in screening. Because screening is aimed at picking up early disease, the sensitivity of most tests is lower in screening than in patients with more advanced disease. Overdiagnosis is less likely in diagnostic situations when symptomatic patients have more late-stage disease.

10.9 **C.** Volunteers for preventive care are more compliant with advice about medical care and usually have better health outcomes than those who reject preventive care. This effect is so strong that it is seen even when volunteers are taking placebo medications.

10.10 **B.** The incidence method is particularly useful when calculating sensitivity for screening tests because it takes into account the possibility of overdiagnosis. The gold standard for screening tests almost always involves a follow-up interval. The first round of screening picks up prevalent as well as incident cases, inflating the number compared to later screening rounds.

10.11 **E.** Cost-effectiveness should be estimated in a way that captures all costs of the preventive activity and all the costs associated with diagnosis and treatment, wherever they occur, to determine the costs of the preventive activity from a societal perspective. All costs that occur when prevention is not done are subtracted from all costs when prevention is done to estimate the cost for a given health effect.

CHAPTER 11   CHANCE

11.1 **C.** Although subgroup analyses risk false-positive and false-negative conclusions, they provide information that can help clinicians as long as their limitations are kept in mind

11.2 **C.** The P value describes the risk of a false-positive conclusion and has nothing directly to do with bias and statistical power or the generalizability or clinical importance of the finding

11.3 **E.** The P value is not small enough to establish that a treatment effect exists and provides no information on whether a clinically important effect could have been missed because of inadequate statistical power.

11.4 D. The result was statistically significant, if one wanted to think of the role of chance in that way, because it excluded a relative risk of 1.0. Response D described the information the confidence interval contributes.

11.5 B. Calling P ≤ 0.05 "statistically significant" is a useful convention but otherwise has no particular mathematical or clinical meaning.

11.6 A. Models do depend on assumptions about the data, are not done in a standard way, and are meant to complement stratified analyses, not replace them. Although they might be used in large randomized trials, they are not particularly useful in that situation because randomization of a large number of patients has already made confounding very unlikely.

11.7 C. Of the 12,000 people in the trial, about 6,000 would be in the chemoprevention arm of the trial. Applying the rule of thumb mentioned in this chapter (but solving for event rater, not sample size), 6,000 divided by 3 or a 1/2,000 event rate could be detected with 6,000 people under observation.

11.8 E. Statistical power depends on the joint effects of all of the factors mentioned in A–D. It may vary a bit with the statistical test used to calculate it, but this is not the main determinate of sample size.

11.9 B. Bayesian reasoning is about how new information affects prior belief and has nothing to do with inferential statistics or the ethical rationale for randomized trials.

11.10 D. The results are consistent with a 1% up to a 46% higher death rate, with the best estimate being 22% higher, and excludes a hazard ratio of 1.0 (no effect), so it is "statistically significant." Confidence internals provide more information than a P value for the same data because they include the point estimate and range of values that is likely to include the true effect.

CHAPTER 12 CAUSE

12.1 B. It would be unethical to randomly allocate a potentially harmful activity, and people would probably not accept long-term restrictions on their use of cell phones.

12.2 E. All responses, which reflect Bradford Hill criteria, would be useful in deciding whether cell phones cause brain cancer, but E, a lack of specificity, is weaker than the rest. (Consider how many diseases cigarette smoking causes.)

12.3 C. Figure 12.1 shows how several risk factors act together to cause coronary heart disease. Nearly all diseases are caused by the joint effect of genes and environment. Figure 12.3 shows a huge decline in tuberculosis rate before effective treatment was established in the 1950s.

12.4 B. In the absence of bias, statistical significance establishes that an association is unlikely to be by chance whereas the Bradford Hill criteria go beyond that to establish whether an association is cause-and-effect.

12.5 C. Cost-effectiveness analyses describe financial costs per clinical effects, such as year of life saved, as in this example, for alternative tests and treatments.

12.6 D. When exposure and disease are measured in groups, not individuals, it is possible that the individuals who got the disease were not the ones who were exposed and that people who were exposed were not the ones who got the disease, a problem called the "ecological fallacy."

12.7 B. In a time-series study, a change in the rate of disease after an intervention might be caused by other changes in local conditions at about the same time. This possibility needs to be ruled out before one can have confidence that the study exposure caused the outcome.

12.8 B. Randomized controlled trials, if well designed and carried out, are the strongest evidence for cause and effect. But they are not possible for many suspected causes because it is not ethical to involve people is studies of harm and because they may not be willing to cooperate with such a trial.

12.9 E. The pattern of evidence from all of the Bradford Hill criteria is more powerful than evidence for any one of them.

12.10 D. The confidence interval is so wide that it is consistent with either harm or benefit and, therefore, does not even establish whether there is an association between cell phones and brain cancer, let alone whether cell phones are a cause.

CHAPTER 13 SUMMARIZING THE EVIDENCE

13.1 E. The main advantage of combining (pooling) study results in a systematic review is to have a larger sample size and as a result a more stable and precise estimate of effect size. Although it could be argued that the results are somewhat more generalizable because they come from more than one time and place, generalizability is not the main advantage.

13.2 D. MEDLINE can be searched using both content and methods terms, but it does not include all of the world's journals, searches miss some of the articles in MEDLINE, and they are not a remedy for publication bias since all citations in it are published. These limitations are why reviewers need to use other, complementary ways of searching for articles in addition to MEDLINE.

13.3 B. Although individual studies usually have limited statistical power in subgroups, pooling of several studies may overcome this problem, as long as patients, not trials, are pooled.

13.4 A. B–E are elements of PICO, core components of a specific research question. Covariates are a critical aspect of the research, especially for observational studies and to identify effect modification in clinical trials, but they are about how successfully the question can be answered, not the question itself.

13.5 B. Systematic reviews should include a description of the methodologic strength of the studies to help users understand how strong the conclusions are. Combining individual elements of quality into a summary measure is less well established, perhaps because it is not meaningful to give each element the same weight.

13.6 D. The usual situation is that small negative studies (ones that find no effect) are less likely to be published than small studies that find effects. Large studies are likely to be published no matter what they find.

13.7 B. Narrative reviews can take a comprehensive approach to the set of questions clinicians must answer to manage a patient but that is at the expense of a transparent description of the scientific basis for the evidence cited.

13.8 B. Forest plots summarize the raw evidence in a systematic review. Pooled effect size and confidence interval may or may not be included, depending on whether it is appropriate to combine the study results.

13.9 A. It is not possible to control for a covariate in a study-level meta-analysis, as one might in one of the parent studies or in a patient-level meta-analysis.

13.10 A. Pooling is justified if there is relatively little heterogeneity across studies, as determined by an informed review of the patient, interventions, and outcomes. A statistical rest for heterogeneity is also useful in general, but not in this case, with so few studies, because of low statistical power.

13.11 D. Random effects models take heterogeneity into account, at least if it is not extreme, and, therefore, result in wider confidence intervals, which are more likely to be accurate than the narrower confidence intervals that would result from a fixed effect model.

CHAPTER 14 KNOWLEDGE MANAGEMENT

14.1 C. It is virtually impossible to keep up with all scientifically strong, clinically relevant new research in your field without help from a publication that does that for you.

14.2 D. Journals are a rich source if information on the many aspects of being a physician—the history, politics, science, ideas, experiences, and more—but are not particularly good for finding answers to immediate questions or even surveillance on new developments in your field.

14.3 D. The resources listed in A–C are all excellent for looking up the answers to clinical questions, whereas a recent article, out of context with others of the same question, is of marginal value unless it happens to be much stronger than all the others that preceded it.

14.4 C. PubMed searches are indispensable for finding whether a rare event has been reported. They are one important part of an effort to find all published articles on a specific clinical question and are useful for researchers, but they are too inefficient for most questions at the point of care.

14.5 B. Although peer review and editing make articles better (more readable, accurate, and complete), articles are far from perfect when the process is over and they are published.

14.6 C. Conflict of interest is in relation to a specific activity and does not exist in the general case of investing in medical products not specifically related to colonoscopy.

14.7 A. B–E are all valuable resources for looking up the answers to clinical questions at the point of care (if computers and the relevant programs are available). Medical journals have great value for other reasons, but they are not useful for this purpose.

14.8 D. Patients and clinicians alike might well respect famous experts but should look for more solid footing—the organization that sponsors them, facts and the source of those facts—when deciding whether to believe them.

14.9 A. GRADE has been developed for treatment recommendations, but not other clinical questions.

14.10 E. All are basic elements of a comprehensive knowledge management plan, as described in this chapter.

Additional Readings

1. INTRODUCTION

Clinical Epidemiology

Feinstein AR. Why clinical epidemiology? Clin Res 1972;20: 821–825.

Feinstein AR. Clinical Epidemiology. The Architecture of Clinical Research. Philadelphia: WB Saunders; 1985.

Feinstein AR. Clinimetrics. New Haven, CT: Yale University Press; 1987.

Hulley SB, Cummings SR. Designing Clinical Research. An Epidemiologic Approach, 3rd ed. Philadelphia: Lippincott Williams & Wilkins; 2007.

Riegelman RIC. Studying and Study and Testing a Test, 5th ed. Philadelphia: Lippincott Williams & Wilkins; 2005.

Sackett DL. Clinical epidemiology. Am J Epidemiol 1969; 89:125–128.

Sackett DL, Haynes RB, Guyatt GH, et al. Clinical Epidemiology: A Basic Science for Clinical Medicine, 2nd ed. Boston: Little, Brown and Company; 1991.

Weiss NS. Clinical Epidemiology: The Study of the Outcomes of Illness, 3rd ed. New York: Oxford University Press; 2006.

Evidence-Based Medicine

Guyatt G, Rennie D, Meade M, et al. User's Guide to the Medical Literature: Essentials of Evidence-Based Clinical Practice, 2nd ed. Chicago: American Medical Association Press; 2008.

Hill J, Bullock I, Alderson P. A summary of the methods that the National Clinical Guideline Centre uses to produce clinical guidelines for the National Institute for Health and Clinical Excellence. Ann Intern Med 2011:154:752–757.

Jenicek M, Hitchcock D. Evidence-Based Practice: Logic and Critical Thinking in Medicine. Chicago: American Medical Association Press; 2005.

Straus SE, Glasziou P, Richardson WS, et al. Evidence-Based Medicine: How to Practice and Teach It, 4th ed. New York: Elsevier; 2011.

Epidemiology

Friedman GD. Primer of Epidemiology, 5th ed. New York: Appleton and Lange; 2004.

Gordis L. Epidemiology, 4th ed. Philadelphia: Elsevier/Saunders; 2009.

Greenberg RS, Daniels SR, Flanders W, et al. Medical Epidemiology, 4th ed. New York: Lange Medical Books/McGraw Hill; 2005.

Hennekins CH, Buring JE. Epidemiology in Medicine. Boston: Little, Brown and Company; 1987.

Jekel JF, Elmore JG, Katz DL. Epidemiology, Biostatistics and Preventive Medicine, 3rd ed. Philadelphia: Elsevier/Saunders; 2007.

Rothman KJ. Epidemiology: An Introduction. New York: Oxford University Press; 2002.

Related Fields

Brandt AM, Gardner M. Antagonism and accommodation: interpreting the relationship between public health and medicine in the United States during the 20th century. Am J Public Health 2000;90:707–715.

Kassirer JP, Kopelman RI. Learning Clinical Reasoning. Baltimore: Williams & Wilkins; 1991.

Sox, HC, Blatt MA, Higgins MC, et al. Medical Decision Making. Philadelphia, American College of Physicians, 2006.

White KL. Healing the Schism: Epidemiology, Medicine, and the Public's Health. New York: Springer-Verlag; 1991.

2. FREQUENCY

Morgenstern H, Kleinbaum DG, Kupper LL. Measures of disease incidence used in epidemiologic research. Int J Epidemiol 1980;9:97–104.

3. ABNORMALITY

Feinstein AR. Clinical Judgment. Baltimore: Williams & Wilkins; 1967.

Streiner DL, Norman GR. Health Measurement Scales—A Practical Guide to Their Development and Use, 3rd ed. New York: Oxford University Press; 2003.

Yudkin PL, Stratton IM. How to deal with regression to the mean in intervention studies. Lancet 1996;347:241–243.

4. RISK: BASIC PRINCIPLES

Diamond GA. What price perfection? Calibration and discrimination of clinical prediction models. J Clin Epidemiol 1992;45:85–89.

Steiner JF. Talking about treatment: the language of populations and the language of individuals. Ann Intern Med 1999;130:618–622.

5. RISK: EXPOSURE TO DISEASE

Samet JM, Munoz A. Evolution of the cohort study. Epidemiol Rev 1998;20:1–14.

249

6. RISK: FROM DISEASE TO EXPOSURE

Grimes DA, Schulz KF. Compared to what? Finding controls for case-control studies. Lancet 2005;365: 1429–1433.

7. PROGNOSIS

Dekkers OM, Egger M, Altman DG, et al. Distinguishing case series from cohort studies. Ann Intern Med 2012;156:37–40.

Jenicek M. Clinical Case Reporting in Evidence-Based Medicine, 2nd Ed. New York: Oxford University Press; 2001.

Laupacis A, Sekar N, Stiell IG. Clinical prediction rules: a review and suggested modifications of methodologic standards. JAMA 1997;277:488–494.

Vandenbroucke JP. In defense of case reports. Ann Intern Med 2001;134:330–334.

8. DIAGNOSIS

McGee S. Evidence-Based Physical Diagnosis. New York: Elsevier; 2007.

Ransohoff DF, Feinstein AR. Problems of spectrum and bias in evaluating the efficacy of diagnostic tests. N Engl J Med 1978;299:926–930.

Whiting P, Rutjes AWS, Reitsma JB, et al. Sources of variation and bias in studies of diagnostic accuracy: a systematic review. Ann Intern Med 2004;140:189–202.

9. TREATMENT

Friedman LM, Furberg CD, DeMets DL. Fundamentals of Clinical Trials, 3rd ed. New York: Springer-Verlag; 1998.

Kaul S, Diamond GA. Good enough: a primer on the analysis and interpretation of noninferiority trials. Ann Intern Med 2006;145:62–69.

Pocock SJ. Clinical Trials: A Practical Approach. Chichester: Wiley; 1983.

Sackett DL, Gent M. Controversy in counting and attributing events in clinical trials. N Engl J Med 1979;301: 1410–1412.

The James Lind Library. http://www.jameslindlibrary.org

Tunis SR, Stryer DB, Clancy CM. Practical clinical trials: increasing the value of clinical research for decision making in clinical and health policy. JAMA 2004;291: 1624–1632.

Yusuf S, Collins R, Peto R. Why do we need some large, simple randomized trials? Stat Med 1984;3:409–420.

10. PREVENTION

Goodman SN. Probability at the bedside: the knowing of chances or the chances of knowing? Ann Intern Med 1999;130:604–606.

Harris R, Sawaya GF, Moyer VA, et al. Reconsidering the criteria for evaluation proposed screening programs: reflections from 4 current and former members of the U.S. Preventive Services Task Force. Epidemiol Rev 2011;33:20–25.

Rose G. Sick individuals and sick populations. In J Epidemiol 30:427–432.

Wald NJ, Hackshawe C, Frost CD. When can a risk factor be used as a worthwhile screening test? BMJ 1999;319: 1562–1565.

11. CHANCE

Concato J, Feinstein AR, Holford TR. The risk of determining risk with multivariable models. Ann Intern Med 1993;118:201–210.

Goodman SN. Toward evidence-based statistics. 1: the P value fallacy. Ann Intern Med 1999;130:995–1004.

Goodman SN. Toward evidence-based statistics. 2: the Bayes factor. Ann Intern Med 1999;130:1005–1013.

Rothman KJ. A show of confidence. N Engl J Med 1978; 299:1362–1363.

12. CAUSE

Buck C. Popper's philosophy for epidemiologists. Int J Epidemiol 1975;4:159–168.

Chalmers AF. What Is This Thing Called Science?, 2nd ed. New York: University of Queensland Press; 1982.

Morganstern H. Ecologic studies in epidemiology: concepts, principles, and methods. Ann Rev Public Health 1995;16:61–81.

13. SUMMARIZING THE EVIDENCE

Goodman S, Dickersin K. Metabias: a challenge for comparative effectiveness research. Ann Intern Med 2011;155: 61–62.

Lau J, Ioannidis JPA, Schmid CH. Summing up the evidence: one answer is not always enough. Lancet 1998;351: 123–127.

Leeflang MMG, Deeks JJ, Gatsonis C, et al. Systematic reviews of diagnostic test accuracy. Ann Intern Med 2008;149:889–897.

Norris SL, Atkins D. Challenges in using nonrandomized studies in systematic reviews of treatment interventions. Ann Intern Med 2005;142:1112–1119.

Riley RD, Lambert PC, Abo-Zaid G. Meta-analysis of individual participant data: rationale, conduct, and reporting. BMJ 2010;340:c221.

14. KNOWLEDGE MANAGEMENT

Cook DA, Dupras DM. A practical guide to developing effective Web-based learning. J Gen Intern Med 2004;19:698–707.

Shiffman RN, Shekelle P, Overhage JM, et al. Standardized reporting of clinical practice guidelines: a proposal from the conference on guideline standardization. Ann Intern Med 2003;139:493–498.

Note: Page numbers in *italics* denote figures; those followed by a *t* denote tables.